Science, Faith, & Human Fertility

RICHARD FEHRING &
THERESA NOTARE,

EDITORS

Science, Faith, & Human Fertility

THE THIRD CONFERENCE ON

ETHICAL FERTILITY HEALTH MANAGEMENT

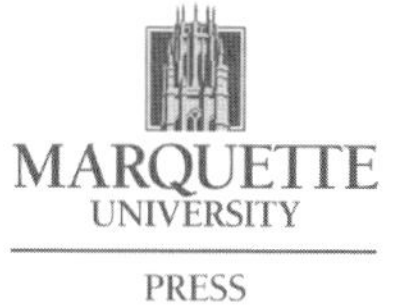

LIBRARY OF CONGRESS CATALOGING-IN-PUBLICATION DATA

Science, faith, & human fertility : the third conference on ethical fertility health management / Richard Fehring & Theresa Notare, editors.
p. cm.
Includes bibliographical references and index.
ISBN-13: 978-0-87462-093-1 (pbk. : alk. paper)
ISBN-10: 0-87462-093-7 (pbk. : alk. paper)
1. Reproductive health—Congresses. 2. Fertility, Human—Moral and ethical aspects—Congresses. 3. Human reproduction—Religious aspects—Catholic Church—Congresses. I. Fehring, Richard J., 1948- II. Notare, Theresa, 1957- III. Title: Science, faith, and human fertility.
RG133.S37 2011
618.1—dc23

2012004476

∞The paper used in this publication meets the minimum requirements of the American National Standard for Information Sciences—Permanence of Paper for Printed Library Materials, ANSI Z39.48-1992.

Marquette University Press
Milwaukee

The Association of Jesuit University Presses

CONTENTS

Panel II: Life-Giving Love in an Age of Technology

Panel III: The Effect of Culture and the Arts on God's Plan for Married Love

ABOUT THE CONFERENCE

Conference Co-Sponsors

The United States Conference of Catholic Bishops, Committee on Laity, Marriage, Family Life and Youth

The Catholic University of America, School of Theology and Religious Studies

The Pontifical John Paul II Institute for Studies on Marriage and the Family at the Catholic University of America

Marquette University, College of Nursing, Institute for Natural Family Planning

Saint Louis University, School of Nursing, Nursing Center for Fertility Education

Co-Sponsor—Science Sessions

Georgetown University, Institute for Reproductive Health

Conference Site

InterContinental Milwaukee Hotel
139 East Kilbourn Avenue
Milwaukee, WI 53202

ABOUT THE CONTRIBUTORS

Melanie Barrett, PhD, Assistant Director, Department of Christian Life, Mundelein Seminary, University of St. Mary of the Lake, , Archdiocese of Chicago

Rev. Robert R. Cannon, MA, MEd, MTh, JCL, Consultant, NFP Program, United States Conference of Catholic Bishops

Jorge Chavarro, MD, ScD, Instructor, Department of Medicine, School of Public Health, Harvard University

Patrick Fagan, PhD, Senior Fellow and Director, Marriage and Religion Research Institute (MARRI), Family Research Council, Washington, DC

Richard Fehring, PhD, RN, FAAN, Professor, Director, Office of Research and Scholarship, Director, Institute for Natural Family Planning, College of Nursing, Marquette University

Lina Guzman, PhD, Program Area Director and Senior Research Scientist, Child Trends, Washington, DC

Victoria Jennings, PhD, Director, Institute for Reproductive Health, School of Medicine, Georgetown University

Rev. William Kurz, SJ, PhD, Professor, Department of Theology, Marquette University

Miriam Labbok, MD, MPH, FACPM, IBCLC, Professor of the Practice of Public Health, Department of Maternal and Child Health, University of North Carolina

Rebecka I. Lundgren, MPH, Deputy Director, Director of Research, Institute for Reproductive Health, School of Medicine, Georgetown University

Daniel McInerny, PhD, Associate Professor of Philosophy, Great Texts Program, Baylor University

Rev. J. Daniel Mindling, OFM Cap, STD, Academic Dean, Professor of Moral Theology, Mount St. Mary's Seminary, Archdiocese of Baltimore

Theresa Notare, PhD, Assistant Director, NFP Program, Secretariat for Laity, Marriage, Family Life and Youth, United States Conference of Catholic Bishops

Bruno Scarpa, PhD, Researcher in Statistics, Department of Statistical Sciences, University of Padua, Italy

Mary Schneider, MSN, FNP-BC, NFPE, Assistant Director, Institute of Natural Family Planning, College of Nursing, Marquette University

Mary Shivanandan, STD, Professor of Theology, John Paul II Institute for Studies on Marriage and the Family at the Catholic University of America, Washington, DC

Irit Sinai, PhD, Senior Research Officer, Institute for Reproductive Health, Assistant Professor, Department of Obstetrics, School of Medicine, Georgetown University

Joseph Stanford, MD, MPH, Associate Professor Medicine, School of Medicine, University of Utah

Paul Whittaker, PhD, Associate Director of Research, Family Planning Council, Inc., Philadelphia, Adjunct Scholar, Epidemiology, Penn State Medicine

Foreword

In 2002, Richard Fehring, PhD, RN, FAAN, Director of the Natural Family Planning Institute of Marquette University College of Nursing invited the Diocesan Development Program for Natural Family Planning (now NFP Program), United States Conference of Catholic Bishops, to co-sponsor an academic conference entitled *Integrating Faith and Science through Natural Family Planning*. Theresa Notare, Assistant Director of the Catholic bishops' NFP program, took this invitation to her supervisors for approval (at the time, the U.S. Bishops' Committee for Pro-Life Activities). The bishops approved the request and noted the appropriateness of the activity. It represented the realization of a long term goal of the bishops' national NFP efforts—to foster serious thinking on the science of Natural Family Planning (NFP) and Catholic teachings which support its use in marriage.

With the publishing of the proceedings of the first conference in 2004 by Marquette University Press, plans began for a second conference. It had been hoped that the second conference would occur within two-years after the first. Due to the nature of scientific research however, time was needed to allow for the development and completion of new studies. The second conference was therefore offered four years later on August 11 and 12, 2006.

The 2006 conference title was changed to: *Human Fertility—Where Faith and Science Meet*, and the site of the event would be the Catholic University of America in Washington, DC. The place of meeting reflected the addition of a new co-sponsor: the Catholic University of America (CUA), the School of Philosophy and the School of Theology and Religious Studies. In addition, a second Catholic university joined the co-sponsors, Georgetown University (GU), Institute for Reproductive Health, School of Medicine. Rev. Kurt Pritzl, PhD, OP, then Dean of the School of Philosophy (CUA), took an active role in setting the agenda for the day of theology and philosophy, while Victoria Jennings, PhD, director of Georgetown's Institute for Reproductive Health, ensured co-sponsorship of the day of science only. This action was in accordance with the federal grant restrictions of the IRH to sponsor only scientific NFP research.

The latest and the third conference, was offered on July 15-17, 2010, and was entitled, *Human Fertility—Where Faith and Science Meet.* Two more Catholic institutions were added as co-sponsors: Saint Louis University, School of Nursing, Nursing Center for Fertility Education and the Pontifical John Paul II Institute for Studies on Marriage and the Family at the Catholic University of America. The third conference also added two additional features: pre-conference workshops on the newer NFP methods (Marquette Model, the Standard Days, and TwoDay methods) and science posters.

Consistent with the original long term goal of the NFP Program of the U. S. Conference of Catholic Bishops, the purpose of these academic conferences is to foster scholarly thinking on the scientific, philosophical, theological, and cultural foundations of the natural methods of family planning. In addition, by providing an academic platform, scholars will be encouraged to explore these topics and enhance the credibility of the methods of NFP while mining the depths of Catholic teachings on married love and life. It is the hope of the co-sponsors that a fourth conference will be scheduled in the not distant future and that other Catholic universities will join in the co-sponsorship of this important work.

Theresa Notare

Introduction

The interdisciplinary conference *Human Fertility—Where Faith and Science Meet* was held at the InterContinental Hotel in Milwaukee, Wisconsin, July 15 to 17, 2010. The mission of the conference was to promote research on the science of Natural Family Planning (NFP) and related issues as well as to foster academic thinking about the Catholic Church's teachings on human sexuality, marriage and family life.

This academic conference has been offered every four years since 2002. The 2010 conference began on the evening of July 15th with a welcome from all of the co-sponsors, a reception, and a concurrent scientific poster session. The posters displayed at the poster session were stimulated by a call for abstracts in 2009 and were selected by a scientific review panel from the co-sponsoring institutions. Twelve abstracts were selected from scientists and scholars who represented a variety of institutions and presented on a variety of topics related to fertility and the provision of NFP services. The scholars and scientists were from the University of Utah, Texas Tech University Health Sciences Center, Marquette University, Georgetown University, British Columbia University, Northeastern State University, and the Couple to Couple League (for the abstracts of the science posters, see Appendix).

The scientific topics were addressed on the first full day of the conference. The topics were presented to meet the objective of reviewing and analyzing current scientific research on the methods of Natural Family Planning (NFP) and related issues. Consequently, the sessions featured current research on the methods of NFP, and notably featured reports from the U.S. Department of Health and Human Services' NFP research grant recipients, among whom were secular family planning researchers.

Related subjects of inquiry included the amenorrheic properties of breastfeeding and the effects of nutrition on human fertility. The opening science session offered a panel on "Optimizing Fertility," beginning with a paper by Jorge Chavarro, MD, ScD (Harvard University) on how nutrition influences fertility. A second paper, presented by Bruno

Scarpa, PhD (biostatistician at the University of Padua, Italy), discussed evidence for optimizing fertility by timing intercourse during the menstrual cycle. Both topics were timely, given the increase in subfertility in the United States, due in part to the delaying of marriage and children to a later maternal age.

Science Panel II offered "Breastfeeding and the Transition to Fertility." This topic is of ongoing importance for those using NFP methods to avoid pregnancy because the transition to fertility is often difficult to monitor. The first presenter was the prominent breastfeeding researcher, Miriam Labbok, MD, MPH, FACPM, IBCLC (University of North Carolina). Dr. Labbok presented on the state of the evidence on lactation amenorrhea, the Lactation Amenorrhea Method (LAM) and the transition to other natural methods of family planning. A doctoral student from Marquette University, Mary Schneider, MSN, FNP-BC, then presented on a new postpartum breastfeeding protocol that involves creating artificial menstrual cycles by use of a hormonal fertility monitor to detect the first post-partum ovulation and the resumption of menstrual cycles. Ms. Schneider included some early results of this protocol in her presentation.

Science Panel III was entitled, "Current NFP Research: Office of Population Affairs (OPA) Grantees: Panel of OPA Sponsored NFP Research in the USA." Representing their institution, presenters were tasked to report on their research design and the status of their projects.

In order to better understand the variety of grantee representatives, we offer a brief background on the guidelines of the OPA NFP grant proposal. In 2008 a call for research on NFP was issued by the federal government's Department of Health and Human Services, Office of Population Affairs. Specifically, the grant requested that research be taken up on why NFP is not utilized by women seeking family planning services at Title X clinics. The grant guidelines also requested that researchers explore how to increase the use of NFP at Title X family planning clinics. Therefore, a variety of family planning researchers in addition to NFP institutions applied for the grants.

Science Panel III presenters included Lina Guzman, PhD (Child Trends Washington, DC), who presented on use of NFP among young adult women and why they would or would not use NFP. Victoria Jennings, PhD (Georgetown University's Institute of Reproductive Health) reported on a planned approach of introducing and expanding the availability of NFP among the Title X clinics by use of the Standard Days Method. Joseph Stanford, MD, MPH (University of Utah), presented his proposal of determining the influence of motivation and intention on efficacy of the Creighton Model method of NFP. Richard Fehring, PhD, RN, FAAN (Marquette University), provided preliminary results of a randomized comparison of two online delivered methods of NFP, i.e., use of an electronic hormonal fertility monitor in comparison to cervical mucus monitoring. The final presenter was Paul Whittaker, PhD (Family Planning Council, Philadelphia), who presented qualitative data on client and provider perspectives on the use of NFP and fertility awareness based methods.

Science Panel IV examined the "Status of NFP: How Many, Who, Why?" It included a presentation by Irit Sinai, PhD (Georgetown University, IRH). Dr. Sinai discussed the state of NFP in the United States and in other nations. Rev. Robert R. Cannon, MA, MEd, MTh, JCL (NFPP consultant, USCCB), discussed the state of, and trends in, NFP use among the Catholic diocesan programs in the United States. A final paper was given by Rebecca Lundgren, MPH, (Georgetown University, IRH), which presented recommendations on how to scale up the use of NFP. Ms. Lundgren based her study on the IRH's experience in scaling up the use of simplified and effective NFP methods in developing countries.

The second full day of the conference (Saturday, July 17th) addressed studies on the topics of human sexuality, fertility and its management, and marriage and conjugal love from the perspectives of faith and culture. Sessions featured papers in the disciplines of theology, sociology, history, literature, and the arts. The first paper, presented by Mary Shivanandan, STD (John Paul II Institute for Studies on Marriage and the Family at the Catholic University of America) discussed an anthropology of love based on the virtues of charity and truth. Dr. Shivanandan provided a foundation for the understanding of human love and the implications for marriage and family life.

The first panel entitled, "Co-creating with the Creator," focused on the elements that comprise a husband and wife's discernment in participation with the Creator in bringing new life into the world. The emphases of the presentations was on Catholic teaching on a husband and wife's "Communion of Persons" in relation to "openness to life" in the conjugal embrace. The first presenter, Rev. William Kurz, SJ, PhD

(Marquette University) addressed this topic from a biblical reflection. The second speaker, Melanie Barrett, PhD (University of St. Mary on the Lake, Mundelein Seminary, Archdiocese of Chicago) offered a theological reflection using the Christian virtues. Both papers stimulated a lively discussion on the topic.

The next panel, "Life-Giving Love in an Age of Technology," examined the difficult topic of infertility and its challenge to marriage. A theological paper, offered by Rev. Daniel Mindling, OFM, Cap, STD (Mount St. Mary's Seminary, MD) looked at the central topic of the child as a gift in marriage, by integrating key concepts in the USCCB document, *Life-Giving Love in an Age of Technology* and the Holy See's *Dignitas Personae*. A sociological paper offered by Patrick Fagan, PhD (Family Research Council, Washington, DC) provided a review of sociological research on the effect of adoption on both parents and children.

The final panel of the day and conference addressed the effect of culture and the arts on God's plan for married love. The first paper, by Theresa Notare, PhD (NFPP, USCCB), addressed how culture, contraception, and religion interacted in the early 20th century to create and stimulate the modern sexual revolution. The final paper by Daniel McInerney, PhD (Baylor University) provided examples of the modern sexual revolution as presented in modern day culture and especially in the modern media.

In addition to the formal conference, a session for NFP scientists and two workshops were offered prior to the opening on July 15. The special session for NFP scientists involved discussion on the state of NFP research over the past ten years (i.e., new methods, efficacy, psychological aspects, fertility monitoring, and special circumstances). Suggestions were offered for future research. One of the workshops involved Marquette University's NFP Institute providing participants with up-dates on the Marquette Model of NFP. A concurrent informational workshop was offered by Georgetown University's Institute for Reproductive Health on the Standard Days Method and the Two Day Method. Conference participants represented a variety of disciplines, including diocesan staff (e.g., marriage and family life directors and NFP diocesan coordinators), NFP teachers, physicians, nurses, Catholic clergy, religious, graduate students (in nursing, medicine, and theology), and professors of various disciplines. Throughout the conference the participants had ample time to discuss the subjects with the speakers and each other. A highlight of the conference was the attendance of Most Rev. Jerome E. Listecki, Archbishop of Milwaukee, who offered encouraging words and his blessings. Appreciation was also extended to Most Rev. George J. Rassas, Auxiliary Bishop of Chicago and member of the U.S. Conference of Catholic Bishops' Committee for Laity, Marriage, Family Life and Youth who participated in the conference. Bishop Rassas celebrated the concluding Mass where he inspired conference participants with an uplifting sermon of the importance of their work in support of marriage and family life.

A conference such as this requires many helpers to ensure its success. The editors wish to extend our gratitude to the many volunteers who helped with the on-site management of the conference. Our deepest gratitude is especially extended to the USCCB's Elizabeth Cortright and Marquette University's Mary Schneider for their administrative help in the months prior to the conference. A special word of appreciation is extended to Mary Schneider for her painstaking work on obtaining continuing education units for nurses and continuing medical education units for physicians. In addition, our sincerest appreciation is extended to Susan Wills, Esq. (USCCB) for her masterful expertise in acting as a style/content editor. It is our hope that the good efforts represented by these Human Fertility conferences will contribute to a deeper appreciation for how wonderfully God has gifted men and women with a capacity to love and co-create according to His divine plan!

Richard Fehring, PhD, RN, FAAN
Theresa Notare, PhD
Editors

PART I

Human Fertility & New Science

PANEL I

OPTIMIZING FERTILITY

1

Diet & Infertility

JORGE E. CHAVARRO, MD, SCD

Assistant Professor of Nutrition, Epidemiology, & Medicine, Harvard School of Public Health & Harvard Medical School

ABSTRACT

The frequency of infertility and impaired fecundity in the United States is substantial and on the rise due to women delaying childbirth to later age and to lifestyle factors (especially obesity) among both women and men. Medical and surgical treatment for infertility can be expensive, not available to all (especially the poor), and some treatments might not be morally acceptable to others. There is growing research that shows dietary and lifestyle factors may be useful in preventing and managing certain types of infertility. Most of the current evidence suggests that infertility due to ovulation disorders and male factor infertility may be susceptible to dietary modification. Furthermore, emerging data suggest that diet may play a role in unexplained infertility. The following paper reviews the evidence for potential dietary and behavioral lifestyle modifications for both male and female infertility. Of particular interest is evidence that high intake of *trans* fatty acids, carbohydrates, low-fat dairy, and higher intake of protein from animal sources were associated with a greater risk of anovulatory infertility. Whereas, folic acid, non-heme iron, high-fat dairy products, and vegetable protein intake were associated with a lower risk of anovulatory infertility. Further research is needed to verify these findings and to prospectively test evidenced based dietary and behavioural treatments, especially among subgroups of women receiving infertility treatments.

INTRODUCTION

Infertility, defined as the failure to conceive after twelve months of intercourse (Practice Committee American Society for Reproductive Medicine 2006), is a common reproductive disorder affecting 1 in 6 couples who attempt to become pregnant at some point during their reproductive lifespan (Hull et al. 1985). As of 2002, more than 7 million women of reproductive age in the United States had decreased fecundity, defined as the inability to get pregnant or carry a pregnancy to term (Chandra et al. 2005), and that by 2025, as many as 7.7 million women could be expected to face this problem (Stephen et al. 1998).

The high frequency of infertility and impaired fecundity is currently coupled with dramatic population-wide shifts in the frequency of well established risk factors for infertility. Between 1970 and 2006 the proportion of women having their first child at age 30 or older increased from 5% to 24% and the proportion of women giving birth to their first child at age 35 or older increased 8-fold (Matthews et al. 2009), clearly indicating a dramatic shift not only in the age at which women get pregnant but also try to get pregnant for the first time. More dramatic trends in delayed childbearing can be seen in some regions of the country. For example, in Massachusetts more than 50% of children are currently born to women older than 30 years and nearly a quarter are born to women older than 35 years (Massachusetts Dept. of Public Health 2008). In addition, the prevalence of overweight and obesity has dramatically increased across the globe. The prevalence of overweight and obesity (Body Mass Index ≥ 25 kg/m^2) among adult women in the United States increased from 41% in 1960-1962 (Flegal et al. 1998) to 64% in 2007-2008 (Flegal et al. 2010). These population-wide trends suggest that the frequency of infertility and impaired fecundity is likely to increase over time if these trends continue.

Although treatment options for infertility are available, only a small proportion of couples who may require assistance to achieve a pregnancy actually do so (Macaluso et al. 2010). Since the gap between offer of fertility treatment services and the demand for these services is so wide, it is worth considering whether other approaches, such as focusing on infertility prevention or identifying modifiable lifestyle characteristics that may improve fertility, could address the population-wide burden of infertility as well as the needs of special populations, such as couples with moral or religious objections to some forms of infertility treatment. This paper reviews the role of diet, a potentially modifiable lifestyle factor, on the prevention of infertility.

CAN DIET PLAY A ROLE IN INFERTILITY PREVENTION?

Among couples who undergo clinical evaluation for infertility, the most commonly identified causes can be broadly classified as ovulation disorders, abnormalities in semen quality, tubal disease and cases without an identifiable cause or unexplained infertility (Barbieri 2004). Clearly, some underlying causes of infertility are not modifiable by dietary factors as is the case of tubal disease; although, in principle, tubal disease is to some extent avoidable by preventing pelvic inflammatory disease through prevention, early detection and treatment of sexually transmitted infections (Macaluso et al. 2010). Nevertheless, since ovulation and spermatogenesis are physiological processes that are responsive to environmental cues, there is the possibility that infertility due to ovulation disorders and defective spermatogenesis could, to some extent, be preventable through dietary modification.

Diet & Infertility Due to Anovulation

THE ROLE OF ENERGY BALANCE

The most convincing evidence for a role of diet on infertility prevention is for infertility due to ovulation disorders. The effects of extreme leanness and vigorous exercise on ovulation have been well characterized. In a series of studies conducted in the 1970's and early 1980's among female athletes and other extremely lean women, Frisch and colleagues convincingly described how a minimal amount of body fat stores were necessary to initiate and maintain ovulatory cycles (Frisch 1987). It is currently known that these effects are caused by hypothalamic dysfunction and decreased gonadotropin secretion possibly due to decreased levels of leptin (ESHRE Capri Workshop Group 2006). Weight loss or decreased availability of food have also been observed to decrease fertility historically during famines and contemporarily among agricultural communities with drastic variations in food supply and body weight in Bangladesh and The Gambia (Prentice et al. 2005).

Excessive body weight is also known to affect ovulation and increase the risk of infertility due to anovulation. For example, Rich-Edwards and colleagues examined the relation between body mass index (BMI) and risk of anovulatory infertility in the Nurses' Health Study II (NHS II) (Rich-Edwards et al. 2002). They observed a U-shaped relation between BMI and risk of ovulatory infertility whereby women with a BMI below 20 kg/m^2 or above 24 kg/m^2 had a significantly higher risk of infertility due to anovulation than women with a BMI of 21kg/m^2. The greater risk of infertility associated with low body weight is consistent with the previous work on hypothalamic amenorrhea whereas the greater frequency of infertility associated with increasing body weight is probably associated with metabolic changes characteristic of the polycystic ovary syndrome (PCOS) and obesity including increased insulin resistance. This in turn lowers circulating levels of sex-hormone binding globulin, causing a secondary increase in circulating androgens (Ehrmann 2005).

It is important to note that an increased risk of infertility was detected at BMI levels within what is considered the normal range of body weight (WHO 1995) and it is therefore unlikely that the increased risk of infertility with increasing body weight can be solely attributed to overt PCOS. Instead, we hypothesized that the steadily increasing risk of anovulatory infertility with increasing BMI was the result of increasing insulin resistance which in turn would be responsible for subclinical phenotypes of PCOS, some of which manifested with anovulation and infertility. Because it was known that dietary and lifestyle factors had a large impact on insulin sensitivity (Diabetes Prevention Program Research Group 2002) we decided to examine whether dietary factors previously associated with insulin resistance or related outcomes (e.g., type 2 diabetes, impaired glucose tolerance, HbA1c levels) were in turn associated to the risk of infertility due to anovulation using data from the NHS II. In addition, we decided to re-examine in this data existing hypotheses regarding the role of dietary factors on the risk of infertility.

THE ROLE OF DIET COMPOSITION

When our team started this group in 2006, the literature regarding diet and fertility consisted of an important number of publications relating intake of alcohol or caffeinated beverages to infertility, a large number of case reports relating deficiencies of specific micronutrients (mostly B vitamins and iron) with infertility, and conflicting evidence regarding a potentially detrimental role of galactose (which is used in animal models to mimic the phenotype of premature ovarian failure (Bandyopadhyay et al. 2003; see also Swarts and Mattison 1998) on human fertility (Cramer et al. 1994; see also Greenlee et al. 2003). We decided to focus our research on three main hypotheses: (1) that dietary factors influencing insulin sensitivity or glucose metabolism (mostly macronutrient intake) were related to the risk of infertility due to anovulation in the same direction of their relation with insulin sensitivity/glucose metabolism; (2) that greater intake of iron and B vitamins was associated with a lower risk of infertility due to anovulation; and (3) that what we termed "gonadal toxicants," namely alcohol, caffeine and dairy foods would be unrelated to infertility due to anovulation. Our last hypothesis, although counter to the preponderance of the evidence available at the moment (at least for alcohol and caffeine intake), was based on the fact that both alcohol and caffeine are known to improve insulin sensitivity (Agardh et al. 2004; Salazar-Martinez et al. 2004; Conigrave et al. 2001; Sierksma et al. 2004) and thus, based on our first hypothesis, these dietary factors would be expected to improve fertility rather than hamper it.

I will first address our findings regarding the gonadal toxicant hypotheses. Our study involved the follow-up of 18,555 married women without a previous history of infertility who, over the period of eight years, accrued 26,971 pregnancies and failed pregnancy attempts. In our study we did not find any relation between intake of alcoholic or caffeinated beverages with subsequent risk of infertility due to anovulation (Chavarro et al. 2009). Although, as previously mentioned, the preponderance of the 29 studies conducted to date on this area suggests that both alcohol and caffeine may impair fertility, very few actually suggest that this purported effect is due to effects on ovulatory function. We have discussed elsewhere (Chavarro et al. 2009) that many of the previous findings could be explained by methodological problems with a large number of studies. Others have also described how retrospective studies and studies of lower methodologic quality are more likely to report a relation between caffeine intake and impaired reproduction (including decreased fertility) than prospective studies (Leviton and Cowan 2002). Similarly, we did not observe an association between lactose intake (the only source of galactose in human diet) and risk of infertility due to anovulation (Chavarro et al. 2007b). Since the levels of galactose intake necessary to affect ovulation in rodent models are beyond the range of usual dietary exposure in humans, we believe our findings are not surprising. In fact, rodents exposed to diets containing lower levels of galactose than those usually used in rodent POF models, do not develop the alterations of ovarian morphology and function observed in rodents exposed to high galactose diets (Lui et al. 2005).

We did, however, discover several dietary factors to be independently associated with the risk of infertility due to anovulation in this population. Intake of *trans* fatty acids (Chavarro et al. 2007b), greater carbohydrate intake and dietary glycemic load (Chavarro et al. 2007d), higher intake of low-fat dairy (Chavarro et al. 2007c), and higher intake of protein from animal sources (Chavarro et al. 2008a), were associated with a greater risk of anovulatory infertility whereas folic acid (Chavarro et al. 2008b), non-heme iron (Chavarro et al. 2006), high-fat dairy (Chavarro et al. 2007c) and vegetable protein intake (Chavarro et al. 2008a) were associated with a lower risk of this outcome. These findings were generally in agreement with our hypotheses and suggest that an overall dietary pattern aimed at increasing the intake of certain micronutrients and improving insulin sensitivity (Lefevre et al. 2005; Murakami et al. 2006; Jeppesen et al. 1997; Gannon et al. 1988; Hubbard et al. 1989; Lavigne et al. 2000). Likewise, our findings for micronutrients, particularly folic acid, are in agreement with studies showing that folate status influences ovarian sensitivity to gonadotropins follicular estradiol synthesis (Thaler et al. 2006; Hecht et al. 2009).

Unexpected findings of our research were our results regarding intake of dairy foods and risk of anovulatory infertility. We found that higher intake of non-fat/low-fat dairy foods was associated to a higher risk of infertility due to anovulation while a higher intake of high-fat dairy, particularly whole milk, had the opposite association (Chavarro et al. 2007c). The association of high-fat dairy with lower infertility risk was observed at very modest intake levels, usually of one daily serving or less, and since very few women in our cohort consumed high-fat dairy products it was not possible to evaluate whether higher intakes had a greater benefit. As mentioned above, our main motivation to examine the relation between dairy intake and infertility was to examine the galactose hypothesis. However, at the time we were conducting the study, some of our colleagues reported an association between intake of low-fat dairy foods, but not high-fat dairy foods, with acne: a clinical manifestation of androgen excess (Adebamowo et al. 2005). Since androgen excess is part one of the components of PCOS (Azziz et al. 2009), a major cause of anovulation in the general population, we decided to examine the relationship between dairy foods and infertility separately for low-fat and high-fat dairy foods. Although unexpected, there are some potential mechanisms that could explain these findings. Low-fat dairy has been associated with greater levels of circulating IGF-I levels (Holmes et al. 2002; Heaney et al. 1999; Giovannucci et al. 2003) which in turn may play a role in the pathogenesis of PCOS and its associated anovulation (Giudice 1992; Duleba et al. 1998). Although there is not an equally compelling mechanism explaining our findings for high fat dairy, some potential mechanisms include the greater content of estrogens in high-fat dairy compared to low-fat dairy (Wolford and Argoudelsi 1979) which could in turn decrease circulating IGF-I levels (Veldhuis et al. 2005; Jorgensen et al. 2004).

After identifying these series of dietary factors associated with infertility risk, we were interested in determining whether an overall dietary pattern including all the separate dietary components, with or without weight control and physical activity, which had been previously associated with lower infertility risk in this population (Rich-Edwards et al. 2002), could prevent anovulatory infertility. We created a diet score to summarize the extent to which each woman in the study adhered to the dietary factors associated with the lowest risk of infertility due to anovulation. Women in the top 20% of adherence to this dietary pattern had a 66% lower risk of infertility due to anovulation compared to women in the lowest 20% of adherence (Chavarro et al. 2007a). Furthermore, this association did not differ across groups of women defined by age, parity or body weight. We also examined whether adding weight control and physical activity within the levels recommended for chronic disease prevention were associated with further risk reduction. Women who adhered to five or more dietary or lifestyle practices within the levels associated with lowest risk of infertility were 84% less likely to experience anovulatory infertility compared to women who adhered to none. Lastly, we estimated that a diet and lifestyle modification on a population level could be expected to prevent approximately two thirds of all cases of infertility due to anovulation (Chavarro et al. 2007a).

DIET & MALE FERTILITY

The role of diet on male fertility, usually evaluated through its relation with conventional semen quality parameters, is relatively understudied. There are, however, two areas where substantial work has been done: the role of body weight and the role of folate metabolism on semen quality.

Body Weight & Male Fertility

It is well established that body weight strongly influences the circulating levels of reproductive hormones in men. Higher body fat stores lead to increased adipose tissue aromatization of androgens into estrogens resulting in higher circulating levels of estradiol (Kley et al. 1980; Longcope et al. 1986). Obesity-related insulin resistance and its resulting hyperinsulinemia decrease SHBG production in the liver (Plymate et al. 1988; Hautamen 2000). Increased body weight also leads to decreased testosterone levels as a result of decreased SHBG binding capacity (Giagulli et al.1994) and, in morbid obesity, impaired functioning of the hypothalamic-pituitary-testicular (HPT) axis (Lima et al. 2000; Vermeulen et al. 1993; Strain et al. 1982) as a result of enhanced negative feedback on gonadotropin secretion by estradiol (Strain et al. 1982; Jarrow et al.1993). More recently, our group (Chavarro, et al., 2010) and others (Jensen et al. 2004; Pauli et al. 2008; Aggerholm et al. 2008; Winters et al. 2006), have also documented an inverse relation between BMI and inhibin B levels, a marker of Sertoli cell function and spermatogenesis.

Yet, it is not entirely clear whether these alterations in reproductive hormone levels necessarily lead to decreased fertility in men. A meta-analysis (Macdonald et al. 2009) and systematic review (Du Plessis et al. 2010) of this topic have been recently published reaching opposite conclusions. In 2004, Jensen and colleagues reported for the first time a U-shaped association between BMI and sperm concentration among young military conscripts in Denmark, whereby young men whose BMI was under 20 kg/m^2 or who were overweight or obese (BMI≥25kg/m^2) had a significantly lower sperm concentration than men in the 20-24.9kg/m^2 BMI range (Jensen et al. 2004). Their report initiated an avalanche of research in this area that, unfortunately, has not completely clarified the role of body weight on male fertility. A few studies have reported a direct relation between male BMI and time to pregnancy or higher frequency of self reported infertility (Ramlau-Hansen et al. 2007; Nguyen et al. 2007; Sallmen et al. 2006). Most of the studies in this area, however, have studied semen quality parameters as a surrogate for male fertility. Findings on the relation between BMI and semen quality have been very inconsistent across studies. Individual studies have reported deleterious effects of higher body weight on sperm concentration (Jensen et al. 2004; Koloszar et al. 2005; Hammoud et al. *in press*; Fejes et al. 2006; Magnusdottir et al. 2005), ejaculate volume (Fejes et al. 2006), total sperm count (Chavarro et al. 2010; Jensen et al. 2004; Magnusdottir et al. 2005; Fejes et al. 2005), motile count (Fejes et al. 2005) and progressive motility (Hammoud et al. 2008). The most consistent positive finding across studies has been lower sperm concentration among overweight and obese men which has been reported by five previous studies (Jensen et al. 2004; Koloszar et al. 2005; Hammoud et al. 2008; Fejes et al. 2006; Magnusdottir et al. 2005) while another four (Chavarro et al. 2010; Pauli et al. 2008; Aggerholm et al. 2008; Qin et al. 2007) did not find this association. Moreover, studies simultaneously examining the effect of BMI on reproductive hormones and semen quality suggest that the association between BMI and semen quality is not mediated by changes in reproductive hormone levels (Chavarro et al. 2010; Qin et al. 2007). Clearly, more research is needed to determine whether a relationship between BMI and male fertility exists.

FOLATE, ONE-CARBON METABOLISM & MALE FERTILITY

Folate-requiring reactions, collectively known as the one-carbon metabolism, encompass a series of related metabolic pathways where one carbon moieties are transferred from donors to intermediate carriers and ultimately used in methylation reactions or as building blocks in the synthesis of DNA (Bailey and Gregory 2006; Lucock 2000). This metabolic pathway has a greater relevance when folate stores are depleted or when folate requirements are heightened, for example due to increased demand for DNA synthesis in gametogenesis (Forges et al. 2007). Because spermatogenesis requires an almost constant DNA synthesis and this pathway is essential for DNA synthesis, it has been subject to some attention on its relation to male fertility and is probably the best understood nutritional or metabolic factor influencing male fertility.

There are multiple lines of evidence linking this metabolic pathway to male fertility. Rodent models of genetic or pharmacologic disruption of this metabolic pathway show its importance in spermatogenesis. In a model of genetic deficiency, male methylenetetrahydrofolate reductase (MTHFR) $^{-/-}$ mice have altered spermatogenesis resulting in a drastic reduction of testicular sperm counts and infertility (Kelly et al. 2005). Interestingly, these effects appear to be partially reversible through dietary interventions (Kelly et al. 2005). Likewise, administration of DHFR inhibitors, to sexually mature mice causes spermatogenic arrest and infertility (Kelly et al. 2005; Kalla et al. 1997; Malik et al. 1995). In humans, common polymorphisms in this pathway have been associated with semen quality parameters. A recent meta-analysis of studies of the common *MTHFR C677T* polymorphism reported pooled odds ratios (OR) (95% confidence interval (CI)) for male factor infertility of 1.39 (1.15–1.69) for *TT* homozygotes and 1.23 (1.08–1.41) for *T* allele carriers (Tüttelmann et al. 2007). Other polymorphic genes in this pathway (*MTR, MTRR*) have also been associated to markers of male fertility among Asians (Lee et al. 2006).

Dietary folates also appear to be important for male fertility in free living populations. Two studies have reported significant associations between low intake of fruits and vegetables, major dietary sources of folates, and male infertility (Wong et al. 2003; Mendiola et al. 2009). In fact, in one of these studies men in the highest tertile of folate intake had an 87% lower risk of oligoteratospermia than men in the lowest tertile of intake (Mendiola et al. 2010). Likewise, seminal plasma levels of vitamin B12 and folate, which are susceptible to dietary modification (Landau et al. 1978), are positively related to sperm concentration (Wallock et al. 2001; Boxmeer et al. 2007) and, among men who have previously fathered a pregnancy and sperm counts above $20x10^6$/mL, seminal plasma folate is inversely related to sperm DNA fragmentation (Boxmeer et al. 2009). Furthermore, folate intake has been associated with a lower frequency of sperm aneuploidy. In a study of healthy non-smoking men, those in the highest folate intake level (722-1150 μg/day) had a lower incidence of disomy X, sex nullisomy, disomy 21 and aggregate aneuploidy in their sperm (Young et al. 2008).

Nevertheless, the therapeutic potential of folic acid supplements on the management of male fertility may be limited. In a randomized trial of folate, zinc, folate + zinc or placebo, subfertile men assigned to the folate + zinc arm had an 74% increase in total normal sperm count compared to pre-intervention values and a 41% increase when compared to post-intervention values in the placebo arm which did not reach statistical significance (Wong et al. 2002). The intervention had no effect on sperm count among fertile men. Moreover, despite the statistically significant increases in sperm counts among subfertile men, the mean post-intervention values for semen quality parameters were still below the WHO cutoff value levels.

CONCLUSION

In order to address the problem of infertility at a population-wide level, as well as the needs of special populations that may not wish to undergo certain forms of infertility treatment even when these are available to them, it is important to identify potentially modifiable risk factors for infertility. There is accumulating evidence that some dietary and lifestyle factors may be useful in preventing and managing certain cases of infertility. Most of the current evidence suggests that infertility due to ovulation disorders and male factor infertility may be susceptible to dietary modification and emerging data suggest that diet may play a role in unexplained infertility (Altmäe et al. 2010) as well as in less common but potentially modifiable causes of infertility such as endometriosis (Missmer et al. 2010). Although these data are encouraging, it is important that these findings are independently reproduced and that related areas of research are expanded, such as investigating the role of diet on outcomes among couples receiving infertility treatments, to get a clearer picture of the potential of diet to prevent and/or manage infertility.

SOURCES CONSULTED

Adebamowo, C. A., D. Spiegelman, F. W. Danby, A. L. Frazier, W. C. Willett, M. D. Holmes. 2005. "High school dietary dairy intake and teenage acne." *Journal of the American Academy of Dermatoloty* 52: 207-214.

Agardh, E. E., S. Carlsson, A. Ahlbom et al. 2004."Coffee consumption, type 2 diabetes and impaired glucose tolerance in Swedish men and women." *Journal of Internal Medicine* 255: 645-652.

Aggerholm, A. S., A. M. Thulsttrup, G. Toft, C. H. Ramlau-Hansen, J. P. Bonde. "Is overweight a risk factor for reduced semen quality and altered serum sex hormone profile?" *Fertility and Sterility* 2008; 90: 619-26.

Altmäe, S., A. Stavreus-Evers, J. R. Ruiz et al. "Variations in folate pathway genes are associated with unexplained female infertility." *Fertility and Sterility*, 2010; 94: 130-7.

Azziz, R., E. Carmina, D. Dewailly et al. 2009. "The Androgen Excess and PCOS Society criteria for the polycystic ovary syndrome: the complete task force report." *Fertility and Sterility* 91: 456-488.

Bailey, L. B., J. F. Gregory III. "Folate." In Bowman, B. A., Russell, R. M. Eds. 2006. *Present Knowledge in Nutrition*. 9th Edition. Washington, DC: ILSI Press; pp.125-137.

Bandyopadhyay, S., J. Chakrabarti, S. Banerjee et al. 2003."Galactose toxicity in the rat as a model for premature ovarian failure: an experimental approach readdressed." *Human Reproduction* 18: 2031-2038.

Barbieri, R. L. 2004. "Female Infertility." In: Straus III, J. F., Barbieri, R. L. Eds. *Yen and Jaffe's Reproductive Endocrinology*. 5th ed. Philadelphia, PA: Elsevier Inc.

Boxmeer, J. C., M. Smit, E. Utomo et al. 2009. "Low folate in seminal plasma is associated with increased sperm DNA damage." *Fertility and Sterility* 92: 548-556.

Boxmeer, J.C., M. Smit, R.F. Weber et al. 2007. "Seminal plasma cobalamin significantly correlates with sperm concentration in men undergoing IVF or ICSI procedures." *Journal of Andrology* 28: 521-527.

Chandra, A., G. M. Martinez, W. D. Mosher, J. C. Abma, J. Jones. 2005. "Fertility, family planning, and reproductive health of U.S. women: Data from the 2002 National Survey of Family Growth." *Vital and Health Statistics* 23: 1-160.

Chavarro, J. E., J. W. Rich-Edwards, B. A. Rosner, W. C. Willett. 2006. "Iron Intake and Risk of Ovulatory Infertility." *Obstetrics and Gynecology*108: 1145-1152.

———. 2007a. "Diet and lifestyle in the prevention of ovulatory disorder infertility." *Obstetrics and Gynecology* 110:1050-1058.

———. 2007b. "Dietary fatty acid intakes and the risk of ovulatory infertility." *American Journal of Clinical Nutrition* 85: 231-237.

———. 2007c. "A prospective study of dairy foods intake and anovulatory infertility." *Human Reproduction* 22: 1340-1347.

———. 2009. "A prospective study of dietary carbohydrate quantity and quality in relation to risk of ovulatory infertility." *European Journal of Clinical Nutrition*. 63: 78-86. EPub 2007 Sep 19.

———. 2008a. "Protein intake and ovulatory infertility." *American Journal of Obstetrics and Gynecology* 198:210.e.1-.e.7.

———. 2008b. "Use of multivitamins, intake of B vitamins and risk of ovulatory infertility." *Fertility and Sterility* 89: 668-676.

———. 2009. "Caffeinated and alcoholic beverage intake in relation to the risk of ovulatory disorder infertility." *Epidemiology* 20: 374-381.

Chavarro, J. E., T. L. Toth, D. L. Wright, J. D. Meeker, R. Hauser, R. 2010. "Body mass index in relation to semen quality, sperm DNA integrity and serum reproductive hormone levels among men attending an infertility clinic." *Fertility and Sterility* 93: 2222-2231.

Conigrave, K. M., F. B. Hu, C. A. Camargo, Jr., M. J. Stampfer, W. C. Willett, E.B. Rimm. 2001. "A prospective study of drinking patterns in relation to risk of type 2 diabetes among men." *Diabetes* 50: 2390-2395.

Cosentino, M. J., R. E. Pakyz, J. Fried. 1990. "Pyrimethamine: an approach to the development of a male contraceptive." *Proceedings of the National Academy of Sciences of the United States of America* 87: 1431-1435.

Cramerm, D. W., H. Xu, T. Sahi. 1994. "Adult hypolactasia, milk consumption and age-specific fertility." *American Journal of Epidemiology* 139: 282-289.

Diabetes Prevention Program Research Group. 2002. "Reduction in the incidence of Type 2 diabetes with lifestyle intervention or Metformin." *New England Journal of Medicine* 346: 393-403.

Duleba, A. J., R. Z. Spaczynski, D. L. Olive. 1998. "Insulin and insulin-like growth factor I stimulate the proliferation of human ovarian theca-interstitial cells." *Fertility and Sterility* 69: 335-340.

Du Plessis, S. S., S. Cabler, D. A. McAlister, E. Sabanegh, A. Agarwal. 2010. "The effect of obesity on sperm disorders and male infertility." *Nature Reviews Urology* 7: 153-161.

D. A. Ehrmann. 2005. "Polycystic ovary syndrome." *New England Journal of Medicine* 352: 1223-1236.

The ESHRE Capri Workshop Group. 2006. "Nutrition and reproduction in women." *Human Reproduction Update* 12: 193-207.

Fejes, I., S. Koloszar, J. Szollosi, Z. Zavaczki, A. Pal. 2005. "Is semen quality affected by male body fat distribution?" *Andrologia* 37: 155-159.

Fejes, I., S. Koloszar, Z. Zavaczki, J. Daru, J. Szollosi, A. Pal. 2006. "Effect of body weight on testosterone/estradiol ratio in oligozoospermic patients." *Archives of Andrology* 52: 97-102.

Flegal, K. M., M. D. Carroll, R. J. Kuczmarski, C. L. Johnson. 1998. "Overweight and obesity in the United States: prevalence and trends, 1960-1994." *International Journal of Obesity Related Metabolic Disorders* 22: 39-47.

Flegal, K. M., M. D. Carroll, C. L. Ogden, L. R. Curtin. 2010. "Prevalence and trends in obesity smong US adults, 1999-2008." *Journal of the American Medical Association* 303: 235-241.

Forges, T., P. Monnier-Barbarino, J.M. Alberto, R.M. Guéant-Rodriguez, J.L. Daval, J.L. Guéant. 2007. "Impact of folate and homocysteine metabolism on human reproductive health." *Human Reproduction Update* 13: 225-238.

Frisch, R. E. 1987. "Body fat, menarche, fitness and fertility." *Human Reproduction* 2: 521-533.

Gannon, M. C., F. Q. Nuttall, B. J. Neil, S.A. Westphal. 1988. "The insulin and glucose responses to meals of glucose plus various protein in type II diabetic subjects." *Metabolism* 11: 1081-1088.

Giagulli, V. A., J. M. Kaufman, A. Vermeulen. 1994. "Pathogenesis of the decreased androgen levels in obese men." *Journal of Clinical Endocrinology and Metabolism* 79: 997-1000.

Giovannucci, E., M. Pollak, Y. Liu et al. 2003. "Nutritional predictors of insulin like growth factor I and their relationships to cancer in men." *Cancer Epidemiology, Biomarkers and Prevention*12: 84-89.

Giudice, L. 1992. "Insulin-like growth factors and ovarian follicular development." *Endocrine Reviews* 13: 641-669.

Greenlee, A. R., T. E. Arbuckle, P. H. Chyou. 2003. "Risk factors for female infertility in an agricultural region." *Epidemiology* 14: 429-436.

Hammoud, A. O., N. Wilde, M. Gibson, A. Parks, D. T. Carrell, W. Meikle. "Male obesity and alteration in sperm parameters." *Fertility and Sterility*, 2008; 90: 2222-5.

Hautanen, A. 2000. "Synthesis and regulation of sex hormone-binding globulin in obesity." *International Journal of Obesity* 24 (Suppl 2): S64-S70.

Heaney, R. P., D. A. McCarron, B. Dawson-Hughes et al. 1999. "Dietary changes favorably affect bone remodeling in older adults." *Journal of the American Dietetic Association* 99: 1228-1233.

Hecht, S., R. Pavlik, P. Lohse, U. Noss, K. Friese, C.J. Thaler. 2009. "Common 677C—>T mutation of the 5,10-methylenetetrahydrofolate reductase gene affects follicular estradiol synthesis." *Fertility and Sterility* 91:56-61.

Holmes, M. D., M. N. Pollak, W. C. Willett, S. E. Hankinson. 2002. "Dietary correlates of plasma insulin-like growth factor I and insulin-like growth factor binding protein 3 concentrations." *Cancer Epidemiology, Biomarkers and Prevention* 11: 852-861.

Hubbard, R., C. L. Kosch, A. Sanchez, J. Sabate, L. Berk, G. Shavlik. 1989. "Effect of dietary protein on serum insulin and glucagon levels in hyper- and normocholesterolemic men." *Atherosclerosis* 76: 55-61.

Hull, M. G., C. M. Glazener, N. J. Kelly et al. 1985. "Population study of causes, treatment, and outcome of infertility." *British Medical Journal* 291: 1693-1697.

Jarrow, J. P., J. Kirkland, D. R. Kotnik, W. T. Cefalu. 1993. "Effect of obesity and fertility status on sex steroid levels in men." *Urology* 42: 171-174.

Jensen, T. K., A-M. Andersson, N. Jorgensen et al. 2004. "Body mass index in relation to semen quality and reproductive hormones among 1,558 Danish men." *Fertility and Sterility* 82: 863-870.

Jeppesen, J., P. Schaaf, C. Jones, M. Zhou, Y. Chen, G. Reaven. 1997. "Effects of low-fat, high-carbohydrate diets on risk factors for ischemic heart disease in postmenopausal women." *American Journal of Clinical Nutrition* 65:1027-1033.

Jorgensen, J. O., J. J. Christensen, M. Krag, S. Fisker, P. Ovesen, J. S. Christiansen. 2004. "Serum insulin-like growth factor-I levels in growth hormone deficient adults: influence of sex steroids." *Hormone Research* 62: 73-76.

Kalla, N. R., S. K. Saggar, R. Puri, U. Mehta. 1997. "Regulation of male fertility by pyrimethamine in adult mice." *Research in Experimental Medicine (Berl)* 197:45-52.

Kelly, T. L. J., O. R. Neaga, B. C. Schwahn, R. Rozen, J. M. Trasler. 2005. "Infertility in 5,10-methylenetetrahydrofolate reductase (MTHFR)-deficient male mice is partially alleviated by lifetime dietary Betaine supplementation." *Biology of Reproduction* 72: 667-677.

Kley, H. K., T. Deselaers, H. Peerenboom, H. L. Krüskemper. 1980. "Enhanced conversion of androstenedione to estrogens in obese males." *Journal of Clinical Endocrinology and Metabolism* 51: 1128-1132.

Koloszar, S., I. Fejes, Z. Zavaczki, J. Daru, J. Szollosi, A. Pal. 2005. "Effect of body weight on sperm concentration in normozoospermic males." *Archives of Andrology* 51: 299-304.

Landau, B., R. Singer, T. Klein, E. S. 1978. "Folic acid levels in blood and seminal plasma of normo- and oligospermic patients prior and following folic acid treatment." *Experientia* 34:1301-1302.

Lavigne, C., A. Marette, H. Jacques. 2000. "Cod and soy proteins compared with casein improve glucose tolerance and insulin sensitivity in rats." *American Journal of Physiology - Endocrinology and Metabolism* 278: E491-500.

Lee, H-C, Y-M Jeong, S. H. Lee et al. 2006. "Association study of four polymorphisms in three folate-related enzyme genes with non-obstructive male infertility." *Human Reproduction* 21: 3162-3170.

Lefevre, M., J. C. Lovejoy, S. R. Smith et al. 2005. "Comparison of the acute response to meals enriched with cis- or trans-fatty acids on glucose and lipids in overweight individuals with differing FABP2 genotypes." *Metabolism* 54: 1652-1658.

Leviton, A., L. Cowan. 2002. "A review of the literature relating caffeine consumption by women to their risk of reproductive hazards." *Food and Chemical Toxicology* 40:1271-1310.

Lima, N., H. Cavaliere, A. Knobel, G. Madeiros-Nieto. 2000. "Decreased androgen levels in massively obese men may be associated with impaired function of the gonadostat." *International Journal of Obesity* 24: 1433-1437.

Longcope, C., R. Baker, C. C. Johnston Jr. 1986. "Androgen and estrogen metabolism: relationship to obesity." *Metabolism* 35: 235-237.

Lucock, M. 2000. "Folic acid: nutritional biochemistry, molecular biology, and role in disease processes." *Molecular Genetics and Metabolism* 71: 121-138.

Lui, G., F. Shi, U. Blas-Machado et al. 2005. "Ovarian effects of a high lactose diet in the female rat." *Reproduction Nutrition Development.* 45:185-192.

MacDonald, A. A., G. P. Herbison, M. Showell, C. M. Farquhar. 2009. "The impact of body mass index on semen parameters and reproductive hormones in human males: a systematic review with meta-analysis." *Human Reproduction Update* dmp047.

Macaluso, M., T. J. Wright-Schnapp, A. Chandra et al. 2010. "A public health focus on infertility prevention, detection, and management." *Fertility and Sterility* 93: 16.e1-.e0.

Magnusdottir, E. V., T. Thorsteinsson, S. Thorsteinsdottir, M. Heimisdottir, K. Olafsdottir. 2005. "Persistent organochlorines, sedentary occupation, obesity and human male subfertility." *Human Reproduction* 20: 208-215.

Malik, N. S., S.A. Matlin, J. Fried, R.E. Pakyz, M.J. Consentino. 1995. "The contraceptive effects of etoprine on male mice and rats." *Journal of Andrology* 16: 169-174.

Massachusetts Department of Public Health. 2008. *Massachusetts Births 2006*. Boston, MA.

Matthews., T. J., B. E. Hammilton. 2009. "Delayed childbearing: more women are having their first child later in life." *NCHS Data Brief* No. 21. Hyattsville, MD: National Center for Health Statistics.

Mendiola, J., A. M. Torres-Cantero, J. M. Moreno-Grau et al. 2009. "Food intake and its relationship with semen quality: a case-control study." *Fertility and Sterility* 91: 812-818.

Mendiola, J., A. M. Torres-Cantero, J. Vioque et al. "A low intake of antioxidant nutrients is associated with poor semen quality in patients attending fertility clinics. *Fertility and Sterility* 2010; 93: 1128-33.

Missmer, S. A., J. E. Chavarro, S. Malspeis et al. 2010. "A prospective study of dietary fat consumption and endometriosis risk." *Human Reproduction* [Epub ahead of print. March 23, 2010].

Murakami, K., S. Sasaki, Y. Takahashi et al. 2006. "Dietary glycemic index and load in relation to metabolic risk factors in Japanese female farmers with traditional dietary habits." *American Journal of Clinical Nutrition* 83: 1161-1169.

Nguyen, R. H. N., A. Wilcox, R. Skjaerven, D. D. Baird. 2007. "Men's body mass index and infertility." *Human Reproduction* 22: 2488-2493.

Pauli, E. M., R. S. Legro, L. M. Demers, A. R. Kunselman, W. C. Dodson, P.A. Lee. 2008. "Diminished paternity and gonadal function with increasing obesity in men." *Fertility and Sterility* 90:346-351.

The Practice Committee of the American Society for Reproductive Medicine. 2006. "Definition of 'Infertility.'" *Fertility and Sterility* 86: S228.

Plymate, S. R., L. A. Matij, R. E. Jones, K. E. Friedl. 1988. "Inhibition of sex hormone-binding globulin production in the human hepatoma (Hep G2) cell line by insulin and prolactin." *Journal of Clinical Endocrinology and Metabolism* 67: 460-464.

Prentice, A. M., P. Rayco-Solon, S. E. Moore. 2005. "Insights from the developing world: thrifty genotypes and thrifty phenotypes." *Proceedings of the Nutrition Society* 64: 153-161.

Qin, D.D., E. Yuan, W. J. Zhou, Y. Q. Cui, J. Q. Wu, E. S. Gao. 2007. "Do reproductive hormones explain the association between body mass index and semen quality?" *Asian Journal of Andrology* 9: 827-834.

Ramlau-Hansen, C. H., A. M. Thulsttrup, E. A. Nohr, J. P. Bonde, T. I. A. Sorensen, J. Olsen. 2007. "Subfecundity in overweight and obese couples." *Human Reproduction* 22: 1634-1637.

Rich-Edwards, J. W., D. Spiegelman, M. Garland et al. 2002. "Physical activity, body mass index, and ovulatory disorder infertility." *Epidemiology* 13: 184-190.

Salazar-Martinez, E., W. C. Willett, A. Ascherio et al. 2004. "Coffee consumption and risk of type 2 diabetes mellitus." *Annals of Internal Medicine* 140:1-8.

Sallmen, M., D. P. Sandler, J. A. Hoppin, A. Blair, D. D. Baird. 2006. "Reduced fertility among overweight and obese men." *Epidemiology* 17: 520-523.

Sierksma, A., H. Patelm, N. Ouchim et al. 2004. "Effect of moderate alcohol consumption on adiponectin, tumor necrosis factor-alpha, and insulin sensitivity." *Diabetes Care* 27: 184-189.

Stephen, E. H., A. Chandra. 1998. "Updated projections of infertility in the United States: 1995-2025." *Fertility and Sterility* 70: 30-34.

Strain, G. W., B. Zumoff, J. Kream et al. 1982. "Mild hypogonadotropic hypogonadism in obese men. *Metabolism* 31: 871-875.

Swarts, W. J., D. R. Mattison. 1998. "Galactose inhibition of ovulation in mice." *Fertility and Sterility* 49: 522-526.

Thaler, C. J., H. Budiman, H. Ruebsamen, D. Nagel, P. Lohse. 2006. "Effects of the common 677C>T mutation of the 5,10-methylenetetrahydrofolate reductase (MTHFR) gene on ovarian responsiveness to tecombinant follicle-dtimulating hormone." *American Journal of Reproductive Immunology* 55: 251-258.

Tüttelmann, F., E. Rajpert-De Meyts, E. Nieschlag, M. Simoni. 2007. "Gene polymorphisms and male infertility a meta-analysis and literature review." *Reproductive BioMedicine Online* 15: 643-658.

Veldhuis, J.D., J. Frystyk, A. Iranmanesh, H. Orskov. 2005. "Testosterone and estradiol regulate free insulin-like growth factor I (IGF-I), IGF binding protein 1 (IGFBP-1), and dimeric IGF-I/IGFBP-1 concentrations." *Journal of Clinical Endocrinology and Metabolism* 90: 2941-2947.

Vermeulen, A., J.M. Kaufman, J. P. Deslypere, G. Thomas. 1993. "Attenuated luteinizing hormone (LH) pulse amplitude but normal LH pulse frequency, and its relation to plasma androgens in hypogonadism on obese men." *Journal of Clinical Endocrinology and Metabolism* 76: 1140-1146.

Wallock, L. M., T. Tamura, C. A. Mayr, K.E. Johnston, B. N. Ames, R. A. Jacob. 2001. "Low seminal plasma folate concentrations are associated with low sperm density and count in male smokers and nonsmokers." *Fertility and Sterility* 75: 252-259.

Winters, S. J., C.Wang, E. Adbdelrahaman, V. Hadedd, M. A. Dyky, A. Brufsky. 2006. "Inhibin-B levels in healthy young adult men and prepubertal boys: is obesity the cause for contemporary decline in sperm count because of fewer Sertoli cells?" *Journal of Andrology* 27: 560-564.

Wolford, S. T., C. J. Argoudelsi. 1979. "Measurement of estrogens in cow's milk, human milk and dairy products." *Journal of Dairy Science* 62: 1458-1463.

Wong, W. Y., H. M. W. M. Merkus, C. M. G. Thomas, R. Menkveld, G. A. Zielhuism, R. P. M. Steegers-Theunissen. 2002. "Effects of folic acid and zinc sulfate on male factor subfertility: a double-blind, randomized, placebo-controlled trial." *Fertility and Sterility* 77: 491-498.

Wong, W. Y., G. A. Zielhuis, C. M. G. Thomas, H. M. W. M. Merkus, R. P. M. Steegers-Theunissen. 2003. "New evidence of the influence of exogenous and endogenous factors on sperm count in man." *European Journal of Obstetrics and Gynecology and Reproductive Biology* 110: 49-54.

World Health Organization. 1995. "Physical Status: The use and interpretation of anthropometry." Report of a WHO Expert Committee, WHO Technical Report Series No. 854. Geneva: World Health Organization.

Young, S. S., B. Eskenazi, F. M. Marchetti, G. Block, A. J. Wyrobek. 2008. "The association of folate, zinc and antioxidant intake with sperm aneuploidy in healthy non-smoking men." *Human Reproduction* 23: 1014-1022.

2

Optimizing Fertility by Timing Intercourse during the Menstrual Cycle

BRUNO SCARPA, PHD

Researcher in Statistics, Department of Statistical Sciences, University of Padua, Italy

ABSTRACT

Optimal timing of intercourse to achieve pregnancy is nowadays an interesting alternative to assisted reproductive therapy (ART). ART procedures are, in fact, usually expensive and convey an increased risk of adverse outcomes for the offspring. It is therefore, advantageous to decrease time to pregnancy by natural methods. One possibility is to time intercourse intentionally during the days of the menstrual cycle having the highest conception probabilities. By using some large and detailed datasets, rules offered by Natural Family Planning (NFP) methods were considered and analyzed in terms of effectiveness, acceptability, and applicability. A biologically based statistical model is used to relate cycle day and biomarkers to conception probability. A methodological approach for searching for optimal rules for timing intercourse based on cycle day, secretions and other information, by using a Bayesian decision theory is also discussed. Good rules result in high conception probabilities while requiring minimal targeted intercourse.

INTRODUCTION

Natural Family Planning (NFP) has been widely used to help couples avoid conception. These methods are based on the identification of simple rules based on self-monitoring of the menstrual cycle and established symptoms of the fertile days (e.g., Stanford et al. 1999). In the last decade, rules to identify potentially fecund days have been similarly used to identify fertile days by couples attempting pregnancy (Stanford et al. 2002).

Most rules are based on the identification of the day of ovulation and its fertile window. Methods of identifying the day of ovulation and the fertile window are traditionally based on basal body temperature (e.g., Marshall 1968), fertility charting of mucus symptom observed at the vagina (e.g., Billings et al. 1972; Hilgers and Stanford 1998; Sinai et al. 1999), and calendar calculations (e.g., Ogino1930; Colombo, Scarpa 1996; Arévalo et al. 1999). It seems reasonable that rules combining calendar, mucus, and temperature are somewhat more effective than methods involving each indicator alone in identifying the fertile window. New methods have been proposed based on serial ovarian ultrasound, monitoring of hormones in urine (e.g., Behre et al. 2000), and monitoring of salivary electrolytes (Fehring 1996).

It is unclear which one of the available rules is the best available option for timing intercourse and achieving pregnancy. Also, it is not clear if some new rule, yet to be defined, could perform better than those proposed. A definition of a "good" rule is also ambiguous since different distinctive features may be required to qualify a method as a good one. Among these features considering methods to achieve conception, are often included: *applicability*, measuring how many cycles or couples could use the method; *easy to use*, depending both on the number of pieces of information needed and on the quantity of operations required to identify the fertile period; *acceptability*, the number of required intercourse acts; *effectiveness*, measuring the effective probability of conception; and *absence of side effects, absence of disturbing psychosexual behavior*, and *low cost*.

As mentioned by Colombo (1998), the shared responsibility on equal footing by men and women is another important feature, unfortunately rarely considered. In fact when natural regulation of fertility is considered simply as a mere technique, this will cause a gross misunderstanding of its deep meaning. In this paper, however, only the simple aspect of analyzing the most measurable features of the natural methods will be analyzed, leaving deeper considerations on responsibility and motivation to others.

The following will discuss different rules widely used in NFP. Also provided is a comparison between the different rules based on recalling a proposal for a methodological background helpful in identifying new rules.

The next section describes the approach followed to compare rules. Section 3 presents the data that will be used for the analysis. Section 4 gives a short draft of the rules compared in this paper. Section 5 shows some results. Section 6 briefly describes the ideas of optimal Bayesian decision framework usable to automatically choose good rules.

A POSSIBLE APPROACH

As indicated by Snick (2005) there are some concerns about the generality of results obtained in studies of couples using NFP methods. Without considering a randomized study (evaluating also the results of a comparison group), it is impossible to definitively show that intentional timing of intercourse with NFP methods causes a reduction in time to pregnancy (TTP). Clearly, the organization of a randomized trial would require a random allocation of each specific rule to a certain number of couples (maybe stratified by some characteristics such age, parity, motivations, education level, etc.). Couples are then followed for a certain period of time and, on the basis of obtained results, one can establish indicators of performance of each rule. Such a framework however, could be very difficult and almost impossible to be implemented for NFP methods. This is due to the great number of rules for avoiding pregnancies. A controlled study would be quite hard to implement. Moreover, the size of the groups needed to obtain reliable results is large—given the great variability observed on the biological phenomena involved. In addition, the motivational and psychological involvement required by the couples is often connected with the specific method proposed by an NFP center or a teacher chosen because of its specific characteristics. Reproducing such an involvement would be difficult to do by randomization. In other words, it would be very difficult for a couple to strictly follow an NFP rule randomly selected, compared to one chosen without coercion.

A different path is needed to compare rules. This is not a proposed methodology to replace a randomized trial, which still is, likely, the only possibility for a fair comparison. This proposed methodology will simply provide a tool for a first classification of the NFP rules used and a possible tool for identifying good rules for timing intercourse to achieve conception. In the interest of simplification, this paper will use the following three characteristics of a viable family planning method: (1) *applicability* of the method, intended as percentage of cycles for which the method enables identification of the fertile window without taking into account the correctness of the latter; (2) *acceptability* of the method, intended as the length of the fertile window; and (3) *effectiveness* of the method, intended as the risk of conception associated with the use of the method.

Of the three criteria listed above, the third one is certainly the most important. The first and second can probably be useful to distinguish between different methods only if these are associated with similar risks. Another important criterion to be considered should be the *ease of use* of a method, but this is gradually losing importance, since even complex procedures can be computerized and used by means of small electronic devices. Comparison of two methods according to the *easy to use* criterion clearly does not require data, while data on actual cycles are needed for comparison of the other criteria.

If observational data are available, about the biometrical characteristics of many cycles and women—such as length, basal body temperature curves, mucus symptom levels, etc.—it would be easy to "simulate" the usage of every single method for each cycle. According to this simulation, evaluation of useful indices to compare two methods by using criteria 1 and 2 does not pose major problems, while the risk of conception associated with the use of a particular method can be estimated by combining the simulation results with information available by using fecundability models similar to those developed by Barrett and Marshall (1968), Schwartz et al. (1980), and Dunson and Stanford (2005). These models provide, for each cycle, the probability of conceiving as a function of the number and instances of intercourse during the cycle, and the length of the post-menstrual period identified from the basal body temperature shift (Marshall 1968) or by mucus peak (Colombo et al. 2006).

Consider one specific rule suggested that will help couples to achieve conception. For a certain cycle it will require sexual intercourse at given days. By applying the day specific probabilities of conception obtained, for example, by Colombo and Masarotto (2000) using the fecundability model developed by Schwartz et al. (1980) to these cycles, it is possible to calculate an estimate of the probability of conception for a couple having sexual intercourse on each day the method considers fertile. The average risk of conception associated with the use of the method considered may then be obtained by averaging probabilities of the different cycles. Clearly, the probabilities thus obtained are somewhat conservative, as they assume intercourse occurs every day considered as fertile. Other intercourse patterns could be evaluated. The delicacy of the subject, and the fact that risk of conception is being estimated deductively and retrospectively, require some prudence in discussing the results.

THE DATA

The simulation of the application of each single NFP method for achieving pregnancy require data on the relevant biometrical measures of a cycle, in addition to the day specific probabilities of conception that we obtained from the Colombo and Masarotto (2000) paper.

The NFP methods considered in this paper are based on the observation of length of cycles, on daily basal body temperature, and on mucus symptoms, at least around the day of ovulation. All this information is available on data from a large European study (Colombo and Masarotto 2000), which enrolled 782 women, during 1992-1996, from seven European centers providing services on fertility awareness using NFP. Information on the study was provided at the participating centers, and women were invited to enroll by their instructors if they satisfied the entry criteria, which included: experienced in use of NFP method, married or in a stable relationship, between 18 and 40 years of age, had at least one menses after cessation of breastfeeding or after delivery, not taking hormonal medication or drugs affecting fertility, and neither partner could have known permanent infertility or illnesses that might cause sub-fertility. The protocol was approved by the International Review Board of Fondazione Lanza (Padua, Italy). In addition, neither partner could have known permanent infertility or illnesses that might cause sub-fertility. It was also required that couples did not use condoms or other barrier methods.

At enrollment the women were given a questionnaire to obtain demographic and reproductive history information. The women were then followed prospectively as they collected detailed daily records of basal body temperature and observations of the mucus, and recorded the days during which intercourse and menstrual bleeding occurred. Because women enrolled were followed for an arbitrary portion of their reproductive lives, they included a mixture of avoiders and achievers, with intention status possibly changing across cycles from the same woman, but no direct information was collected on pregnancy intention in each cycle. The peak mucus day has been used to estimate the day of ovulation within each menstrual cycle (for cycles in which sufficient data are available) as described by Colombo and Masarotto (2000).

The women had received training at the study centers on how to identify different types of sensation and mucus, and were experienced in the use of the method. Teachers and women classified each day of the cycle according to a four-point scale according to the type of mucus symptom described by women: (1) dry, rough and itchy or nothing felt and nothing seen; (2) a damp feeling but nothing is seen; (3) damp feeling and appearance of mucus thick, creamy, whitish, yellowish, not stretchy/elastic, sticky; and (4) wet, slippery, smooth feeling with appearance of mucus transparent, like raw egg white, stretchy/elastic, liquid, watery, reddish. Higher scores indicate higher levels of estrogenic-type mucus and hence conditions more conducive to sperm survival and transport. Day 1 of the menstrual cycle was defined as the first day of fresh red bleeding, excluding any previous days with spotting. A detailed description of the study protocol is available (Colombo and Masarotto 2000).

In order to evaluate the Billings Ovulation Method, it was not possible to use the same data as for the other methods, since mucus is classified by this method in a different way based on symptoms and mucus needs to be observed along all the cycle (not only in the days close to ovulation). For such a method we will use data from an Italian study (Colombo et al. 2004) that enrolled 193 women during 1993-1997, from four centers providing services on fertility awareness using the Billings Ovulation Method (Billings et al. 1972). This study was very similar to the European one and information on the study was provided at the participating centers. Women were invited to enroll by their instructors if they satisfied the entry criteria, which where similar to the other study except for the NFP method of which couples were required to be expert, that in this case was the Billings Method. Only 33 of 193 women had used hormonal contraception before entering the study, with only 1 woman stopping use within 3 months of the first cycle in the study.

Mucus in this study was classified in a five-point scale according to the type of mucus symptom described by the women. As discussed in Colombo et al. (2004), the two most fertile types of mucus score are very similar clinically. Therefore, we collapsed these into one category, resulting in the following four-point scale: (1) dry; (2) a humid or damp feeling; (3) thick, creamy, elastic, whitish moist mucus; and (4) slippery, stretchy, watery, clear mucus. Even if it is difficult to evaluate the reliability of the reported mucus classification, the women enrolled in this study were in the habit of routinely recording mucus symptoms on a daily chart. In addition, women were informed about the aims of the study and about the importance of recording mucus. They understood that carefully recording this information would lead to more reliable study results, which would potentially help them personally. In addition, a teacher was responsible for the women, monitoring their data collection and checking in to verify that they had recorded the daily information. A detailed description of the study protocol is available in Colombo et al. (2004).

Clearly the use of a different dataset does not provide the possibility to have a fair comparison between the Billings and the other methods, but the following results allow some rough evaluation of performance of different methods.

As already discussed, a fecundability model is needed to evaluate effectiveness. The Schwartz et al. (1980) model was used to estimate the parameters obtained by Colombo and Masarotto (2000). In order to use exactly the same fecundability model for all the methods, it was decided to consider the mucus peak as the indicator of ovulation, so that the model could be applied the same for both of the discussed datasets. Peak of mucus seems to be defined in very similar ways by the two protocols. Colombo and Masarotto (1980, Table 9) provided estimates of the parameters of the model considering the mucus peak as ovulation indicator.

SOME NFP METHODS

This section briefly discusses some of the NFP method rules for achieving pregnancy. Some rules are direct modification of simple avoiding method instructions, others are rules that, in practice, NFP center staff suggest to couples interested in achieving pregnancy. These methods will be compared with respect to the features of interest in the following Section.

Ogino-Knaus

The most widely known calendar rule to avoid conception can be reverted by requiring acts of intercourse on all days in the windows defined by the length of shorter previous cycle minus 19 days and the length of longer cycle minus 9 days (Ogino 1930). This method was applied by considering only the 12 cycles before the one analyzed: therefore, it excluded from the analysis all cycles observed in the first year since a woman entered in the study.

Standard Days Method

The reverse of the Standard Days Method (Arévalo et al. 1999) for avoiding conceptions requires simply having intercourse every day between day 8 and day 19 of the cycle for women with a regular cycle (12 previous consecutive cycles between 26 and 32 days).

Two Day Method

The reverse of the Two Day Method (Arévalo et al. 2004) requires intercourse in the days when mucus is observed and in the following ones. For this method it is necessary that the woman is able to recognize mucus, so that cycles when mucus is observed for less than 5 days or for more than 14 days are discarded.

Sympto-Thermal Röetzer

In his book, Röetzer (2007) suggests that couples who wish to achieve pregnancy begin acts of intercourse almost at the end of the days of mucus of best quality, up to the first day of high temperature after the basal body temperature shift. Type 4 mucus of the European study was identified as the "best quality" and interpreted as the "almost at the end" rule as two days before the temperature shift if mucus in these days was fertile.

Sympto-Thermal Camen

A different implementation of the Sympto-Thermal method proposed by centers Camen (Milan, Italy) suggests having intercourse from the first day of transparent and stretchy mucus until the first day of high temperature after the basal body temperature shift.

The type 4 mucus for this method was identified as the transparent and stretchy type mucus.

Billings Ovulation Method

An official book for the Billings Ovulation Method (see, Billings and Westmore 1991), provides couples with a set of rules to achieve pregnancy. They are:

- Intercourse on alternate evenings is required at the beginning of the cycle to be able to identify the starting day of the mucus symptom;
- When change occurs (that is, the beginning of the mucus symptom is observed), delay intercourse until a slippery sensation develops;
- The days of the mucus slippery sensation are recommended for the best chance of achieving pregnancy;
- Conception is claimed to be common when couples have a single act of intercourse that occurs just as the slippery peak symptom is changing to sticky and/or clear fluid cervical mucus is becoming thick and cloudy. According to Billings, it may be necessary to wait until a definite change in sensation occurs before having intercourse.

These method rules were applied by considering alternating acts of intercourse at the beginning of the cycle, and every day when mucus of type 4 and 5 (by using the Italian dataset).

COMPARISONS AND RESULTS

Table 1 (next page) shows mean indexes of applicability, acceptability and effectiveness obtained by simulating the pattern of intercourse, as described above, by using the observed lengths of cycles, basal body temperatures and mucus classification. As expected, in general, rules requiring more acts of intercourse also have a higher probability of conception; however, it seems that the simple Two Day method, requiring only 35% of days with intercourse in a cycle (about 10 days in a regular cycle of 28 days) presents quite a high effectiveness measure.

More sophisticated methods such as Symtho-Thermal and the Billings Ovulation Method present a lower probability of conception (between 50 to 70 percent of the maximum of the probability). Among these methods it seems that the Camen method presents the interesting feature of requiring less than 20% of days with intercourse (about 5 days in a regular 28 days cycle) while not showing a dramatic drop in effectiveness.

In order to take into account the variability observed among cycles and evaluate possible errors due to usage of the estimates of the fecundability model as the plug in evaluating effectiveness, Table 2 shows some descriptive statistics of the distribution of probabilities of

Table 1: Comparisons of some indicators of performance of some methods of NFP

	Applicability	Acceptability	Effectiveness	
	% of cycles applicable	*% of days with intercourse*	*Average probability of conception*	
			Intercourse every day	*Intercourse 1/7th of days*
Standard Days	60.01	42.07	19.34	7.99
Two Day	62.29	35.83	19.26	8.11
Ogino	22.98	56.12	19.88	8.69
Roetzer	73.57	50.89	11.24	4.93
Camen	71.21	18.87	14.77	6.93
Billings*	65.25	61.19	16.81	6.94
Everyday	-	-	20.20	-

* *Indicators for the Billings method have been obtained by using data from the Italian study*

conception. Variability seems to be less relevant for methods based on a single quantity (calendar or mucus). Higher variability is observed for the more sophisticated methods.

A DIFFERENT APPROACH

In the previous sections conception probabilities were obtained as measures of effectiveness by plugging in point estimates of fecundability parameters into a statistical model (Schwartz et al. 1980). Clearly this strategy, even if it is good as a first approximation, could give misleading results by ignoring estimation uncertainty. Different approaches could be proposed in order to overcome this drawback of this type of analysis. A possibility proposed by Scarpa, et al. (2007) is based on a formal Bayesian decision theoretic approach. Such a procedure uses Markov Chain Monte Carlo methods to make calculations feasible, and removing the unknown parameters by integrating them out (for details of the algorithm see Scarpa and Dunson 2007). They also used a simpler model of fecundability requiring the estimation of a much smaller number of parameters, considering the effect of the

Table 2: Summary of the distribution of cycle specific probability of conception for each method considered

	mean	*sd*	*1st quartile*	*Median*	*3rd quartile*
Standard Days	19.34	2.35	19.71	20.15	20.17
Two Day	19.26	1.54	18.83	19.92	20.12
Ogino	19.88	1.33	20.17	20.17	20.2
Roetzer	11.25	5.38	6.41	10.61	14.56
Camen	14.77	4.37	12.61	15.88	18.67
Billings	16.81	3.44	14.56	17.47	19.71

type of mucus not changing in different days around ovulation. By following such an approach they compared a large number of simple rules based on mucus symptom observations and defined the optimal one, once defined, they determined the level of importance of effectiveness with respect to acceptability. Once again, mucus seems to be the most important indicator of changes in hormones during the menstrual cycle, and it is interesting to observe how, in order to identify the most fertile days in a cycle, it seems more reliable to base observations on that single indicator, more than on a mixture of different signals.

SOURCES CONSULTED

Arévalo, M., I. Sinai, V. Jennings. 1999. "A fixed formula to define the fertile window of the menstrual cycle as the basis of a simple method of natural family planning." *Contraception* 60:357-360.

Arévalo, M., V. Jennings, M. Nikula, I. Sinai. 2004. "Efficacy of the new TwoDay Method of family planning." *Fertility and Sterility* 82:885-892.

Barrett, J. C., J. Marshall. 1969. "The risk of fecundability on different days of the menstrual cycle." *Population Studies* 23:455–461.

Behre, H. M., J. Kuhlage, C. Gassner, B. Sonntag, C. Schem, H. P. Schneider, E. Nieschlag. 2000. "Prediction of ovulation by urinary hormone measurements with the home use ClearPlan Fertility Monitor: comparison with transvaginal ultrasound scans and serum hormone measurements." *Human Reproduction* 15:2478–2482.

Billings, E. L., J. J. Billings, J. B. Brown, H. G. Burger. 1972. "Symptoms and hormonal changes accompanying ovulation." *Lancet* 1:282–284.

Billings, E., A. Westmore. 1991. *The Billings Method: Controlling Fertility without Drugs or Devices*. Makati, Philippines: St. Paul Publications.

Colombo, B. 1998. "Evaluation of fertility predictors and comparisons of different rules." *Genus* 54:53-167.

Colombo, B., G. Masarotto. 2000. "Daily fecundability: first results from a new data base." *Demographic Research* 3:5.

Colombo, B., B. Scarpa. 1996. "Calendar methods of fertility regulation: a rule of thumb." *Statistica* LVI:3-14.

Colombo, B., A. Mion, K. Passarin, B. Scarpa. 2006. "Cervical mucus symptom and daily fecundability: first results from a new data base." *Statistical Methods in Medical Research* 15:161–180.

Dunson, D. B., J. B. Stanford. 2005. "Bayesian inferences on predictors of conception probabilities." *Biometrics* 1:126–133.

Fehring, R. J. 1996. "A comparison of the ovulation method with the CUE ovulation predictor in determining the fertile period." *Journal of American Academy of Nurse Practitioners* 8:461–466.

Hilgers, T. W., J. B. Stanford. 1998. "Creighton-Model NaProEducation Technology for avoiding pregnancy." *Journal of Reproductive Medicine* 43:495-502.

Marshall, J. 1968. "A field trial of the basal body-temperature method of regulating births." *The Lancet* 2:8–10.

Ogino, K. 1930 "Ovulationstermin und Konzeptionstermin." *Zentralbl Gynakol* 54:464-479.

Röetzer, T. 2008. *Naturliche Geburtenregelung der Partnershaftliche Weg*. Wien, Osterrerich: Herder & Co.

Scarpa, B., D. B. Dunson. 2007. "Bayesian methods for searching for optimal rules for timing intercourse to achieve pregnancy." *Statistics in Medicine* 126:1920-1936.

Scarpa, B., D. B. Dunson, E. Giacchi. 2007. "Bayesian selection of optimal rules for timing intercourse using calendar and mucus." *Fertility and Sterility* 88:915-924.

Schwartz, D., P. D. M. MacDonald, V. Heuchel. 1980. "Fecundability, coital frequency and the viability of ova." *Population Studies* 34: 97–400.

Sinai, I., V. Jennings, M. Arévalo. 1999. "The TwoDay algorithm: a new algorithm to identify the fertile time of the menstrual cycle." *Contraception* 60: 65-70.

Snick, H. K. A. 2005. "Should spontaneous or timed intercourse guide couples trying to conceive?" *Human Reproduction* 10:2976-2977.

Stanford, J. B., P. B. Thurman, J. C. Lemaire. 1999. "Physicians' knowledge and practices regarding natural family planning." *Obstetrics and Gynecology* 94:672-678.

Stanford, J. B., G. L. White, H. Hatasaka. 2002. "Timing intercourse to achieve pregnancy: current evidence." *Obstetrics and Gynecology* 100:1333–1341.

PANEL II

BREASTFEEDING AND THE TRANSITION TO FERTILITY

3

The Development & Use of the Lactational Amenorrhea Method (LAM): Transitioning to Other Natural Methods

MIRIAM LABBOK, MD, MPH, FACPM, IBCLC

Professor of the Practice of Public Health
Department of Maternal and Child Health, University of North Carolina

ABSTRACT

Breastfeeding contributes to the health and survival of both mothers and children. Exclusive breastfeeding for the first 6 months of life, followed by continued breastfeeding while complementary foods are being introduced, is associated with significantly improved child health and survival. This same pattern of infant feeding contributes to maternal postpartum recovery and to reductions in breast and other cancers later in life. Birth spacing also supports health and survival; short birth intervals are associated with increased risk of birth-related problems for mother and child, as well as with nutrition and health risks for the child.

While there are many Natural Family Planning (NFP) methods shown to be effective during regular menstrual cycles, their use during breastfeeding has always required additional considerations and rules, and is considered a 'special case.' Methods that depend on signs and symptoms of the fertile period may be difficult to use at this time, demanding skilled interpretation and/or long periods of abstinence to ensure high efficacy. Today, with the majority of women in the United States practicing the healthy global normative behavior of initiating breastfeeding in the postpartum period, breastfeeding can no longer be considered a "special case." Rather, it is the normal postpartum practice in virtually every country.

Women have long experienced and observed that they were less likely to become pregnant during breastfeeding, but breastfeeding *per se* is not a form of family planning. Over the last 35 years or so, the physiology of breastfeeding has undergone increased study, and we have learned the signs of fertility return related to breastfeeding. From this, the natural, introductory method of family planning known as the Lactational Amenorrhea Method, or LAM, was developed. Following three criteria—amenorrhea, full or nearly full breastfeeding, and six months (as the time when regular complementary feeding should commence)—a woman experiences less than a 2% chance of pregnancy, a level of efficacy comparable to some of the most efficacious spacing methods; however, the period of time after these criteria no longer apply, i.e., after menses first returns or after breastfeeding is reduced, constitutes a period of difficult transition for many NFP methods. This article provides background on the importance of breastfeeding, the development and testing of LAM, and discusses issues associated with the transition to periodic abstinence/NFP methods.

INTRODUCTION

Breastfeeding and adequate birth intervals contribute to both maternal and child health and survival (Rutstein 2005; Conde-Agudelo et al. 2007). Short birth intervals are associated with increased risk to both maternal and child birth outcomes, and later child health; families should be encouraged to space their births at least two, preferably three years apart. While there are many approaches to Natural Family Planning (NFP) that have been shown to be effective during regular menstrual cycles, use of these methods during breastfeeding has always been considered a "special case." NFP methods that depend on fertility signs and symptoms may be difficult to use, demanding skilled interpretation or demand long periods of abstinence (Labbok et al.1994; Kennedy et al.1991). Today, with the majority of women in the United States as well as worldwide initially breastfeeding in the postpartum period, breastfeeding can no longer be considered a "special case" but rather as the normal postpartum practice.

The Lactational Amenorrhea Method (LAM) was developed to serve as an introductory method for use during breastfeeding in the postpartum period. LAM provides a period of infertility aiding in guarding the mother's health against a too short interval before her next pregnancy. LAM also is useful during a reproductive time when symptoms and signs of fertility return may be difficult to interpret. LAM has been studied for efficacy and acceptability around the world. Studies consistently find high efficacy and good levels of acceptability in multiple countries, socio-economic strata, and cultures. Nonetheless, LAM is not seen as a mainstream method by many NFP providers (or contraceptive and reproductive health interest groups).

This paper will review the history and development of LAM, efficacy studies, transition to other natural methods, and related research issues. It will also treat the current understanding and use (misunderstanding and misuse) of LAM, globally and in the United States of America.

RATIONALE FOR SUPPORTING BREASTFEEDING

Breastfeeding is the biological normal resolution of pregnancy for mother and child. Therefore, it is not surprising that lack of breastfeeding, especially lack of exclusive breastfeeding, is associated with measurable risks (Ip et al. 2007; AHRQ 2009; McNiel et al. 2010; Horta et al. 2007; Jonas et al. 2008; Negishi et al.1999; Mezzacappa 2005; Ward et al. 2004). Children who are not breastfed, or less than optimally breastfed, experience significantly more non-specific gastroenteritis, asthma, obesity, type 1 and type 2 diabetes, childhood leukemia, sudden infant death syndrome (SIDS), necrotizing enterocolitis, pneumonia, ear infections, atopic dermatitis, high blood pressure, high cholesterol, and lower scholastic performance. Mothers who do not breastfeed experience a higher risk of type 2 diabetes, breast cancer, ovarian cancer, maternal postpartum depression, high blood pressure, slower uterine involutions, increased postpartum blood loss, increased maternal stress, modified nutrient and calcium metabolism, and earlier fertility return. Given this extraordinary list of health benefits, parents who wish to give their child the best start on life should be counseled to breastfeed as close to the optimal patterns as possible.

For optimal health impact, the World Health Organization (WHO) and others advise: (1) early initiation of breastfeeding within the first hour, facilitated by immediate placement of the baby skin-to-skin with the mother; (2) exclusive breastfeeding for the first six months; and (3) continued breastfeeding with age appropriate complementary feeding for up to two years or longer. Exclusive breastfeeding at the breast conveys the most responsive physiological relationship, provides an ever-changing milk supply, and allows the infant to control the amounts ingested. The milk consumed at each feed starts out thinner and becomes more and more fatty, in this manner, each breastfeeding proceeds from "soup" to "dessert." Feeding expressed human milk is the next best approach; however, the advantages from direct breastfeeding, including the child-controlled satiety in response to ingesting the fatty hindmilk, are lost. Also, when the mother and child are separated, the infectious agents they are exposed to differ, and the mother may not be producing all the immune factors the baby may need. Non-human milks are a far third among feeding choices. Commercial formula consists of watered-down cow milk with additives and emulsifiers; this mixture cannot approximate the hundreds of components and living cells found in human milk (Labbok et al. 2004).

HISTORY OF THE SCIENCE OF BREASTFEEDING AND ITS RELATIONSHIP TO FERTILITY

Research in the last 50 years has confirmed the "old wives tale" that breastfeeding delays fertility return postpartum. Hence, breastfeeding not only provides the best healthy start on life, but also helps to preserve birth spacing. The World Fertility Surveys and national studies confirmed that, without family planning used, the median number of months until the next pregnancy occurs is significantly longer in breastfeeding populations; however, those that attempted to find a direct mathematical association between the duration of breastfeeding and the duration of amenorrhea—a proxy for fertility return—were frustrated by the variability they found. It was not until the 1970s that researchers began to consider that the pattern of breastfeeding (frequency, amount of other food or fluids, rapidity of weaning) would influence the relationship between total duration of breastfeeding and the timing of menses return. Two seminal studies found that varying feeding pattern are associated with varying health outcomes and varying fertility return, with best health and survival, and greatest suppression of fertility, associated with the more intensive patterns of breastfeeding (Victora et al. 1987; Perez et al. 1971). Concurrently the independent studies of John Tyson and Richard Chatterton were beginning to shed some light on the relationship between breastfeeding and fertility. Researchers responsible for additional studies during the 1980s (Howie et al. 1982; Family Health International 1988; Gray et al.1990; Diaz et al.1988) were gathered at the Rockefeller Bellagio Center on Lake Como to explore whether it might be possible to identify factors associated with fertility return during breastfeeding. This group identified three variables that, together, were predictive of fertility return among breastfeeding women. "Women who are not using family planning, but who are fully or nearly fully breastfeeding and amenorrheic, are likely to experience a risk of pregnancy of less than 2% in the first six months after delivery"(Kennedy et al.1989). [see next page]

The three variables identified from the research were then codified as an algorithm defining the method of family planning, the Lactational Amenorrhea Method (or LAM). LAM, presented as an algorithm (Labbok et al. 1994), was developed by a group of family planning and Maternal Child Health program leaders at Georgetown University's Institute for Reproductive Health (IRH). At that time, and still today, the Institute for Reproductive Health is tasked with the study of Fertility Awareness-Based Methods, or the Natural Family Planning methods that rely on identifying potentially fertile days when intercourse is most likely to result in a pregnancy. During the post-partum period women who are practicing LAM may also be considered users of an NFP method.

Following this codification as an algorithm, LAM then underwent clinical study for acceptance, effectiveness, and efficacy. Other studies offered the three criteria as general information to inform the timing of the introduction of another family planning method. The dozens of studies of LAM and of the three criteria that are found in the literature consistently confirm that the potential of an unplanned pregnancy is less than 2%, and often less than 1%.

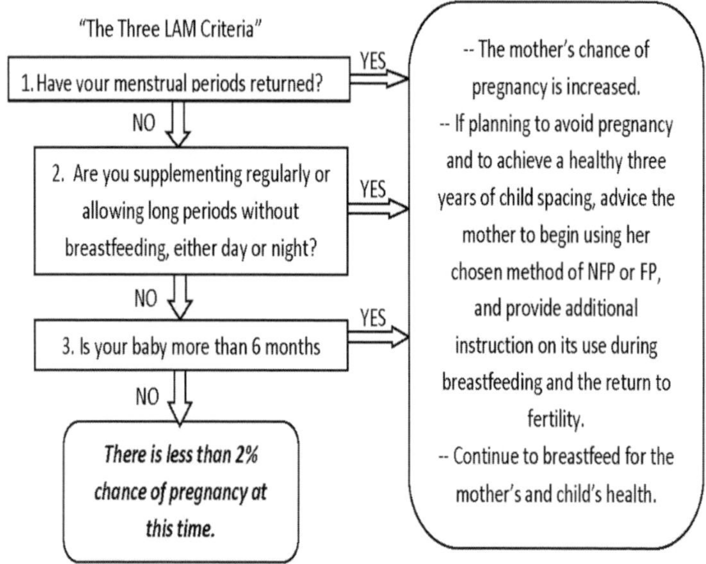

The Lactational Amenorrhea Method – LAM
Ask the mother, or advise her to ask herself, these three questions:
"The Three LAM Criteria"
1. Have your menstrual periods returned?
YES
NO
2. Are you supplementing regularly or allowing long periods without breastfeeding, either day or night?
YES
NO
3. Is your baby more than 6 months
YES
NO
There is less than 2% chance of pregnancy at this time.
-- The mother's chance of pregnancy is increased.
-- If planning to avoid pregnancy and to achieve a healthy three years of child spacing, advice the mother to begin using her chosen method of NFP or FP, and provide additional instruction on its use during breastfeeding and the return to fertility.
-- Continue to breastfeed for the mother's and child's health.

Subsequent studies not only confirmed the efficacy of LAM, but also that the effectiveness was not dependent on education, religion, or geographic location. Further, research confirmed that more than 80% of LAM acceptors began to use another family planning method (including NFP methods) in a timely manner. Over the years, LAM has been used in more than 40 countries around the globe.

A WORD ABOUT COMPLEMENTARY FAMILY PLANNING OPTIONS FOR BREASTFEEDING WOMEN

In general, research confirmed that users of LAM were more likely to transition to another family planning method and to remain non-pregnant at 12 months postpartum (Hardy et al. 1998). Family planning methods, including NFP, have been used during breastfeeding with varying results. As may be seen in Table 1, during Ovulation Method (OM) use, breastfeeding and full breastfeeding were associated with lower fertility than method use in the postpartum period when there was no breastfeeding (Labbok et al. 1991).

Table 1. Ovulation Method efficacy during breastfeeding: life table pregnancy rates				
Month	All Women	No BFing	Any BFing	Full BFing
N	378	198*	367	339
	% (S.E.)	% (S.E.)	% (S.E.)	% (S.E.)
6	3.5 (1.0)	8.2 (2.6)	2.3 (0.9)+	1.2 (0.8)+
9	7.2 (1.5)	12.6 (2.4)	5.3 (2.1)+	**
12	11.1(19)	15.3 (2.6)	**	**

* Each woman entered the life table in the month that she was no longer breastfeeding
** Numbers too few for analysis

These life table pregnancy rates reveal the following three outcomes of note: (1) the months following cessation of breastfeeding are a time when a higher rate of pregnancy occurs; (2) similar rates of unplanned pregnancy occurred among all women post menses return regardless of their breastfeeding status: 14 among breastfeeders, and 15.3 among non-breastfeeders; and (3) rates were also elevated at the time when infant feeding supplementation began. These findings underscore the importance of the menses return criteria as predictive of fertility return.

The research also found that these increases in unplanned pregnancy were not directly attributable to non-adherence to the OM rules; in fact, there was some indication that adherence to the rules actually increased during those months. Further analysis showed that sensation, rather than observations, served as slightly better predictors of menses return during lactation. In sum, it is clear that women practicing OM in the postpartum period should take special care with these transition periods if they wish to avoid pregnancy. Another concern was that some women reported mucus symptoms during this time that were often unrelated to estrogen production and would indicate times for abstinence that were not necessarily related to adequate ovarian activity.

We conclude from these findings that OM use among breastfeeding women who wish to delay the next pregnancy might benefit from:

- increased support for breastfeeding to allow longer use of LAM
- Education on increased potential for unplanned pregnancy when (a) supplementation starts or (b) when menses returns (Labbok et al.1991)
- If the OM method is used during these higher risk periods, it may be that sensation might better predict fertility return than observation of mucus.

Study of the Symptom-Thermal methods found that the first cycle that occurs has up to a 4 day difference between the estimated date of Basal-Body-Temperature (BBT) and the luteinizing hormone (LH) peak + 1 day. In addition, the luteal phase lasted only 10 days on average, indicating that this first cycle was probably not adequate for conception to occur (Zinaman et al.1991).

In sum, for the postpartum breastfeeding woman, LAM use, rather than other NFP methods, allows avoidance of unnecessary abstinence and provides a highly effective acceptable natural method; however, the period following the end of LAM use—when breastfeeding changes or when menses returns—is a period of increased potential for an unplanned pregnancy, even when there is careful adherence to the method rules. While users themselves reported no issues with transition from LAM to NFP, "danger" points were identified. The recommendation that emerged was that if a couple is interested in using these fertility awareness based methods, it may be best to teach or re-teach the NFP method during breastfeeding and LAM use and have a refresher when menses return and/or when breastfeeding changes or complementary foods are introduced.

CONCLUSIONS

The Lactational Amenorrhea Method (LAM) is based on the physiology of breastfeeding. Its use supports breastfeeding, adequate child spacing, and maternal and child health, nutrition and maternal and child survival. When used with other NFP or fertility awareness based methods, LAM contributes to a longer period of infertility, hence, a longer inter-birth interval. The advantages to the mother's and child's health from both breastfeeding and birth spacing have been well documented.

LAM has been found "do-able" and efficacious in multiple settings worldwide; it supports optimal breastfeeding, and identifies the time for the introduction of the next method chosen by the couple to support healthy birth spacing and, as desired later, pregnancy achievement.

SOURCES CONSULTED

AHRQ *Guide to Clinical Preventive Services*, 2010-2011; available at www.ahrq.gov/clinic/pocketgd1011/gcp10s2e.htm#Breastfeeding; accessed May 23, 2011.

Chantry et al. "Lactation among adolescent mothers and subsequent bone mineral density." *Archives of Pediatrics & Adolescent Medicine* 158 (July):650-656.

Conde-Agudelo, A., A. Rosas-Bermudez, A. C. Kafury-Goeta. 2007. "Effects of birth spacing on maternal health: a systematic review." *American Journal of Obstetrics and Gynecology* 196 (April):297-308.

Diaz, S., G. Rodriguez, O. Peralta, P. Miranda, M. Casado, A. Salvatierra, C. Herros, A. Brandeis, H. Croxatto. 1988. "Lactational amenorrhea and the recovery of ovulation and fertility in fully nursing Chilean women." *Contraception* 38:53-67. Family Health International. 1988. "Breastfeeding as a family planning method." *Lancet* 2:1204-205.

Gray, R., O. Campbell, R. Apelo, S. Eslami, H. Zacur, R. Ramos, J. Gebret, M. Labbok. 1990. "The risk of ovulation during lactation." *Lancet* 335:25-29.

Hardy, E., L. C. Santos, M. J. Osis, G. Carvalho, J. G. Cecatti, A. Faundes. 1998. "Contraceptive use and pregnancy before and after introducing lactational amenorrhea (LAM) in a postpartum program." *Advances in Contraception* 14 (March):59-68.

Horta, B., R. Bahl, J. Martinés, C. Victora. 2007. "Evidence on the long-term effects of breastfeeding: systematic reviews and meta-analysis." Geneva: World Health Organization; available at www.who.int/child-adolescent-health/publications/NUTRITION/ISBN_92_4_159523_0.htm; accessed May 23, 2011.

Howie, P., A. McNeilly. 1982. "Effect of breastfeeding patterns on human birth intervals." *Journal of Reproductive Fertility* 65:545-557.

Ip, S. et al. 2007. "Breastfeeding and Maternal and Infant Health Outcomes in Developed Countries. Evidence Report/Technology Assessment No. 153." AHRQ Publication No. 07-E007. Rockville, MD: AHRQ; available at www.ahrq.gov/clinic/tp/brfouttp.htm; accessed May 23, 2011.

Jonas, W., E. Nissen, A. Bansjo-Arvidson, I. Wiklund, P. Henriksson, K. Uvnas-Moberg. 2008. "Short- and long-term decrease of blood pressure in women during breastfeeding." *Breastfeeding Medicine* 3 (June):103-109.

Kennedy, K., S. Parenteau-Carreau, A. Flynn, B. Gross, J. Brown, C. Visness. 1991. "The natural family planning-lactational amenorrhea method interface: observations from a prospective study of breastfeeding users of natural family planning." *American Journal of Obstetrics and Gynecology* 165 (6 Pt 2):2020-2026.

Kennedy, K., R. Rivera, A. McNeilly. 1989. "Consensus statement on the use of breastfeeding as a family planning method." *Contraception* 39:477-496.

Labbok, M., D. Clark, A. Goldman. 2004. "Breastfeeding: maintaining an irreplaceable immunological resource." *Nature Reviews Immunology* 4 (July):565-572.

Labbok, M., A. Perez, V. Valdes, F. Sevilla, K. Wade, Vh. Laukaran, Ka. Cooney, S. Coly, C.

Sanders, Jt. Queenan. 1994. "The Lactational Amenorrhea Method (LAM): A postpartum introductory family planning method with policy and program implications." *Advances in Contraception* 10:93-109.

Labbok, M., R. Stallings, F. Shah, A. Perez, H. Klaus, M. Jacobson, T. Muruthi. 1991. "Ovulation method use during breastfeeding: is there increased risk of unplanned pregnancy?" *American Journal of Obstetrics and Gynecology* 165 (6 Pt 2):2031-2036.

McNiel, M., M. Labbok, S. W. Abrams. 2010. "What Are the Risks Associated with Formula Feeding? A Re-Analysis and Review." *Birth* 37:1.

Mezzacappa, E. S., R. M. Kelsey, E. S. Katkin. 2005. "Breast feeding, bottle feeding, and maternal autonomic responses to stress." *Journal of Psychosomatic Research* 58 (April):351-365.

Negishi, H., T. Kishida, H. Yamada, E. Hirayama, M. Mikuni, S. Fujimoto. 1999. "Changes in uterine size after vaginal delivery and cesarean section determined by vaginal sonography in the puerperium." *Archives of Gynecology and Obstetrics* 263 (November):13-16

Perez, A., M. Labbok, D. Barker, R. Gray. 1988. "Use-effectiveness of the ovulation method initiated during postpartum breastfeeding." *Contraception* 38:499-508.

Perez, A., P. Vela, R. Potter, G. Masnick. 1971. "Timing and sequence of resuming ovulation and menstruation after childbirth." Po*pulation Studies* 25:491-503.

Rutstein, S. O. 2005. "Effects of preceding birth intervals on neonatal, infant and under-five years mortality and nutritional status in developing countries: evidence from the demographic and health surveys." *International Journal of Gynaecology and Obstetrics* 89 Suppl 1:S7-24.

Victora, C. G., P. G. Smith, J. P. Vaughan, L. C. Nobre, C. Lombardi, A. M. Teixeira, S. M. Fuchs, L. B. Moreira, L. P. Gigante, F. C. Barros. 1987. "Evidence for protection by breast-feeding against infant deaths from infectious diseases in Brazil." *Lancet* 2: 319-322.

Ward et al. 2005. *Current Opinion in Obstetrics and Gynecology* 17 (August): 435-439.

Zinaman, M., W. Stevenson. 1991. "Efficacy of the symptothermal method of natural family planning in lactating women after the return of menses." *American Journal of Obstetrics and Gynecology* 165 (6 Pt 2):2037-2039.

4

Efficacy of a Protocol for Avoiding Pregnancy during Breastfeeding Transition

MARY M. SCHNEIDER, MSN, FNP-BC, NFPE

Assistant Director, Institute for Natural Family Planning
College of Nursing, Marquette University

RICHARD J. FEHRING, PHD, RN, FAAN

Director, Institute for Natural Family Planning
College of Nursing, Marquette University

ABSTRACT

The transition from amenorrhea to the commencement of ovulation and the first three menstrual cycles postpartum is a time when women who use Natural Family Planning methods (NFP) often unintentionally become pregnant. The purpose of this research was to test the efficacy and acceptability of a breastfeeding protocol to avoid pregnancy that utilized electronic hormonal fertility monitoring (EHFM) to create artificial menstrual cycles and to track fertility.

The outcomes for this study were unintended pregnancy rates and acceptability based on a 10 item measure with scores ranging from 10-70, with the higher score indicating more acceptability.

In terms of the method used, 95 women were recruited (mean age 30.0) who sought to avoid pregnancy while breastfeeding and who entered into a Web site that provided NFP instructions, an electronic charting system, a special breastfeeding protocol, and support from professional nurses. The protocol involved creating 20 day artificial menstrual cycles and monitoring urinary estrogen rises with the EHFM device. The participants were assessed for acceptability of the protocol at 1 and 3 months. Correct use and total unintended pregnancy rates were determined by survival analysis.

The results of the study yielded 4 unintended pregnancies, all due to incorrect use, among 61 participants who were charting online. The 12 month correct use unintended pregnancy rate was 0.00 per 100 users (Std. Error = 0.00) and the 12 month total unintended pregnancy rate was 14.0 per 100 women users (Std. Error = 0.07). Mean acceptability scores of the protocol to avoid pregnancy were not statistically different at one (42.7), and three months of use (46.5).

It is the conclusion of the researchers that the Web based breastfeeding protocol was highly effective when used correctly. Acceptability of the nurse supported online system of providing NFP services to postpartum breastfeeding women increased with use.

INTRODUCTION

Breastfeeding and breastfeeding weaning can be one of the most precarious times of a woman's reproductive life. It can be a time of joy or a time of great trepidation as she tries to interpret her signs of fertility. Women who use natural signs of fertility to plan their families during the breastfeeding transition often have difficulty identifying their fertile and infertile time resulting in long periods of abstinence and/or unplanned pregnancies. Hatherly (1985) and Brown, Harrison and Smith (1985), found there was an increase in the unintended pregnancy rate in women who used Natural Family Planning (NFP) methods during breastfeeding and suggested the increase in unintended pregnancies is due to the women's inability to clearly identify their fertile and infertile days. Brown et al. (1985) compared mucus and temperature signs to urinary hormones of 55 post-partum breastfeeding women and found a disassociation between the secondary sign of the urinary reproductive hormones and the tertiary signs of mucus and temperature about 40% of the time. Hatherly (1985) suggested that this might be the reason why experienced NFP users choose not to use natural signs of fertility while breastfeeding. A more recent article by Stanford and Howard (1999) also found when reviewing pregnancies for a mucus only method "total pregnancy probabilities were higher among the breastfeeding couples on days that were considered fertile (23.8 per 100 couples at one year for breastfeeders vs. 17.1 for all couples)" (Stanford and Howard 1999, p. 399).

To date there are very few studies that investigate the efficacy of NFP methods during breastfeeding, suggesting that although this is a very important area of research in NFP it is also the most neglected. It is precisely this reason why researchers at the Marquette University Institute for NFP have chosen to focus on the breastfeeding transition phase of fertility. The goal is to increase the number of couples using NFP as well as prevent premature discontinuation of breastfeeding during the breastfeeding weaning phase by helping couples feel more confident they will be able to avoid an unintended pregnancy.

In a preliminary review of ten breastfeeding women, Fehring, Schneider and Barron (2005) evaluated a protocol that used a hormonal monitoring device to detect two pre-ovulatory hormones from the woman's first morning urine. The monitor is used in conjunction with fertility charts to track fertility. They found that when couples used the monitor to track their fertile signs, days of abstinence were 17% of the total days of the cycle (first day of charting through the first menstrual cycle) compared to almost 50% of the days for mucus only (Fehring et al. 2005, p. 806). This monitor provides the couple with an additional objective sign of fertility that helps them feel more confident in identifying times of fertility and infertility. The Marquette Method Breastfeeding Weaning Protocol combines the monitor and fertility charts with simple instructions where the couple trigger artificial cycles after every twenty days of testing until ovulation is detected. It is a simple and user friendly program. The purpose of this pilot research study was to test the efficacy and acceptability of this breastfeeding protocol.

BENEFITS OF BREASTFEEDING

There is no debate as to whether or not breastfeeding the baby for at least six months has benefits to both mother and baby. The literature is filled with the many benefits to mother, baby, family, and the community at large. Despite this positive evidence, the number of women who exclusively breastfeed for at least six months is low. The problem is multifactorial, stemming from the lack of support for the mother, baby, and family unit to the lack of support from health care providers and healthcare systems.

The health benefits to the baby from breastfeeding have been well documented. Ladomenou, Moschandreas, Kafatos, Tselentis and Galanakis (2010) followed infectious episodes of 926 infants for twelve months and found that when women breastfed their infants exclusively there was a significantly lower rate of otitis media, necrotizing enterocolitis, gastroenteritis, acute respiratory infections and sepsis, compared to those women who partially breastfed or bottle-fed their infants. Bartick and Reinhold (2010) did a comprehensive cost analysis of these same infant diagnoses and found that if "90% of U.S. families could comply with medical recommendations to breastfeed exclusively for six months the United States would save $13 billion per year and prevent 911 infant deaths" (Bartick and Reinhold 2010, p. 1048). The National Health and Nutrition Examination Surveys showed that from 2005-2006, 77% of women initiated breastfeeding, exceeding the goal of 75% set by Healthy People 2010. By six months however, only 35% of them were still exclusively breastfeeding, a figure that is well below the 50% goal of Healthy People 2010. Of note, the goal for Healthy People 2010 has been retained for Healthy People 2020.

PROMOTING BREASTFEEDING

If a woman is able to exclusively breastfeed until the baby is six months old and she hasn't had a return to menses, she falls within the protocol of the Lactation Amenorrhea Method (LAM). The chance of getting pregnant during this time according to the LAM protocol is less than 2%. Despite this strong protocol and despite the benefits of breastfeeding, according to the Breastfeeding Report Card 2010, the number of women who actually do continue to exclusively breastfeed is "stagnant and low."

Today it is very rare for couples to be able to afford raising children on just one income, making it difficult, if not almost impossible, for working mothers to exclusively breastfeed once they return to work. Mothers often return to work before the baby is six months old. This directly impacts their ability to exclusively breastfeed and they are no longer able to use the LAM protocol. A small subset of working mothers who have successfully breastfed up to the point of returning to work may choose to pump the breast during working hours and nurse the baby when they return home. Pumping the breast produces fluctuation in signs of fertility and makes it difficult for many couples to interpret the signs of fertility.

A return to fertility that occurs with the fluctuation of nursing is directly affected by the estrogen level, which also affects cervical mucus and temperature signs. A hormone called prolactin is released during the suckling action by the baby at the breast and suppresses estrogen. Estrogen is a primary pre-ovulatory hormone that is released by the growing follicle. One of its actions is to act on the cervix and cervical crypts to produce fertile type mucus. When prolactin is low, due to decreased suckling at the breast, estrogen levels begin to rise and follicular growth is stimulated. When suckling is resumed the estrogen level is suppressed and follicular growth is halted. Thus, the fluctuation in suckling, as seen during breastfeeding weaning, produces confusing signs of fertility for the couple. A return to fertility can be expected whenever the mother decreases suckling time at the breast, such as when she returns to work or naturally as the infant grows and solid foods are introduced into the diet.

For most American women the amount of time the baby suckles at the breast or the intensity of the suckling at the breast is not enough to suppress fertility. Thus, a fluctuation in the signs of fertility is expected and couples using NFP experience a variable return to fertility leading to a higher unintended pregnancy rate. Use of the mucus or temperature sign during this time can create immense anxiety-provoked ambivalence for the couple, which often leads to long periods of unnecessary sexual abstinence, surrender to passions or use of a contraceptive. And for many Catholic couples, contemplation of surrendering to passions or the use of a contraceptive method may provoke anxiety. This anxiety may also be compounded by the length of the breastfeeding experience, which can last from a few days to years. It may be a time, marked by different stages, where the couple is unable to establish any pattern of fertility. It is no wonder that couples using NFP become frustrated and seek expert advice from their NFP teacher and even clergy consultants.

PROPOSED THEORETICAL STAGES OF BREASTFEEDING

The stages of breastfeeding and breastfeeding weaning can be divided into four distinct areas. Stage one is the time from the birth of the baby until the first ovulation marked by the estrogen rise and follicular development. Stage two is from the first ovulation until the first menses which according to Brown et al. (1985) may consist of a short luteal phase of "less then eleven days and even as short as eight days"

(Brown et al.1985, p. 20). Stage three is the first three to six menstrual cycles after the birth of the child where often cycles have delayed ovulation and are characterized by long cycles. Finally, stage four is when the woman resumes regular menstrual cycles six months after returning to cycles. It is the variability and unpredictability of the first three stages that causes anxiety for couples using NFP. These are also the targeted stages for the Marquette Method Breastfeeding Weaning Protocol.

Researchers and teachers at the Marquette Institute for NFP have developed a protocol that uses a urinary hormonal fertility-monitoring device that is available over the counter for about $200. The device, known as the Clearblue Easy Fertility Monitor, provides the couple with an objective sign of fertility from the woman's first morning urine. The monitor detects two primary pre-ovulatory hormones: estrone-3-glucuronide (E3G) and Luteinizing Hormone (LH). Couples using this device along with a breastfeeding weaning protocol, developed by the Institute for NFP, have been very successful in avoiding pregnancy during the breastfeeding weaning transition phase.

METHODS

The method used for the research was a prospective, one-group intervention study. We proposed to have fifty to one-hundred total and partial breastfeeding women for the study. The participants were recruited by e-mail notifications, fertility and breastfeeding blogs, and social online media. The most important method of recruitment had been through the "snowball" effect of breastfeeding women notifying other breastfeeding women of the protocol and the online NFP support system.

The breastfeeding participants were instructed to register online. At that time, they were asked to consent to follow the breastfeeding postpartum protocol and contribute a minimum of six online charting system menstrual cycles. Participants were anonymous and received a username that was unique to them when they registered. This study has received human rights approval through the Marquette University Office of Research Compliance.

The online NFP delivery and support system consists of a fertility charting system and an active online discussion forum where users get answers on a daily basis to their questions from Marquette NFP professional nurses. Couples using the online charting system can easily access the charting system once they login. When they want to record their observation in the charting system they simply put their cursor over the day they are charting and a picture menu appears. The woman then uses these pictures to help match her fertility sign of the mucus and/or the electronic fertility monitor. She clicks on her correct observation and it shows up on her chart.

Couples using the breastfeeding weaning protocol also create artificial cycles with the monitor after every twenty days of testing (see Addendum for protocol and Figure 1). When the monitor does not detect estrogen (shown as a single bar or "low") the woman tests every other day. When a threshold of E3G has been reached, indicating follicular activity characterized by two bars or "high," the woman tests daily. When the monitor indicates an estrogen threshold has been detected, daily testing can be expected until the LH surge has been found or the couple resets the monitor and the woman returns to "low" fertility. The couple will continue to use the breastfeeding protocol until they experience a peak on the monitor indicating the LH surge has been identified. When the LH surge is detected the couple does not reset the monitor. They let it continue to advance each day until the woman has her first menses post-partum. When she has her menses she resumes regular cycle instructions by testing daily until she sees the LH surge.

OUTCOME MEASURES

Pregnancy Outcomes

The electronic charting system is designed to automatically trigger a notification to the user when the luteal phase is longer than 17 days for couples in regular cycles. For couples anticipating ovulation using the breastfeeding protocol this does not apply because they do not have a peak (LH) surge each charted cycle. However, this is not a problem because every time the couple completes a chart online (i.e., each artificial cycle) they are asked if they achieved pregnancy that cycle. If "yes" is chosen, the woman has immediate access to the pregnancy evaluation that takes only a few minutes to complete. The woman can expect a response within a short period of time after she submits the evaluation from specially trained NFP nurses who are notified electronically of a pregnancy. All pregnancies are reviewed by two professional NFP nurses for the days of fertility, the days of recorded intercourse and for the couple's intention to achieve or avoid a pregnancy. If the reviewers have any questions there is a response section for them which when completed will trigger an e-mail to the user to return to the site and review comments.

Each pregnancy was classified (with agreement of the couple) according to the following classification system as recommended by Lamprecht and Trussell (1997): (1) pregnancies were classified as intentional only when a couple reports prior to the pregnancy cycle an intention to use the method to become pregnant; (2) all unintentional pregnancies were used in the analysis of pregnancy risk during typical use; and (3) all unintentional pregnancies occurring during cycles in which NFP rules were followed were used in the analysis of pregnancy risk during correct use.

Acceptability

Acceptability of the online protocol was assessed by a ten-item, seven point Likert scale evaluation tool (1 = not satisfied and 7 = very satisfied) that was automatically e-mailed to the woman at one, three and six months of use, triggered from the first day of registration. The evaluation is a modified version of the acceptability and ease of use tool developed by social psychologists, Severy and Robinson (2004) to assess how couples operationalize the use of family planning methods. Analysis of the acceptability results for this study showed an internal consistency (Cronbach's Alpha) equivalent to 0.83 – 0.91.

PRELIMINARY RESULTS

Demographics

At this time, ninety-five participants are primarily Caucasian (88%) and Catholic (92%). They have a mean age of 30.0 (*SD* = 4.5) and have been married a mean of 5.0 years (SD = 3.6) and have a mean of 2.8 children (*SD* = 1.5; range 1-9).

Unintended Pregnancies

Of the 95 breastfeeding participants, 61 contributed 1-12 months of use for a total of 385 months. Currently, there are 4 unintended pregnancies all due to incorrect use among the 61 breastfeeding women who have utilized the protocol for 6-12 months and charted online. The 12 month correct use unintended pregnancy rate is 0 per 100 users at 12 months of use (Std. Error = 0.00). The twelve month total unintended pregnancy rate was 14 (Std. Error = 0.07).

Acceptability

Mean acceptability scores were not statistically different at one (N = 37; Mean = 42.7; SD = 9.13) and three months of use (*N* = 14; Mean = 46.5; SD = 9.80).

DISCUSSION

Unintended Pregnancy

The unintended pregnancy results of the post-partum breastfeeding protocol are promising and comparable to the efficacy of those who are in regular menstrual cycles, especially when used correctly and with the use of the hormonal monitor (Fehring, Schneider and Raviele 2011). Furthermore, the results appear to be better than past studies that indicate NFP increases the unintended pregnancy rate and use of cervical mucus only methods (Hatherley 1995; Howard and Stanford 1999). However, to determine if there is an improvement of this protocol over other NFP methods, cohort or randomized comparison studies would need to be carried out. Furthermore, these results are only preliminary.

Although preliminary results indicate that the breastfeeding protocol has been effective, a review of the unintended pregnancies revealed they occurred during the transition between stage two to the first full cycle post-menses, or the beginning of stage three. Confusion after returning to cycles occurs due to moving from the breastfeeding protocol instructions to regular cycle instructions. After the monitor has detected an LH surge followed by a menses the couple is instructed to return to regular cycle instructions and test daily when the monitor requests a test regardless if the monitor results are low. The women who experienced an unintended pregnancy continued to use the breastfeeding protocol during this transition time, testing every other day until high. Thus, these pregnancies occurred during the pre-ovulatory phase of the first full cycle of stage three.

Acceptability

Results at this time show there is no statistically significant difference in acceptability at one, and three months of use. At one and three months the couples' mean acceptability scores were 42.7. At three months the mean acceptability scores rose slightly to 46.5. This suggests that couples entering the study start out with high expectations that do not change over three months of use; however, only 37 of the 95 participants reported their acceptability at one month of use and 14 at three months of use. There were not enough participants and statistical power to determine differences. Furthermore, to get a full understanding of couples' satisfaction a one-year evaluation should be offered. These acceptability scores however, are not that different from the acceptability scores of the non-breastfeeding participants (Fehring, Schneider, and Raviele, 2011). In fact they seem to be better than the acceptability scores of the randomized comparison study of two online methods of NFP that is reviewed in these proceedings (see Fehring and Schneider 2011). A one year evaluation would provide a calmer reflection on the use of the protocol, i.e., outside of the anxiety of going through the breastfeeding transition.

Limitations and Future Research

Ideally we would like couples to provide a year's worth of charting that starts from the time the lochia has subsided through the sixth cycle to better understand the dynamics of the breastfeeding phases. In reality, couples entering this study register and chart at different times during the breastfeeding stages making evaluation of acceptability difficult to interpret; yet, the information collected so far is valuable and will be used to design future research.

Other improvements being considered are: a revision of the protocol that highlights instructions during the transition from stage two to stage three and an updated website that specifically supports the breastfeeding protocol and charting. Finally, thought will be given to creating web-based instructions and charting that are more accessible to individuals who do not have ready access to the Internet.

Although internet access to vital information, like learning about how to live with one's fertility as a married couple, is a way to meet the needs of hundreds and even thousands of couples, only a small percentage of women/couples who are using NFP during the breastfeeding stages are being reached. A large percentage of minority and low income women/couples do not have easy access to the Internet.

The majority of participants at this time are primarily Caucasian Catholics. Nine percent of participants have registered as Hispanic. Only a few participants are actively charting their cycles. McDowell, Wang and Kennedy-Stephenson (2008) reported findings from the National Health and Nutrition Examination Survey and found that among women surveyed the group that has the highest breastfeeding rate is that of the Hispanic community. Efforts must continue to focus on developing NFP instructions that meet their needs.

A New Fertility Algorithm

From the information gathered so far it can be seen that when couples enter stage three of the breastfeeding weaning phase and are not in regular cycles, ovulation is delayed. This delay in ovulation presents an opportunity to update the protocol and adjust the current instructions (which states the fertile window starts on day six for the first six cycles in stage three) to begin on day ten after the first menses and taper down one day each month. This would mean that for cycle two the fertile window would start on day nine, cycle three the fertile window starts on day eight and so on until cycle five when the start of the fertile window becomes day six again and regular cycle instructions can be resumed. Further clarification of the stages of breastfeeding will help us know if adaptation is possible.

A Virtual Community of Support

About a third of the women registered on the Marquette NFP website (*http://nfp.marquette.edu*) are using the breastfeeding protocol. The website however, was originally designed for couples in regular cycles. This means that there is not a translation of the breastfeeding protocol to the electronic charting system so it is not ideal for breastfeeding couples. Women who use the website are informed of this and are instructed to download and/or print the breastfeeding protocol to use as their guide. They are told to disregard the electronic fertility window that is automatically calculated on every chart and follow the breastfeeding protocol. This is not ideal. Another concern is that although the charting is online and daily access to an NFP teacher is possible about one-third of the registered participants have actually provided 3-12 months of usable charting. Retention of couples is a problem for most NFP methods both in person and online. Although online methods are more convenient they still may be considered cumbersome to some couples.

Inadvertently a virtual community has been created on the Marquette NFP website due to the presence of breastfeeding women who use the website for instructions and blogs. The online forums have created a community of NFP users who rely on professional NFP nurses, NFP only physicians, bioethicists and each other for support and guidance. The online forums provide a safe haven, a place where couples can comfortably ask questions and learn more about their fertility. The online teaching site is also a rich environment for current and future research. Presently, there is evidence of the efficacy of this protocol. Supporting this early evidence are the testimonies from women who have found a community of support, a community of hope. Below is a testimonial from one of the participants on the discussion forum about her experience with the protocol, website and professional feedback. This is only one of many such discussions occurring on the website almost weekly.

"Totally agree with you! When I hear other people in NFP forums that make a person feel guilty for wanting to space-let alone limit, I get so irritated. Maybe some people are cut out to be like the Duggars and have 19 kids, but we are not all called to do the same thing! I only have 3, but mine are 3 (will be 4 in May), 28 mo., and one year (today!). They were all 16 and a half months apart or less. And I got pregnant with each one while I was still nursing the baby! I feel so overwhelmed at times and I know I couldn't handle another one, let alone another surprise!!! So for us it was either abstinence till I started cycles again, which I only started this month! Or artificial birth control, and then I found this method and I feel so much better about NFP in general. I too am so happy to hear that I am not alone in this fertility/family planning journey!"

SOURCES CONSULTED

Bartick, M., A. Reinhold. 2010. "The burden of suboptimal breastfeeding in the United States: A pediatric cost analysis." *Pediatrics* DOI: 0.1542/peds.2009-1616.

Brown, J., P. Harrison, M. Smith. 1985. "A study of returning fertility after childbirth and during lactation by measurement of urinary oestrogen and pregnanediol excretion and cervical mucus production." *Journal Biosocial Science*, Supplement 9, 5-23 Department of Health and Human Services.

Breastfeeding Report Card 2010. www.cdc.gov/breastfeeding/data/report-card.htm.

Fehring, R., M. Schneider, M. Barron. 2005. "Protocol for determining fertility while breastfeeding and not in cycles." *Fertility and Sterility* 84 (3) 805-807. DOI: 10.1016/jfertnstert.2005.03.042.

Fehring, R., M. Schneider, K. Raviele. 2011. "Pilot Evaluation of an Internet-based Natural Family Planning Education and Service Program." *Journal of Obstetrics, Gynecology, and Neonatal Nursing*. 40(3): 281-91.

Fehring, R., M. Schneider. 2011. "Randomized Comparison of Two Internet-Supported Natural Family Planning Methods: (Preliminary Findings)." In Fehring, R. and Notare, T. Eds. *Human Fertility; Where Faith and Science Meet. Proceedings of an Interdisciplinary Conference, August 15-17, 2010.* Milwaukee: Marquette University Press.

Hatherly, L. 1985. "Lactation and postpartum infertility: The use-effectiveness of natural family planning (NFP) after term pregnancy." *Clinical Reproduction and Fertility* 3: 319-334.

Howard, M., J. Stanford. 1999. "Pregnancy probabilities during use of the Creighton Model Fertility*Care* system." *Archives Family Medicine* 8:391-402.

Ladomenou, F., J. Moschandreas, A. Kafatos, Y. Tselentis, E. Galanakis. 2010. "Protective effect of exclusive breastfeeding against infections during infancy: a prospective study." *Archives of Disease in Childhood* 10:1136/adc.2009.169912.

McDowell, M., C.Y. Wang, J. Kennedy-Stephenson. 2008. "Breastfeeding in the United States: Findings from the National Health and Nutrition Examination Surveys, 1999–2006." U.S. Department of Health and Human Services Centers for Disease Control and Prevention National Center for Health Statistics, (NCHS, Data Brief, no. 5, April 2008).

Lamprecht, V., J. Trussell. 1997. "Effectiveness studies on natural methods of natural family planning." *Advances in Contraception* 13(2/3): 155-165.

Severy, L., J. Robinson. 2004. "Psychological aspects of achieving or avoiding pregnancy." In Fehring, R. and Notare, T. Eds. *Integrating Faith and Science Through Natural Family Planning*. Milwaukee: Marquette University Press, pp. 111-133.

MARQUETTE UNIVERSITY INSTITUTE FOR NATURAL FAMILY PLANNING - BFW Sample chart

LAST 12 CYCLES SHORTEST_____ LONGEST_____ EARLIEST DAY OF PEAK IN LAST 6 CYCLES______ DATE FOR BEGINNING THIS CHART: ________________

CYCLE DAY	1	2	3	4	5	6	7	8	9	10	11	12	13	14	15	16	17	18	19	20	21	22	23	24	25	26	27	28	29	30	31	32	33	34	35	36	37	38	39	40
Cyle 1 Date																																								
Clearblue Recording		L		L		L		L		L		L		L		L		L		L																				
Intercourse = I				I				I		I						I																								
Cycle 2 Date																																								
Clearblue Recording	L		L		L		L		L		L		L		L		L		L																					
Intercourse = I	I				I						I								I																					
Cycle 3 Date																																								
Clearblue Recording	L		L		L		L		L		L		L		L		L		L	L																				
Intercourse = I					I				I						I					I																				
Cycle 4 Date																																								
Clearblue Recording	L		L		L		L		L		L		L	H	H	H	H	H	H	H																				
Intercourse = I	I		I		I				I				I						I																					
Cycle 5 Date																																								
Clearblue Recording	L		L		L		L		L		L	H	H	H	H	H	H	P	P	H1	L2	L3	L	L	L	L	L													
Intercourse = I					I				I																	I														
Cycle 6 Date																																								
Clearblue Recording	1	2	3	2	1	L	L	L	H	H	H	H	H	H	H	H	P	P	H1	L2	L3	L	L	L	L	L	L	L												
Intercourse = I																								I		I	I	I												

TO AVOID PREGNANCY: Do not have intercourse during fertility-*Regular Cycles ONLY!*

1. Fertility BEGINS on day 6 during the first 6 cycles; After 6 cycles of charting
2. Fertility BEGINS on the earliest day of Peak during the last 6 cycles minus 6 days
3. Fertility ENDS on the last Peak day plus THREE full days; After 6 cycles of charting
4. Fertility ENDS on the last Peak day of the last 6 cycles plus 3 days
5. Do not have intercourse on any HIGH or PEAK reading on the monitor

Clearblue Coding System:

Low Fertility = Green Color
High Fertility = Blue Color
Peak Fertility = Blue with a "P"
Menses = Red Color

Couple Intention Recording: (Place a check next to your intention before beginning each cycle)

Cycle 1: Avoid__x___ Achieve_____ Cycle 2: Avoid__x___Achieve_____
Cycle 3: Avoid__x___ Achieve_____ Cycle 4: Avoid__x___Achieve_____
Cycle 5: Avoid__x___ Achieve_____ Cycle 6: Avoid_____Achieve__x___

MARQUETTE UNIVERSITY UNIMARKER CHART - CPEFM EXAMPLE CHART

Figure 1: Example breastfeeding protocol chart that uses the electronic fertility monitor to track fertility by creating 20 day artificial cycles until ovulation is detected by the LH surge and Peak monitor reading.

ADDENDUM

MARQUETTE UNIVERSITY COLLEGE OF NURSING INSTITUTE FOR NATURAL FAMILY PLANNING

Breastfeeding Protocol for the Clearblue Fertility Monitor Protocol for couples who want to avoid a pregnancy

NOTE: After reviewing basic instructions for the monitor you are ready to apply the breastfeeding weaning instructions. Always use the first morning urine. You must have at least four hours between voids (4 hour concentration) for the monitor to accurately detect your fertility. If you get up more frequently during the night, you will have to collect the urine and test it during the monitor test window. There is no need to refrigerate your collected sample. Remember the Clearblue Fertility Monitor is marketed for couples who want to achieve a pregnancy. This protocol has not been approved by Unipath Diagnostics. If you have any questions please contact your Marquette Model Teacher.

- The breastfeeding protocol is as follows:
- Trigger a cycle by pushing the "M" button on the monitor
- Fast forward the monitor to day 5
- The next 20 days the monitor will ask for a test
- Test your first morning urine every other day
- When a "high" is recorded test the urine everyday
- Re-trigger the monitor and fast forward every 20 days
- ***Continue steps 1-6 until you detect a Peak reading and resume menses.***
- Intercourse instructions are:
- To avoid pregnancy, avoid intercourse on High and Peak days and three full days after the last Peak day.

PANEL III

CURRENT NFP RESEARCH

OFFICE OF POPULATION AFFAIRS GRANTEES
PANEL OF OPA SPONSORED NFP RESEARCH IN USA

5

FABM Use among Young Adult Low-Income Minority Women

LINA GUZMAN, PHD

Program Area Director & Senior Research Scientist, Child Trends, Washington, DC, with

SELMA CAAL, MANICA RAMOS, & JENNIFER MANLOVE

The findings presented here are based on preliminary analysis and are subject to change. Please direct questions to Lina Guzman, lguzman@childtrends.org.

ABSTRACT

The purpose of this study is to learn how low-income minority women use fertility awareness based methods (FABM) using semi-structured qualitative interviews. The research is focused on studying FABM among low-income African-American and Hispanic women, given their higher rates of unintended pregnancies.

Fertility awareness methods can be a viable option for birth control for low-income minority women because they involve little or no cost. The following five general research questions guide this study:

(1) what type of FABM users are they; (2) why are women choosing to use FABM; (3) how (well) are women using FABM; (4) what do women know about FABM and where do they get their information; and (5) what factors are barriers and facilitators to their using FABM.

The sample consists of 58 African-American (52%) and Hispanic (48%) women aged 18 to 29. These preliminary findings indicate that women use FABM in a variety of ways. Some women in the sample use FABM as their primary method of family planning; others use FABM as a back-up method when their primary birth control is not available, and others use it in conjunction with other birth controls some or most of the time.

In our sample, women chose FABM for various reasons including its ease of use, because it provides an alternative to synthetic hormones or provides an added level of birth control; and because its use was encouraged by people in their lives. The majority of women in our study track their cycle using a calendar method and many had been tracking their cycle since they began menstruating.

While women have obtained information about FABM from a range of sources, many were not well informed. Indeed, although the majority of women were abstaining or using barrier contraceptives during what they perceived to be their fertile period, many were not using FABM correctly because they could not identify their fertile window.

Women liked that FABM helped them to feel empowered and in touch with their body and provided a hormone-free alternative to family planning. The most common barrier to FABM use reported by women was that it provided an inadequate level of protection against pregnancy and sexually transmitted infections (STIs). Differences are examined across key subgroups including race/ethnicity, income, education, and religion.

INTRODUCTION

Reports of unintended pregnancies and childbearing suggest that almost half (49%) of pregnancies in the United States are classified as unintended (mistimed or unwanted) (Finer and Henshaw 2006). In 2001, women aged 20-24 reported the highest rates of unintended births, followed by women between the ages of 15-19. Similarly, low income women had the highest unintended pregnancies in that year (Finer and Henshaw 2006). Research examining associations between pregnancy intentions and child outcomes has shown unintended births to be linked with suboptimal outcomes for children and parents.

As such, two of the objectives of the Healthy People 2010 initiative are to increase the proportion of intended pregnancies by 70% and to increase the proportion of females at risk of unintended pregnancy to use a method of family planning by 100% (State Family Planning Administrators 2001). The nation's Title X National Family Planning Program seeks to provide safe and effective family planning and related health care services for little or no cost, particularly targeting low-income, uninsured and underinsured individuals (Fowler et al. 2008).

Among the family planning methods promoted by Title X are fertility awareness based methods (FABM). FABM involves identifying potentially fertile days during each menstrual cycle and avoiding sexual intercourse during the fertile window to avoid unintended pregnancy. FABM does not require regular visits to health care providers. Because many of the clients served by Title X do not regularly visit a health care provider (Fowler et al. 2008; Hatcher et al. 2003; Ryder and Campbell 1995), FABM may represent a useful option to offer Title X clients. Yet, less than 1% of both female and male clients served by Title X in 2006 reported that their primary family planning method was fertility awareness-based (Fowler et al. 2008). These low numbers suggest that more can be done to educate clients about FABM to provide them with an alternative to artificial methods.

The purpose of this study is to learn about FABM use among minority women. Specifically, the research addresses five questions: (1) what type of FABM users are low-income minority women; (2) why are low-income minority women choosing to use FABM; (3) how (well) are women using FABM; (4) what do women know about FABM and where do they get their information; and (5) what factors are barriers and facilitators to their using FABM.

DATA AND METHODS

Data

This study is based on 58 interviews conducted with Hispanic and African American women living in an urban mid-sized city area in the mid-Atlantic region who had ever used FABM. Using purposive sampling techniques, we segmented the sample to ensure the inclusion of participants with characteristics identified in the literature as related to FABM use, such as relationship type and nativity status. Additionally, we targeted low-income women because this is a target group of Title X and rates of unintended pregnancy are higher among those with lower income. Women were eligible to participate if they met the following criteria: (1) Hispanic or African American; (2) between the ages of 18 and 29; (3) were not pregnant and not planning pregnancy within the next year; (4) had an annual income of $55,000 or below; and (5) reported having ever used FABM to avoid a pregnancy.

Recruitment

We recruited participants through three community reproductive health clinics serving low-income Hispanic and African-American women as well as study ads posted on Craigslist. Designated program staff in each clinic administered an initial screener questionnaire (developed by the study investigators) during their intake process, to identify women who had ever used FABM. The screener included a series of questions and follow-up probes to ensure that our target population (i.e., ever used FABM) was identified and that under-reporting of FABM was minimized (see Addendum A). Women who were identified as possible FABM users by program staff were then asked to provide their contact information or asked to contact the study center. Once contacted, study staff did additional screening to confirm their FABM use status and to ensure eligibility into the study based on the other (demographic based) criteria. A total of 735 women were screened by clinics, of whom 116 women were identified as potential FAM users and were furthered screened by our study staff. A total of 72 women were found eligible and recruited and 65 completed interviews. Seven women were determined not to be FABM users during the interview. The analysis presented below is limited to those 58 women who had ever used FABM.

Procedure

Interviews were conducted using semi-structured exploratory interviewing techniques in which discussions were guided through open-ended questions and targeted probes designed to gather information about FABM use, relationship status and pregnancy intentions, knowledge, attitudes and beliefs about contraception including FABM and fertility awareness, sexual intercourse and contraceptive use, past pregnancies, receipt and access of services; and background information. The 1.5 hour interviews were conducted in English and Spanish and took place in clinics, the study center, at a semi-private public location or at the participant's home. All procedures and materials received IRB review and approval.

Data Analysis

A brief summary of each interview was drafted upon its completion and interview audio recordings were transcribed. Throughout the field period, study team members met in a series of debriefing sessions to review interview summaries and notes. The summaries and transcriptions were also reviewed by senior study staff. The focus of these debriefings and reviews was to identify initial themes and findings that then served as the basis of a coding scheme used to conduct a systematic analysis of the data. After the coding scheme was developed, the interviews were coded. The coded data were then entered into a SPSS database in order to explore patterns and variation by race/ethnicity, nativity status, etc. We also used Nvivo, a qualitative data analysis software, to identify themes and quotes.

KEY FINDINGS

Sample

The sample was divided roughly equally between African-American (52%) and Hispanic (48%) women. Just over one-third of participants were born outside the United States. The average age of participants was 24.5 (*SD* = 3.2). Just over two-thirds of women in the sample (67%) earned less than $25,000 in the last year and about one in five had a high school diploma or less education. Thirty-three percent were in a residential union (married or cohabiting) and 67% were in a dating nonresidential union. Slightly under half of the women (45%) were mothers. Thirty-three percent of the women in the sample were Catholic. Sixty percent of the participants reported they were using FABM at the time of the interview; the remainder had used FABM in the past.[1]

Five main themes emerged from our interviews, as follows: (1) women vary in the way they use FABM; (2) women choose FABM for various reasons; (3) the majority of women use FABM by tracking their cycles with the help of a calendar; (4) women obtain FABM information from various sources, but they are not well informed of the various aspects of FABM; and (5) women's inaccurate perceptions of the effectiveness of FABM serve as barriers to their use of the methods.

FABM USERS ARE NOT ONE SIZE FITS ALL

Preliminary findings indicate that FABM users are not a monolithic group. They use FABM in various ways and degrees and (as described in detail below) arrive at the use of FABM for a variety of reasons. Three common types of users are identified by the research. Among the FABM users the most common are those who use FABM "in conjunction" with another method—that is, they use FABM along with one or more other methods most or all of the time (rather than just during their fertile time). Close to one-half (47%) of the women in the sample fall into this category. The vast majority in this group reported using FABM along with condoms and/or withdrawal in order to provide an added level of protection against pregnancy and STIs (see Addendum B, exhibit 1 for a profile of a typical "in conjunction with" user).

The second group identified includes women for whom FABM serves as their "primary" or sole method of birth control (26%). The third group of FABM users, which consists of 28% of the sample, could be characterized as "back-up" users. Although women in this group often reported having a primary method of family planning, they tend to rely on a range of other methods, including FABM, depending on what they have available at the moment. For example, they use a patchwork approach to contracepting and rely on other methods when they forget to refill their prescription or when they do not have money to do so. In short, this group uses FABM on an "as needed" basis and sometimes as a last resort, as described by this African American respondent:

> *INT: ... Do you use withdrawal or condoms, simultaneously with the family planning, is all of this at once, or do you use one when you forget the other?*
>
> *R: Use one when I forget the other.*
>
> *INT: In what kind of situation would that be?*

R: When I can only get [buy] the Nuva ring in that time when I'm on my menstrual cycle. If I go beyond that point, I can't use it, so I would have to … use condoms …

INT: And when do you use withdrawal?

R: I guess when you're just in that moment and you're not thinking clearly about using condoms or… if I didn't have the chance to get the birth control [Nuvaring].

INT: So if you don't have the Nuvaring you use condoms and if you don't have the Nuvaring or condoms you use withdrawal. And when do you use Natural Family Planning?

R: …That's the last one [FABM] of them [methods].

Differences in type of use across key subgroups

Several differences emerge when we compare type of use across key characteristics. A slightly higher percentage of Hispanics are "primary" users (29%) compared with African Americans (23%). Thirty percent of African American women are using FABM in a "hodgepodge" (30%) manner compared with one-quarter of Hispanic women. A roughly equal percentage of Hispanic and African American women reported being "in conjunction" users (47%, 46% respectively). A higher percentage of women with some college (50%) or a bachelor's degree (BA; 50%) reported using FABM "in conjunction" with other methods, compared with women who have a high school diploma or less education (33%). On the other hand, a higher percentage of women with a high school diploma (42%) reported using FABM as their primary method relative to women who had some college (29%), and women who have a BA or higher (11%). As expected, a higher percentage of women who have a residential partner (37%) reported using FABM as their primary method, compared with those who were dating (21%). A higher percentage of women who earned $25,000 or more reported using FABM "in conjunction" or as a "back-up" compared with women earning less than $25,000 (79%, 72%, respectively). No differences were found across religious groups in type of FABM use.

Variations over time

We also observed a variation in the type of FABM women were using during their reproductive life-cycle. For example, several women moved from being one type of user to another type of user (e.g., primary to "in conjunction") depending on economic and family circumstances. Additionally, while some women have used FABM continuously for a period of time (52%), others have used it sporadically during their sexual life time (29%) and others have used it only once or twice (19%) (see Addendum B, exhibit 2 for an example of this variation in FABM use). The average length of use of FABM among the women in our sample is 2.2 years.

WHY ARE MINORITY WOMEN USING FABM?

We asked women to describe why they chose to use FABM. Most women often reported more than one reason, and their reasons are varied but could be categorized into the following four broad groups: (1) ease of use; (2) concerns about the use of synthetic hormones; (3) a desire to have an additional means to avoid pregnancy; and (4) social and structural reasons. Almost half of the women (41%) reported choosing FABM because it is "easy to use." As noted by this 20-year-old Hispanic woman, FABM has "*no doctor's visits, no medications, nothing to remember except your days[and] no side effects.*" Participants also noted that it allows for a better sensation than condoms.

Forty-five percent of our sample reported that they choose to use FABM because they have concerns about using "synthetic hormones." Many in this group were adamant about using a family planning method that is "hormone free" or "natural." Some women in this group want to avoid having side effects from the use of hormonal methods. Others, such as this 21-year-old Hispanic woman, had prior bad experiences with hormonal methods, including headaches, mood swings, and irregular menstrual periods.

> INT: *Okay. And what do you like most about the Rhythm Method?*
>
> R: *It's natural and you don't get pregnant, there's no medicine.*
>
> INT: *And why don't you want to take something that isn't natural?*
>
> R: *I don't like to take a lot of medicine, it gives me a headache.*
>
> INT: *So because of the side effects?*
>
> R: *Yes, they scare me.*

Almost three quarters (73%) of the sample reported that they chose FABM because it provides "protection against pregnancy." It is important to note here that all women in the sample were using FABM to avoid pregnancy, a criterion to be part of the study. Many of those, however, who reported that they were using FABM because it provides a means to avoid pregnancy also reported using FABM in conjunction with another method. In short, they see their use of FABM as maximizing their chances of avoiding a pregnancy. Others in this group believe that FABM is the best and most reliable method with which they are familiar.

One quarter of the sample (25%) stated that they use FABM due to social (e.g., partners) and structural influences (e.g., insurance and religion). For example, a small number of women (n= 6) reported having turned to FAM after they lost their health insurance or because FABM (n=5) is endorsed by their religion. A few women reported that their use of FABM was driven in part by their relationship. For example, their partner viewed FABM as a good compromise given a desire to avoid side effects from hormonal methods as well as the lessened sensation from the use of condoms.

Differences across Groups

A number of differences emerged in the reasons why participants reported using FABM. A higher percentage of Hispanics (54%) choose to use FABM because of concerns with synthetic hormones, compared with African-Americans (37%). Likewise, a higher percentage of foreign-born women than native-born women reported choosing FABM because they are concerned about using synthetic hormones (65% vs. 37%) or because it provides (additional) protection against pregnancy (82% vs. 68%). A higher percentage of women with some college education (64%) followed by women with a high school diploma or less (58%) reported using FABM because of its ease of use compared to women with a BA or above (44%). In contrast, a higher percentage of women with higher levels of education (some college, 50%; college degree or more, 56%) reported using FABM because of a desire to avoid hormonal side effects, compared with women with a high school degree or less (17%). A higher percentage of women with high school diploma or less (33%) reported structural/social factors to be the reason as to why they use FABM, compared to their counterparts with higher levels of education (some college, 21%; BA or higher, 24%). There were no differences in reasons participants reported using FABM for Catholics versus non-Catholics.

HOW ARE MINORITY WOMEN USING FABM?

We asked women to describe how they used FABM, in particular how they tracked their cycle and identified their fertile window, what they did during their fertile period (e.g., abstain, use other forms of birth control, etc), how consistently they tracked their cycle and refrained from having sexual intercourse during their fertile window. We used this information to assess their accuracy of use as well as the consistency with which they used FABM.

Women reported tracking their cycle in one of three ways: using a calendar method, medical detection, or what we termed, "the short cut method." The majority of women in our sample tracked their cycle using a calendar method (90%). Indeed, many women (including some that were later determined to be non-users of FABM) noted that they have been tracking their cycle since they began menstruating, and some FABM users who rely on other methods to track their cycle still map their cycle with a calendar. While some women use a traditional paper calendar or count days[2] to determine their fertile period, others use new technology to map their cycle. For example, some women reported using applications on their cellular phones or internet-based software to determine their fertile period, and others, such as these two African-American women: the first, a 24-year-old, used an application on her cell phone and the second, a 25-year-old, used an electronic calendar.

> *R:... I prefer to look at my phone, I enter when I got my period and it says when you're ovulating, when you have sex.*
>
> *INT: Is this an iPhone or something?*
>
> *R: My husband's.*
>
> *INT: Is this a specific [phone] application?*
>
> *R: ...Yeah... I can't remember the name of it, I have to show you, I don't understand I just enter it on my phone like this cannot be good. The first one is my days, yeah my days and you see down here they have like what today is, the start of your period and you press it in and next, you know your next period...it will tell you if you have sex you put it in here, so it kind of calculates all of that. And then the next one, so that's the new one so the next one that I was using before that one came is called the P O calendar.*
>
> *INT: So how do you keep track of your cycle?*

R: …I use like outlook email calendar, save it there, the number of days I'm on [my period]. Then I use the web MD ovulation calendar.

Only a couple of women reported using a medical detection method, including monitoring of cervical mucus secretions and basal body temperature. A third method used in our sample was the 'short cut method" (21%) which includes two distinct approaches to identifying infertile (safe) and fertile (unsafe) periods of their menstrual cycle. The first group is referred to as "safe zone by period." Women in this group determine when they could have sexual intercourse based on when they menstruate rather than on when they ovulate. That is, they identify a window (in most cases) before and after their menstrual period during which they perceive it to be "safe" to have sexual intercourse without the use of a contraceptive barrier because they believe they are infertile. Implicitly, the assumption is that for the remainder of their cycle, it is "unsafe" to have sexual intercourse (without the use of a contraceptive barrier), though women tended not to explicitly establish their fertile window. The second group within the "short cut method" included women who reported that they were able to determine their fertile window because they could feel when they were ovulating. It is worth noting that a little over a quarter of women (28%) reported using more than one method to track their cycle, as illustrated by this 27-year-old Hispanic woman.

INT: ….So in the past year how have you kept track of your cycle and the days that it's safe and not safe to have sex?

R: …Pretty much in my head, I would do the calendar but I remember my days so I don't do it….. but if I do need to… count, I'll be like well I started that day and do that sort of thing. Mostly I just do my temperature like with my finger and then like discharge and that's how I guess like the change in discharge for me.

A little over half (53 %) of the women in our sample are using FABM accurately. Women were considered to be using FABM accurately if they are able to correctly identify their fertile period and abstained, or had some form of birth control during their fertile period. When we teased apart these two components of accuracy of FABM use, we found that women appeared to have more trouble identifying their fertile period than abstaining or having some form of birth control during their fertile window. Specifically, 90% of women in our sample reported that they abstained from sex or had some form of birth control during what they perceived to be their fertile window; however, 40% of women could not correctly identify their fertile period. While women reported abstaining or using contraceptives during their fertile period, many also had trouble doing so consistently. Sixty percent of women consistently abstained or had some form of birth control all the time during what they perceived to be their fertile window.

Differences across Group

A higher percentage of Hispanic women (70%), compared with their African American counterparts, accurately use FABM (70% vs. 43%) and identify their fertile window (70% vs. 54%). Likewise, a higher percentage of foreign-born women (75%) accurately use FABM, compared with native-born women (49%). Interestingly, a higher percentage of back-up (63%) and primary users of FABM (60%) were determined to be accurately using FABM, compared to "in conjunction with" users (50%). Sixty-five percent of women who reported using FABM because of concerns with side effects and the use of hormonal methods were accurately using FABM compared with women who were using FABM primarily for contraceptive reasons (53%). A higher percentage (63%) of women earning more than $25,000 use FABM accurately, compared with women earning less than $25,000 (53%). Women with higher levels of education (BA or more, 69%) accurately use FABM, compared with those who had lower levels of education (some college, 52%; HS or less 50%). Catholic women were more likely to accurately use FABM (68%), compared with non-Catholic women (50%). Fewer differences were found in consistency of use. Over half of the women with a high school degree or less (58%) consistently use FABM and consistently track their cycle, compared with 43% of women with some college or 35% of women with a BA or more. Non-Catholic women (64%) and those with more income (68%) were more likely to consistently use FABM, compared with their Catholic (53%) and lower-income (56%) counterparts.

WHAT DO MINORITY WOMEN KNOW ABOUT FABM?

Central to women's ability to use FABM accurately is knowledge, perhaps more so than with other methods of family planning. Yet, unlike other forms of family planning, FABMs are often not taught in school or discussed in clinical settings. To assess their level of knowledge, we asked women to describe what they know about FABM as well where they had learned about FABM, and what they had learned. Women reported learning about FABM from multiple sources that could be grouped into two broad categories of information resources: (1) social and (2) media. Sixty-two percent of women reported getting their information from family, friends, their partners, doctors, and teachers, and (among the foreign-born) from their home country. About half of the sample (47%) also reported obtaining information about FABM from the Internet, television, pamphlets, and magazines. The vast majority (88%) of the women reported that they had received information about the effectiveness of FABM, and how to map their menstrual cycle and determine their fertile period (69%) as well as how the method works (45%). Interestingly, although one-third of women in the sample received information from their doctor, this information was typically intended to discourage women from using FABM. As the quote below from a 25-year-old African American woman illustrates, women in our sample often note that their doctors would try to dissuade them from using FABM by pointing out FABM's "ineffectiveness" against preventing pregnancy, in particular compared with hormonal methods.

> *INT: ....What did you ask your doctor in particular.....*
>
> *R: What she thought about it [FABM].*
>
> *INT: Alright, and what did she say?*
>
> *R: She said it wasn't safe to use.*
>
> *R: Not if I didn't want to get pregnant... she wanted me to take hormonal birth control.*

Although women have received information about FABM from varying sources, their level of knowledge ranges from very informed to somewhat informed to not at all informed. We assessed participants' knowledge across these key areas: how to use FABM, how it works, and its effectiveness.[3]

Thirty-eight percent of participants were found to be very informed, 36% were somewhat informed, and 26% were found to be not at all informed. In general, women in the sample tended to be least informed about their fertile window. For example, while some might be aware that they have a fertile window, they are not aware that they ovulate during this period, that this is when they can become pregnant, or about the basic physiological processes that take place during their menstrual cycle. This finding reflects other patterns reported above, including the use of "safe zone" by the period and lower accuracy in the identification of the fertile window. Other women (38%) are aware that ovulation is associated with their fertile window but cannot identify it, as illustrated by the quote below from a 28-year-old African American woman.

> INT: *You said you also track you period. How do you do that?*
>
> R: *... Well I do come on like every 12th of the month, so I avoid sex a week before and a week after.*
>
> INT: *And that's your fertile period a week before and week after your period?*
>
> R: *Yeah.*
>
> INT: *....And who taught you that, how to track that way?*
>
> R: *I read about it, I've read about it before*

Almost half of the sample (47%) underestimate the effectiveness of this method, assessed as reporting an effectiveness level of less than 75%.[4] Furthermore, more than half of the women (57%) have low scores in their knowledge of women's fertility.[5]

In sum, although women obtained information about FABM from varying sources, for the most part, they are not well informed about various aspects of FABM.

Differences across Groups

Some key subgroup differences emerged in knowledge about FABM. In general, a higher percentage of Hispanics (43%), compared with African-Americans (33%), and foreign-born, compared with native born (32%), are very informed about FABM. A higher percentage of low income women (41%, less than 25K) and those with higher levels of education (BA or higher, 44%; some college, 36%) are well informed about FABM, compared to their high income (32%, $25,000 or more) and lower education counterparts (33%, HS or less). The same pattern held for general fertility awareness, with one exception.

Women with lower levels of education have higher levels of fertility awareness (42%, high school or less) than women with higher levels of education (33%, BA or more). A higher percentage of Catholics (47%) were found to be very informed, compared with non-Catholics. We did not find differences between Catholics and non-Catholics in terms of levels of fertility awareness.

BARRIERS AND FACILITATORS TO FABM USE

The barriers women experience using FABM may contribute to the accuracy and consistency of use, as well as to continued use over time. Likewise, the extent to which women find FABM easy to use, see benefits to its use, and/or enjoy using it may facilitate its accurate, consistent, and continued use. We asked women about what they most liked and disliked about using FABM.

Barriers

Women reported disliking FABM for a number of reasons. Among the most common complaints, however, was what was perceived as "inadequate" protection against pregnancy and STIs (67%) and difficulty using FABM (28%). Many women in our sample worry that they might become pregnant while using FABM, as illustrated by this 22-year-old Hispanic female.

INT: ...And what did you most dislike about using the calendar?

R: Just that I was kind of never really felt secure that it...standing alone it would prevent pregnancy.

Women's reports about difficulty in using FABM included difficulty in tracking their cycle, difficulty gaining their partner's cooperation, and difficulty abstaining from sex during their fertile period, as described by this 28-year-old African American woman.

INT: And what do you most dislike about tracking your cycle?

R: It can be sometimes annoying because....

INT: How so? Annoying how?

R: Like if you wanted to do something [sexual] but you know you got to stay away from those days.

Differences across groups

About one-third of African American women reported that FABM is difficult to use (33%), compared with Hispanic women (21%). Close to three-quarters of Hispanic women (79%), compared with their African-American counterparts (57%), reported that they do not feel that FABM provides sufficient means to avoid pregnancy or protection against STIs. A higher percentage of Catholic women (42%) perceive FABM as difficult to use (42%), compared with non-Catholics (21%). Interestingly, about one-third of women with higher levels of education (BA or more, 33%; some college, 32%) reported that FABM is hard to use and that it does not offer enough protection against STIs or sufficient means to avoid pregnancy (72%, 71% respectively), compared with women who have a high school diploma or less (8%, 50%, respectively). A higher percentage of Catholic women (42%) thought FABM is hard to use, compared to their non-Catholic counterparts (21%).

Facilitators

The aspect that women reported they most liked about using FABM is that they feel empowered through its use and that it allows them to feel more in touch with their body (45%), as illustrated by this 24-year-old African American woman.

> INT: *What do you like most about using Natural Family Planning?*
>
> R: *… It helps you stay in tune with your body a lot better… It teaches you how to listen to your body and you're on top of things. ….If you're in tune with your body and something goes wrong then you'll be in tune with it from day one.*

The next most common feature they like is its ease of use (41%). Some women like that it is easy to use. Others like that it is a "low maintenance" method, for example, there is no need for doctor visits or prescriptions. The following quote from a 28-year-old Hispanic woman provides an example of this:

> INT: *And you said that you think it's pretty easy to use …. Can you tell me more about that?*
>
> R: *[There are] no doctor's visits, no medications, nothing to remember except your days, no side effects.*

Other reasons that woman reported liking FABM include that it is hormone free and has no side effects (40%); it prevents pregnancy (21%); and their partner likes it or doesn't have to use condoms (19%).

Differences across groups

The aspects of FABM that women reported most liking vary by race/ethnicity, nativity status, religious affiliation, and education. A higher percentage of African American women reported liking FABM because they feel empowered and like that it helps them feel in touch with their body (53%) and because their partner likes it or does not want to use a condom (23%), compared with Hispanic women (36% and 14%, respectively). In contrast, a higher percentage of Hispanics (32%) reported liking FABM because of its contraceptive properties, compared with their African American counterparts (10%). A higher percentage of Hispanic women (39%) reported liking FABM because it helps them avoid side effects from hormonal methods compared with African American women (17%). Likewise, a higher percentage of foreign-born women reported liking FABM because it has no hormones or side effects (53%), because it is easy to use (47%) and because of its contraceptive properties (32%), compared with native-born women (34%, 39%, 10% respectively). A higher percentage of Catholics than non-Catholics reported liking FABM because of its contraceptive properties (42% compared to 10%). A higher percentage of women with higher levels of education (BA or above) reported liking FABM because it has no hormones or side effects (56%) compared with women with less education (high school degree or less, 17%). In contrast, a higher percentage of women with lower levels of education (high school degree or less, 25%), compared with women with higher levels of education (BA or more, 11%), reported that one of the qualities they most like about FABM is that their partner likes it and it allows their partner to not use a condom.

DISCUSSION

In this study we explored the use of FABM among low-income minority women. Our findings help fill a critical gap in our understanding of FABM use in the United States, in particular among Hispanic and African American women. The preliminary results of the research show that FABM users are not a homogenous group. The women in our sample use FABM in a number of ways. While some women use it as their primary method, most use it either "in conjunction" with another method of birth control, or as a "back-up" when their typical method is not available. Additionally, our findings suggest that a woman's use of FABM is not static over time. Some women in our study use FABM sporadically over time, returning to and leaving its use as their needs and circumstances change. Additionally, the way in which they use it (e.g., primary vs. in conjunction with another method) also appears to vary over time.

The women in our sample turned to FABM for a range of reasons. Our results indicate that many turn to FABM because of its ease of use. While our findings suggest that only a small number of women turned to FABM because they lost their insurance, our discussions with women also suggest that FABM's no-to-low cost is attractive to women and in some (small number) of cases a main reason for choosing to use FABM. This suggests that for some, the use of FABM may signal an unmet need.

The preliminary results also suggest that a nontrivial percentage of women are turning to FABM as an alternative to hormonal methods. This group of women appears to differ from other FABM users and may include two distinct groups of women—those who have used hormonal methods and experienced side effects, and those who are skeptical about using synthetic hormones. The latter group appears to include highly educated women, as well as Hispanic and foreign-born women whom past research suggests have less experience with hormonal methods. Nonetheless, these women appear to be rejecting hormonal methods of family planning.

The findings regarding accuracy of use and knowledge of FABM are both sobering and encouraging. On the one hand, our results indicate that a substantial percentage of women in our sample are not using FABM accurately. When we dissect accuracy of use into its two components, however, we find that the vast majority of women are abstaining or using another method of birth control during what they perceive to be their fertile window. Two in five women in our study, however, cannot accurately identify their fertile window. These findings are encouraging because it suggests that the behavioral components of accurate FABM use are already present and what is lacking is knowledge. This is promising because behavior is often harder to change. Nonetheless these findings indicate a clear gap in knowledge of FABM, and women's fertility awareness in general, and have important implications for service providers. Indeed, just over one quarter of women in the sample were found not to be informed at all about FABM, and the biggest knowledge gaps relate to the women's fertile window and ovulation. Irrespective of what method of family planning women are using, this is important information that will aid women in understanding their bodies and managing their fertility.

Additionally, our preliminary findings regarding knowledge, coupled with our findings about the ways in which FABMs are used and variations over time, suggest that it may be useful for reproductive health care providers to inquire about women's use of FABM even if they are currently using other methods of contraception. While women who are currently coupling FABM use with hormonal methods or condoms may not be perceived as being in high need of instruction of FABM use, their needs may change over time.

Lastly, these preliminary findings clearly suggest that FABM is an attractive option to some women and speaks to the need to discuss and better inform women of how to use FABM. This may be particularly important as our findings hint to the possibility that many women may turn to FABM as a method of birth control at some point in their lifetime but may be doing so lacking critical information. Moreover, many women noted that they had been mapping their cycle on a calendar since they began menstruating. In short, to a large degree there may be a latent demand and ability to use FABM. Our findings also suggest that some women may be using FABM because of a lack of options—either they have lost their health insurance, cannot afford other methods of birth control, or their partner does not want to use condoms. These may represent an important group to target.

Our study has some limitations worth noting. First, it includes a relatively small sample of minority and low-income women drawn from a mid-Atlantic urban city. Given likely racial/ethnic and income variations in the use of FABM, the study should be replicated in other parts of the country and with other racial/ethnic groups. Thus, we acknowledge that our findings are not necessarily generalizable to a nationally representative sample of minority women. Indeed, a next step in this project is to conduct a survey with a nationally representative sample of young adult women to examine their use and knowledge of FABM and fertility awareness.

END NOTES

1. Women who reported using FABM in the past were asked to describe their most recent time they used FABM,including their relationship status, how they used it and why they chose to use FABM. As such, for past users the data about FABM use reported here refers to their most recent episode of FABM use.
2. Only 1 woman reported using Cycle Beads to track her cycle.
3. In general, women were assessed as not being very informed if they lacked knowledge about all three pieces; somewhat informed if they possessed knowledge of 2 out of the three components; and very informed if they had knowledge about all three pieces. Further adjustments in assessments were made based on other information provided during the interview.
4. These methods are 75–99% effective at preventing pregnancy. (Centers for Disease Control and Prevention 2009).
5. Fertility awareness was gauged by a series of close-ended questions, such as,"A woman is safe from getting pregnant 7 days before her period starts and 7 days after her period ends,""Ovulation is always 14 days after menstruation," and "If a woman's menstrual cycle is irregular she cannot become pregnant."

ADDENDUM A

Please tell me if you have EVER done this, even if it was just once or a long time ago.

1. Have you EVER used Natural Family Planning? This is sometimes called the Calendar Method, the Rhythm Method, safe period by temperature or the cervical mucus test. Have you EVER used any of these methods?

.. Yes

.. No

2. Couples can avoid having sex on certain days of the month when the woman is more likely to become pregnant. Have you EVER avoided having sex during the days in the month you were more likely to become pregnant?

.. Yes

.. No

3. Have you EVER tracked your menstrual cycle:

a. To know when it is safe to have sex without using other types of birth control?

.. Yes

.. No

b. To know when you will be getting your period or to know when your period is late?

¨ Yes

¨ No

c. To know when you need to avoid having sex?

¨ Yes

¨ No

d. To know when you need to use birth control in order to NOT get pregnant?

¨ Yes

¨ No

IF NO TO 3A, 3C, AND 3D, GO TO STOP SCREENER

ADDENDUM B

Exhibit 1. A Typical "In Conjunction With" FABM User

PRECAUTION IS PRIORITY

Chevonne is a 27-year-old African American who has been casually dating her partner for about six months, although they do not regularly have sex. Chevonne is Christian and attends services regularly and turns to her religion for emotional support and guidance. Chevonne does not have children and is not sure she wants to. Chevonne does not like to take any type of medication including synthetic hormones because she does not "want to take anything that I have to worry about … [including] side effects or what else it could be doing to me." She used oral contraceptives, but discontinued using them because she experienced negative "side effects," such as weight gain and feelings of sluggishness. Chevonne uses FABM in conjunction with condoms because she wants to avoid hormonal methods and wants an added level of protection to avoid pregnancy and STIs. Chevonne learned about FABM in her health class while attending a Catholic high school and is well informed about FABM and women's fertility. Chevonne refers to FABM as the "Calendar method" and has used it consistently and accurately for 3 years. She likes FABM because she does not "actually have to take any [medication]," and because she wants to do "things the natural way." The one thing that Chevonne dislikes about FABM is that it is not 100% effective.

Exhibit 2. Variation of FABM Use over Time

LACK OF KNOWLEDGE MAY LEAD TO METHOD FAILURE

Christina is a 22-year-old Hispanic woman who was born in Latin America. She has a fourth grade education and lives with her partner of four years with whom she has two children—a 3-month-old and a 6-year-old. She would like to wait several years to have another child. Christina has used oral contraceptives, condoms, withdrawal and FABM in the past. Her preferred, and current, method is condoms. Christina began using FABM four years ago when she began her relationship with her partner. At first, she used it in conjunction with condoms and withdrawal and about a year ago began using it as her primary method until she became pregnant. After having her second child, Christina returned to using condoms because she worries that her partner may be cheating on her. Although she likes condoms, she and her partner feel they are very expensive and place a financial burden on them. For this reason, she may return to using FABM someday. While Christina reports having received information about FABM from her doctor back home including how to identify her fertile window, what to do during her fertile period, and how effective FABM is, she has a poor understanding of women's fertility. In fact, she uses FABM incorrectly, abstaining during her menstrual period when she believes she is fertile. During the rest of her cycle she has non-contraceptive sex.

SOURCES CONSULTED

Centers for Disease Control and Prevention. "Unintended Pregnancy Prevention: Contraception." Division of Reproductive Health: Atlanta, GA www.cdc.gov/reproductivehealth/unintendedpregnancy/contraception.htm (accessed June 13, 2011).

Finer, Lawrence B., Stanley K. Henshaw. 2006. "Disparities in Rates of Unintended Pregnancy in the United States, 1994 and 2001." *Perspectives on Sexual and Reproductive Health* 38:90-96.

Fowler, C. I., J. Gable, J. Wang. 2008. "Family Planning Annual Report: 2007 National Summary." Research Triangle Park, NC: RTI International.

Hatcher, Robert, W. Rinehart, R. Blackburn, J. Geller, J. Shelton. 2003. "Fertility Awareness-Based Methods Including Periodic Abstinence." In Robert Hatcher et al., eds. *The Essentials of Contraceptive Technology.*

Baltimore: The Johns Hopkins Bloomberg School of Public Health, Population Information Program.

Ryder, Bob, Hubert Campbell. 1995. "Natural Family Planning in the 1990s." *Lancet* 346: 233.

State Family Planning Administrators. 2001. *Healthy People 2010-Reproductive Health*. Seattle: Project from the Office of Population Affairs, Department of Health and Human Services.

6

Creighton Model Effectiveness, Intentions, Behavior Assessment (CETBA)

JOSEPH B. STANFORD, MD, MPH

Professor of Medicine, School of Medicine, University of Utah

CHRISTINA A. PORUCZNIK, PHD, MSPH

Assistant Professor of Medicine, School of Medicine, University of Utah

DAISY KRAKOWIAK-REDD

Participant Coordinator

ABSTRACT

One facet of all types of Natural Family Planning that doesn't translate well to research methods generally used for 'contraceptives' is the ability to use the method both to avoid a pregnancy and to achieve a pregnancy. In typical contraception research, women planning to avoid pregnancy for a year are recruited into the study, given the method to be researched, and every pregnancy is considered to be a failure of the method. Researchers at the University of Utah are conducting an institutional review board-approved international study to evaluate the effectiveness of the Creighton Model for users wanting to avoid pregnancy at seventeen FertilityCare Centers and a projected 300 couple participants. While past studies have shown that the Creighton Model is a highly effective method, this study will use new ways to measure how well it works. This is important because the knowledge gained will improve comparisons between the Creighton Model and other family planning methods. The study will also explore intentions and behaviors of couples to avoid or achieve a pregnancy.

INTRODUCTION

The purpose of this paper is to describe the Creighton Model Effectiveness, Intentions and Behavior Assessment (CEIBA), an ongoing multi-center observational cohort study. The authors will introduce the study team, describe the study's aims, explain the reasons for the study's design, review the progress of the study, and discuss the implications of the study. Overall, the study is critical in advancing knowledge about the effectiveness of the Creighton Model to avoid pregnancy, and may be of interest in understanding the general motivations and behaviors of Natural Family Planning users.

STUDY TEAM

The following people have collaborated in the design and implementation of the study: Christy Porucznik, PhD, Co-Investigator, collaborator on the study design and operations; Xiaoming Sheng, PhD, Co-Investigator, advisor about the statistical calculations that can be performed with the gathered data; Thomas W. Hilgers, MD, creator of the Creighton Model and therefore primary consultant; Warren Miller, MD, and James Trussell, PhD, consultants (Dr. Miller is an expert in studying pregnancy intentions while Dr. Trussell is an expert in studying family planning effectiveness).

The staff who run the study on a day-to-day basis include the following: Becky Crockett, the study coordinator; Michael Lowe, the IRB specialist; Daisy Krakowiak, participant coordinator; and Nirupma Singh, research assistant. While the study is headquartered in Salt Lake City, Utah, this study would not be possible without the participation of 13 (and counting) Fertility*Care*™ Centers across the United States and Canada. The Fertility*Care*™ Practitioners involved in the study work very hard in enrolling participants from their clientele and scanning and sending their records to us. The study team is grateful for their ongoing participation in this research.

STUDY AIMS

As the name suggests, the goal of the Creighton Model Effectiveness, Intentions and Behaviors Assessment (CEIBA) is to study how well the method works to avoid pregnancy in the context of couples' *wishes and desires* to avoid or achieve pregnancy, as well as their *behaviors* to avoid or achieve pregnancy. More specifically, the study has four aims:

Aim 1: To evaluate Creighton Model pregnancy rates during "perfect" and "typical use" to avoid pregnancy in a way that is directly comparable to the approach used in family planning effectiveness studies.

This aim is important because it will allow couples and their health-care providers to directly compare how effective the Creighton Model is to other methods of family planning and will help them make an informed decision in choosing a method. Because this directly comparable information is not available as of yet, the Creighton Model is overlooked as an effective family planning method and is often misunderstood in medical circles.

In the analysis, pregnancies *and cycles* will be classified. Only cycles of perfect use to avoid pregnancy (and at least some sexual activity) will be included in the risk set for perfect use pregnancy rates; similarly only segments of imperfect use to avoid pregnancy will be included in the risk set for imperfect use pregnancy rates (Trussell, Grummer-Strawn 1991; Trussell 2004). Couples may transition between these states. For example, one couple might complete their first cycle with imperfect use to avoid pregnancy, the second and third cycles with perfect use to avoid, and the fourth cycle again with imperfect use to avoid. Sensitivity analyses will be done for different definitions of perfect and imperfect use to avoid pregnancy.

Aim 2: To evaluate pregnancy rates by the Creighton Model behavioral classifications, as done with the six prior Creighton Model effectiveness studies.

In addition to calculating "perfect" and "typical use," we will calculate pregnancy rates as has been done in past Creighton Model studies so that we can compare those rates across time and see if there have been any trends in effectiveness since the prior studies (Doud 1985; Fehring, Lawrence et al. 1994; Hilgers, Stanford 1998; Howard, Stanford 1999). The way pregnancy rates are classified in the Creighton Model is based on behavior rather than on stated intention (see Table 1). The Creighton Model pregnancy classifications are achieving related

Table 1. Creighton Model Pregnancy Classification

Code	Category	Description
I	Achieving related pregnancy	From the available information, the method was used as a method of avoiding pregnancy, and the woman became pregnant.
II A	Avoiding- method related pregnancy	From the available information, the method was used correctly as a method of avoiding pregnancy, and the woman became pregnant.
II B	Avoiding- using related pregnancy	From the available information, the method was used incorrectly (but taught correctly) as a method of avoiding pregnancy, and the woman became pregnant.
II C	Avoiding- teaching related pregnancy	From the available information, the method was taught incorrectly (but used correctly according to instruction) as a method of avoiding pregnancy, & the woman became pregnant.
II D	Avoiding- using/teaching related pregnancy	A combination of using related & teaching related.
III	Unresolved pregnancy	From the available information, the circumstances of the pregnancy cannot be placed into any of the above classifications.
NR	Not CrM-related pregnancy	Pregnancy did not occur during use of the CrM, but rather during the use of another method, such as condoms or withdrawal.

pregnancies (due to proceptive behavior), avoiding related pregnancies (subdivided into method-related, using-related, teaching-related, both using/teaching-related), unresolved pregnancies (due to insufficient information for classification), and pregnancy unrelated to the CrM (pregnancy did not occur during use of the CrM, but during use of another method, such as condoms). In prior CrM effectiveness studies, the same denominator of all couples was used for all these rates, but in this study we will refine this approach and include cycles with only that particular type of use in the denominator. This will be done with life table analysis. For example, to calculate the avoiding related pregnancy rate, only those cycles where the method was behaviorally used to avoid pregnancy will be included.

Aim 3: To evaluate the intention status of all pregnancies during Creighton Model use according to standard measures, recognizing the conceptual limitations of those measures.

There are two widely used measures for unintended pregnancy. The first is based on prospectively stated intentions (Lamprecht,Trussell 1997). If a woman (or couple) states that she plans to avoid pregnancy for the next month, or cycle, or year, all subsequent pregnancies are considered unintended until a new declaration is made. The second approach, usually used retrospectively, and used in the U.S. National Survey of Family Growth (NSFG), is to ask whether the woman wanted a pregnancy at the time it occurred or sooner (an intended pregnancy), would have preferred that it occur later (a mistimed pregnancy), or not at all (an unintended pregnancy). Pregnancies will be classified by these measures so that they may be directly comparable to other family planning studies that include pregnancy intentions. At the same time, the relationships between these measures and more detailed measures (aim 4) and behaviors to explore the implications and limitations of the assumptions underlying these measures of intention will be analyzed.

Aim 4: To explore the multiple dimensions of pregnancy motivations, intentions, and behaviors during CrM use by newer detailed measures.

There is growing consensus among researchers in the field that current measures of pregnancy intention are simplistic at best, and at worst, can be very misleading (Kaufmann, Morris et al. 1997; Luker, Sable et al. 1999; Sable 1999; Campbell, Mosher 2000; Joyce, Kaestner et al. 2000; Klerman 2000; Sable, Libbus 2000; Santelli, Rochat et al. 2003). Because of the limitations to standard measures of pregnancy intention, we are gathering measures of pregnancy happiness, childbearing motivations, child postponing motivations, sexual behavior, contraceptive behavior, and proceptive behavior (Miller 1995; Sable, Libbus 2000; Miller, Severy et al. 2004).

Figure 1. Hypothetical model of couples using the Creighton Model through time with varying intentions and behavior and how pregnancy rates can be calculated with various assumptions

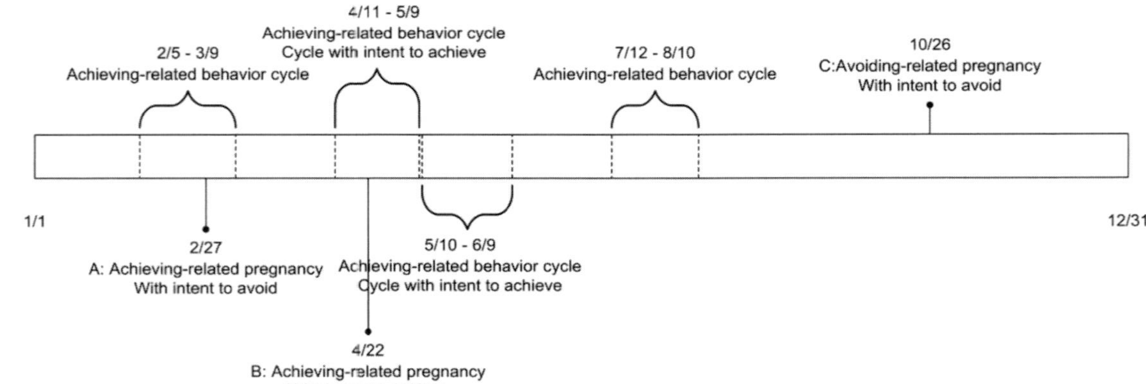

All cycles with intent to avoid pregnancy and avoiding behavior unless otherwise noted

Traditionally, pregnancy rate would include all cycles and all pregnancies
Pregnancy rate = Pregnancies A, B & C / All Cycles

Perfect use pregnancy rate can be calculated by taking into account the reported behaviors
Avoiding-Behavior Pregnancy Rate = Pregnancy C / Avoiding Behavior Cycles
Achieving-Behavior Pregnancy Rate = Pregnancies A& B / Achieving Behavior Cycles

Pregnancy rates may be calculated considering the stated intention:
Avoiding-Intent Pregnancy Rate = Pregnancies A & C / Avoiding Intent Cycles
Achieving-Intent Pregnancy Rate = Pregnancy B / Achieving Intent Cycles

STUDY DESIGN AND ANALYSIS

To achieve our aims, the study is designed as a prospective cohort of 300 new Creighton Model users. Thirteen of 190 Fertility*Care*™. Centers are actively screening and recruiting clients for the study. The study does not change the way the Creighton Model is taught, rather the study follows the clients through time and observes their intentions and behaviors with regard to avoiding or achieving a pregnancy. In the beginning, participants are asked about their childbearing motivations. Pregnancy intentions are asked at the beginning of each cycle, which is particularly important because, like all methods of Natural Family Planning, the Creighton Model can be used either to avoid or achieve a pregnancy. These questions are asked of the man and woman with confidential and secure online questionnaires.

ANALYSIS

The most important part of our study is to classify cycles according to intentions of *not wanting* to become pregnant versus *wanting* to become pregnant, and how the method was used. Fundamentally, we are asking which cycles should be categorized as perfect use of the method or imperfect use of the method based on how well couples adhered to the method according to their intentions. Our prospective study allows us to answer this question in more than one way and to compare the results from those approaches.

Since the main aim of our study is to determine the effectiveness of the Creighton Model to avoid pregnancy, the main outcome we are looking at is pregnancy. In the past, pregnancy rates for the Creighton Model were calculated by taking all or sometimes selected pregnancies and dividing them by all cycles. Note how all cycles were counted the same, even though intentions to achieve or avoid and behavior to achieve and avoid vary. Figure 1 is a hypothetical model to illustrate how different people with different intentions and behaviors can vary across time, but how their cycles are counted the same way in the calculation. Thus, a conception cycle with a couple wanting to *achieve* and using the system to do so and a conception cycle with a couple wanting to *avoid* and using the system to do so are counted the same way. We lose not only what behaviors couples have, but also their intentions.

In order to calculate a pregnancy rate during perfect use of the method to avoid pregnancy, cycles need to be better classified. For example, when assessing the rate of perfect use (or method-related) pregnancies, only cycles of consistent method use to avoid pregnancy (perfect use to avoid pregnancy) should be included in the denominator (see Figure 1). That way, a rate can be calculated that reflects pregnancies that occur only in cycles that were used accurately and consistently to avoid pregnancy.

As discussed, the Creighton Model classifies pregnancies based on behavior rather than on intention. In prior CrM effectiveness studies, the same denominator of all couples was used for all these rates, but in this study we will refine this approach to analyze rates on the denominator of the cycles with only that particular type of use. Thus, when calculating achieving related pregnancies, only cycles with achieving related behavior will be included in the denominator (see Figure 1). That way, we will have a more accurate measure of pregnancies occurring during cycles in which couples had achieving related behavior. I have previously outline the plan for these analyses in similar detail in the 2004 textbook of NaProTechnology (Stanford 2004).

In addition to calculating pregnancy rates based on behavior, we can calculate pregnancy rates based on intentions. In the study, we ask both the man and the woman at the beginning of each cycle if they intend to achieve or avoid and the strength of that intention. We can therefore group cycles in which couples tell us that they are intending to avoid pregnancies and calculate the pregnancy rates that occur during the cycles with that intention (see Figure 1). As may be noted, even though the intention is to avoid pregnancy, couples may exhibit either avoiding related behavior or achieving related behavior. Thus, we are able to determine the pregnancy rate of couples who stated that their intention is to avoid.

STUDY PROGRESS

Our study got off to a bit of a late start as our research team received a delayed notice of the funding award in October 2008. We met with the funding agency and our study consultants in January 2009. In the following months, we worked diligently on finalizing the study protocol, questionnaires, and manual of procedures, which were completed by May 2009. In July 2009, the University of Utah IRB approved the study; however, since there are 13 separate sites involved in the study, each one had to go through the IRB approval process. The sites received approval at varying times from July 2009 to July 2010.

Enrollment of couples began as sites received IRB approval and we are continually enrolling new participants. Thus far (July 2010), we have 56 enrolled couples.

We conducted a brief interim analysis of the couples we have so far to provide an idea of who is in the study. The average age of women in the study is 26.9, with ages ranging from 22 to 41. The majority of study participants are engaged (n=29, 52%). Married couples also constitute a large portion of the study participants (n=24, 43%) whereas couples who are not engaged or married (i.e. single) make up just a small portion (n=3, 5%). Most of the women in the study are White non-Hispanic (n=47, 84%).

Currently, we have 152 completed women's cycle questionnaires. Table 2 displays the number of cycles with the varying degrees of intentions to achieve or avoid a pregnancy. The majority of cycles have the woman's stated intention to try to avoid pregnancy or to try as hard as possible to avoid, followed by cycles where the woman's intention is to abstain from all genital contact (the latter category is usually chosen by engaged couples).

Table 2. Pregnancy intentions by cycle (149 cycles)

Intention	**Number of cycles**
Trying to get pregnant	1
Neither trying nor not trying	6
Trying to avoid	46
Trying as hard as possible to avoid	40
Abstaining from all genital contact	56

Table 3 [next page] displays the number of cycles with women's responses to the question "How would you feel if you were to find out you were pregnant right now?" This question was only asked of couples who were planning sexual intercourse in the next cycle. The majority of cycles had the woman's stated response of being happy or very happy, followed by having mixed feelings. Only 12 cycles had the woman's stated response of being unhappy or very unhappy.

Overall, our study has been successful in screening for couples who are initially using the Creighton Model to avoid pregnancy. In addition, our study is already finding that even with stated intentions to avoid pregnancy, the majority of women would still be happy if they were to find out they were pregnant. However, these data are preliminary. As the study continues and concludes, we look forward to analyzing our data further.

Table 3. Hypothetical pregnancy question responses by cycle (91 cycles)

Response to "How would you feel if you were to find out you were pregnant right now?"	Number of cycles
Very unhappy	4
Unhappy	8
Mixed	25
Happy	45
Very happy	

STUDY IMPLICATIONS

The results from this study may have several implications. First, the results will provide us with insight into relations between pregnancy intentions, behaviors, and outcomes in a way that is more sophisticated than previous studies. At the same time, the results will report "perfect" and "typical" use pregnancy rates for the Creighton Model, which will be directly comparable with other family planning methods. These two implications combined will increase the clarity about the effectiveness of the Creighton Model. This scientific clarity will be stronger than normative judgments that are made by critics against the Creighton Model and other NFP methods.

In focusing the discussion on scientific results, the Creighton Model, along with other NFP methods, may break through barriers of misunderstanding and may become more widely adopted. With this new information, health professionals may become more aware and better understand NFP and provide it as an option to their patients. In turn, we hope there may be an upswing in NFP utilization by couples. Not only will more couples practice a safe, natural, and effective method that is individually beneficial to them, but our society may recognize the values of responsible sexuality and parenthood by using NFP. While these implications may seem lofty, we believe that our study, as well as other NFP studies, can be a part of a movement towards increased understanding and usage of NFP.

SOURCES CONSULTED

Campbell, A. A., W. D. Mosher. 2000."A history of the measurement of unintended pregnancies and births." *Maternal Child Health Journal* 4:163-169.

Doud, J. 1985. "Use-effectiveness of the Creighton Model of NFP." *International Review of Natural Family Planning* 9:54-72.

Fehring, R. J., D. Lawrence et al. 1994. "Use effectiveness of the Creighton-Model Ovulation Method of natural family planning." *Journal of Obstetrics and Gynecology and Neonatal Nursing* 23:303-309.

Hilgers, T. W., J. B. Stanford. 1998. "The use-effectiveness to avoid pregnancy of Creighton model NaProEducation technology: a meta-analysis of prospective trials." *Journal of Reproductive Medicine* 43:495-502.

Howard, M. P., J. B. Stanford. 1999. "Pregnancy probabilities during use of the Creighton Model Fertility Care System." *Archives of Family Medicine* 8:391-402.

Joyce, T., R. Kaestner et al. 2000. "The stability of pregnancy intentions and pregnancy-related maternal behaviors." *Maternal and Child Health Journal* 4:171-178.

Kaufmann, R. B., L. Morris et al. 1997. "Comparison of two question sequences for assessing pregnancy intentions." *American Journal of Epidemiology* 145:810-816.

Klerman, L. V. 2000. "The intendedness of pregnancy: a concept in transition." *Maternal Child Health Journal* 4:155-162.

Lamprecht, V., J. Trussell. 1997. "Natural family planning effectiveness: evaluating published reports." *Advances in Contraception* 13:155-165.

Luker, K. C., M. R. Sable et al. 1999. "Contraceptive failure and unintended pregnancy." *Family Planning Perspectives* 31:248-253.

Miller, W. B. 1995. "Childbearing motivation and its measurement." *Journal of Biosocial Science* 27:473-487.

Miller, W. B., L. J. Severy et al. 2004. "A framework for modelling fertility motivation in couples." *Population Study* (Cambridge) 58:193-205.

Sable, M. R. 1999."Pregnancy intentions may not be a useful measure for research on maternal and child health outcomes." *Family Planning Perspective* 31:249-250.

Sable, M. R., M. K. Libbus. 2000."Pregnancy intention and pregnancy happiness: are they different?" *Maternal Child Health Journal* 4:191-196.

Santelli, J., R. Rochat et al. 2003. "The measurement and meaning of unintended pregnancy." *Perspectives on Sexual and Reproductive Health* 35:94-101.

Stanford, J. B. 2004. "Measuring effectiveness and pregnancy rates of the CrMS." In, *The Medical and Surgical Practice of NaProTechnology*, 215-231. T. W. Hilgers. Ed. Omaha: Pope Paul VI Institute Press.

Trussell, J. 2004."Contraceptive failure in the United States." *Contraception* 70:89-96.

Trussell, J., L. Grummer-Strawn. 1991. "Further analysis of contraceptive failure of the ovulation method." *American Journal of Obstetrics amd Gynecology* 165 (6 Pt 2): 2054-2059.

7

Meeting Clients' Needs for Family Planning without Hormones: Opportunities for Introducing SDM/CycleBeads

VICTORIA JENNINGS, PHD

Director, Institute for Reproductive Health, School of Medicine, Georgetown University

KATHERINE LAVOIE CAIN, MPH

Independent Consultant

REBECKA LUNDGREN, MPH

Deputy Director, Director of Research Institute for Reproductive Health, School of Medicine, Georgetown University

ABSTRACT

Despite their efficacy and safety, availability and use of fertility-awareness based family planning methods (FABM) are low in U.S. Title X clinics. The Standard Days Method® (SDM) is a simple yet effective FABM that can be taught in a short time. Introducing SDM into clinic programming represents a feasible way to mainstream FABM and expand choice by providing an alternative to hormonal methods. SDM is appropriate for women who get their periods every 26 to 32 days and is used with a color-coded visual tool called CycleBeads®. A study is being conducted to develop and test a process to introduce SDM in four clinics in California and Massachusetts. The process pioneers the World Health Organization's Strategic Approach for family planning method introduction in a U.S.-based project and calls for the integration strategy to be developed through a participatory process focusing on client needs and quality services. This paper presents the results of the needs assessment phase that assesses the demand for SDM and identifies opportunities and barriers for SDM introduction. Methods included community focus groups to assess potential demand for SDM; provider interviews to assess knowledge, attitudes, and practices with regard to FABM and SDM; and a site assessment to identify operational and logistical considerations to adding SDM to services. Results suggest that SDM appeals to potential clients who desire a non-hormonal family planning method and providers are amenable to offering it. This paper also describes the components of the subsequent phases to the project—namely, the introduction and evaluation phase, and the research utilization and dissemination phase—and how the results from the needs assessment were used to tailor the integration strategy to each clinic's setting.

INTRODUCTION

In spite of the wide range of family planning options available in the United States, each year approximately half of pregnancies in this country are unintended (Henshaw 1998; see also Finer and Henshaw 2006). In the United States, some 7% of women (15-44) who do not use a method of family planning are at risk of unintended pregnancy amounting to over 4.3 million women. It is important to consider strategies to reach these women.

Fertility awareness-based methods (FABM)—sometimes referred to as Natural Family Planning (NFP)—are safe and effective, yet they are underutilized in the United States. These methods include Rhythm/Calendar, Standard Days Method® (SDM), Basal Body Temperature, Cervical Mucus, Sympto-Thermal, and electronic hormonal methods. Among perfect users of NFP, the percentage of women experiencing an unintended pregnancy during the first year of use ranges from two to five percent, depending on the method. For pregnancy avoidance, the effectiveness of many of the NFP methods, with perfect use, is equal to or more effective than many contraceptives, including the contraceptive sponge, male and female condom, diaphragm, and cervical cap.

The U.S. government provides funding for family planning services under Title X of the Public Health Act, which authorizes grants "to assist in the establishment and operation of voluntary family planning projects which shall offer a broad range of acceptable and effective family planning methods and services (including natural family planning methods, infertility services, and services for adolescents)." Although Natural Family Planning (NFP) methods are explicitly referenced in the Title X statute, the utilization of NFP methods remains low among clients seeking services in Title X-funded clinics. Recent data from the Family Planning Annual Report (FPAR) show that in 2008, less than one percent of female Title X clients (10,409 females) relied on fertility awareness based methods as their primary method of pregnancy prevention (Fowler et al. 2009).

To explore the potential of expanding the availability of FABM in the United States, the Department of Health and Human Services' Office of Population Affairs has provided funding through Georgetown University to evaluate whether integrating SDM in selected Title X clinics helps to increase FABM availability and use. Specifically, this study aims to identify factors which constrain and facilitate FABM availability and use; develop and test a process to introduce the SDM within a framework of expanded choice; and assess acceptance, correct use, and satisfaction.

The Standard Days Method is a fertility awareness-based family planning method developed by researchers at Georgetown University, which was designed to be simple to teach, easy to use, and feasible to mainstream into programs. The SDM specifies a fixed fertile window of days 8-19 during a woman's menstrual cycle. The method is appropriate for women with menstrual cycles between 26 and 32 days and is typically used with CycleBeads®, a color-coded string of beads, which helps a woman track her cycle days, identify when she is fertile, monitor her cycle length, and communicate with her partner about pregnancy prevention. The SDM was tested in a multisite efficacy study, which found a first-year pregnancy rate of 4.8 per 100 woman-years of correct use (Arévalo et al. 2002).

International research suggests that integration of SDM is a promising strategy to help expand availability and use of FABM. From 2001-2007, SDM was introduced through 14 pilot studies around the world by ministries of health, family planning associations, and community organizations. Results showed the following: SDM appeals to a broad range of women; women use it correctly; both men and women report a high level of satisfaction with the method; and SDM counseling can fit within the normal time allotted for a family planning counseling session in most programs (Gribble et al. 2008).

The World Health Organization (WHO) recognizes SDM as an evidence-based practice (WHO 2002, 2007), and the method is available in over 30 countries around the world. Currently, Georgetown University's Institute for Reproductive Health (IRH) is working with ministries of health in over five countries to scale-up SDM at national and sub-national levels.

Like other fertility awareness based methods, the SDM is not yet available on a wide scale in the United States. Although CycleBeads have been on the market since 2002, and many individuals, clinics, and retail outlets have purchased CycleBeads, SDM is not part of many programs. In addition, CycleBeads are not covered by most U.S. state health departments or private insurance plans.

Preliminary experience introducing the SDM in a U.S. context indicated the potential for this method to benefit secular family planning programs. As part of broader service delivery research on a couple-focused approach to family planning counseling that took place in 2007-2008, IRH worked with providers in three Planned Parenthood clinics and one community-based health center in California to integrate the method into services. Though SDM was not the main focus of the research, it was the first time SDM was included in U.S.-based research efforts, and lessons learned from this experience informed the design of the current SDM-focused study.

Results suggested that providers and counselors found SDM easy to teach and that women were interested in learning about the method. They also found it to be an empowering tool for women to help them learn about their fertility. The community-based health clinic reported over 100 SDM users during the first year it was offered, suggesting that the method met a client need.

STUDY DESIGN

Following these promising pilot experiences, the next step was to conduct a study with the explicit purpose of evaluating SDM integration in U.S. Title X clinics. For this research, Georgetown University collaborated with two Title X Regional Training Centers: the Center for Health Training (Oakland, CA); and the JSI Research and Training Institute based in Boston, MA (a non-profit affiliate of John Snow, Inc., a public health research and consulting firm). These were the primary research and training partners. Service delivery partners included two clinics in California (one Planned Parenthood clinic and one community-based health center), and two Health Quarters reproductive health clinics in Massachusetts, all of which receive Title X funds. Three out of the four service delivery sites serve a largely low-income, Hispanic clientele. Additional sites were added one year into the study but are not described in this paper.

In order to maximize the potential benefit of SDM introduction, this research utilizes the World Health Organization's Strategic Approach to contraceptive introduction as a guiding framework. According to the Strategic Approach (Simmons et al. 1997; Fajans et al. 2006), the decision to offer a new method should be based on needs perceived by stakeholders—including providers and clients—for such a method. The strategy for providing the method, including who offers it, counseling protocols, how it is described to clients, how information about it is shared with potential users, and how it is supported by the service delivery system, should be developed through a participatory, transparent process that focuses on client needs and quality services (as defined by Bruce 1990). This approach has been used successfully internationally (Simmons et al. 1997; Fajans et al. 2006), and this project represents the first time it has been applied in the U.S.

The Strategic Approach has three stages: the strategic assessment of need, the research stage during which the method is introduced and evaluated, and the third stage in which research results are used for policy and planning (Simmons et al. 1997; Fajans et al. 2006). This paper describes the first stage, the needs assessment component, and the second (research) stage, which is currently underway. The study design is depicted in Figure 1 [see next page]. The Georgetown University Institutional Review Board approved the study.

The purpose of the needs assessment was to assess potential clients' knowledge, needs, and interest in FABM; provider knowledge, attitudes, and practices regarding FABM; service delivery systems and outreach activities; and opportunities and challenges to adding SDM to the method mix. In accordance with the Strategic Approach, a participatory process was used to gather this information, which included a site assessment, staff interviews, and community-based focus group discussions.

Figure 1: Study Design

<table>
<tr><th></th><th colspan="2">Phase I
Needs assessment</th><th colspan="4">Phase II
SDM integration & evaluation</th><th>Phase III</th></tr>
<tr><th>Data elements</th><th colspan="2">Pre SDM integration</th><th></th><th colspan="2">Process evaluation</th><th>Outcome evaluation</th><td rowspan="8">Use of research results for policy and planning</td></tr>
<tr><td>Site assessment</td><td>√</td><td rowspan="6">Tailor SDM integration activities</td><td rowspan="6">Integrate the SDM into existing services</td><td></td><td rowspan="6">Modify integration activities</td><td></td></tr>
<tr><td>Provider & staff interviews</td><td>√</td><td></td><td>√</td></tr>
<tr><td>Client focus groups</td><td>√</td><td></td><td></td></tr>
<tr><td>Simulated clients</td><td></td><td>√</td><td></td></tr>
<tr><td>Waiting room questionnaire</td><td>√</td><td></td><td></td></tr>
<tr><td>Client follow up</td><td></td><td></td><td>√</td></tr>
<tr><td>Service statistics</td><td></td><td></td><td></td><td></td><td></td><td></td></tr>
</table>

RESULTS

The results of the needs assessment are described below. These results were used to tailor the integration plan to each clinic's specific context.

Site Assessment

As part of the site assessment, study staff collected the service statistics for each of the participating clinics for 2008 (Table X). These data indicate that the number of FABM users from each of the participating clinics is negligible. Specifically, in 2008, the clinics reported a total of two FABM users out of a total of 13,501 female family planning users. However, since some providers reported teaching about FABM and/or distributing CycleBeads, FABM use was likely underreported.

Managers were interviewed to assess the feasibility of SDM integration. Study staff discussed a range of issues with the managers including role of each type of staff in SDM integration, how SDM would fit into family planning counseling, what forms would be used or created to document and/or consent SDM users, type and duration of SDM training, how SDM may be incorporated into educational materials and outreach activities, paying for SDM clients, CycleBeads storage, and how clinic relationships with external organizations could help or hinder the integration process.

No manager anticipated significant problems to integrate the method into systems. Existing multi-method educational materials do not include SDM. These methods are currently not in billing forms, so the forms would need to be modified to ensure FABM/SDM users are properly tracked. Written protocol and consent forms may need to be developed and integrated, but this would also be feasible. Financing was not an issue at this time because clinics could be reimbursed for counseling time for SDM, and because CycleBeads were donated by IRH. However, CycleBeads procurement was identified as an obstacle to future integration and scale up because they are not covered by insurance plans.

Staff Interviews

A total of 24 staff involved in providing family planning services to clients were interviewed from the study clinics. This group included 8 clinicians, 3 nurses, and 13 non-clinical staff who served as counselors and health educators. These interviews revealed that FABM availability at the clinics was limited. At all of the clinics, the counselors and health educators lacked information about FABM and therefore were not able to offer them. In the case that a client requested a natural method, the counselor would refer the client to the clinician. Most of the clinicians indicated they had some experience offering FABM/NFP but did not offer them on a regular basis. Some clinicians have their own way of teaching how to use NFP and have calendars they can give to patients to track their menstrual cycle. Two clinicians had undergone training on SDM and had given out a couple sets of CycleBeads.

In general, staff at all of the clinics were in favor of offering a FABM—and in particular, the SDM—in order to meet the needs of their clients seeking such a method. "The more options available to our clients, the better," was a sentiment echoed by staff at all of the sites. Nearly all providers said they would be very comfortable offering SDM and having their clients use it, as long as the client was adequately informed about the method and how to use it.

In particular, the Planned Parenthood site seeks to serve a large Hispanic and Catholic population among whom staff felt the SDM would be well accepted. Planned Parenthood staff also mentioned that the SDM might appeal to migrant workers because the method requires no follow-up or resupply. At one of the Health Quarters sites in Massachusetts, staff mentioned that there were many myths about birth control and fear of side effects, particularly among the first generation Latino immigrant community and therefore they might be interested in the SDM in particular. Outreach staff at this site said they had already been talking about the method in community talks and found that it has sparked interest, saying "people are always very eager to hear about it when I bring it up."

Staff cited various factors that may inhibit FABM availability and uptake. Some providers were skeptical about the effectiveness of FABM, and one provider said that she would offer FABM only to someone who couldn't use hormones or was seeking pregnancy. Staff also had concerns about client's interest in and ability to use the SDM. They thought that lower effectiveness rates for FABM might discourage potential users, and that clients' general lack of fertility awareness might result in a lack of confidence in the method. Some providers thought that the method would not work for some women who might forget to track their menstrual cycle daily using CycleBeads, or who had multiple partners. One mentioned that the people who would most likely want the method would not be likely to visit the clinic. More than one provider thought that the method might not be appropriate for teens due to their maturity level.

Community-Based Focus Groups

A total of seven focus group discussions were conducted with community members living in the areas served by the clinics. Four groups were conducted in English, and three were conducted in Spanish. The total number of participants was 45, with a mean age of 31. Criteria for participation included that the participants (all female) were in a relationship, wanted to avoid pregnancy, and were either not using family planning or not satisfied with their current method. Approximately 65% of them reported to be currently using a family planning method.

Participants in all the focus groups said they knew of some if not many women who wished to avoid a pregnancy but were not using a family planning method. The main reasons they stated for this included fear or dislike of side effects caused by hormonal methods, lack of confidence in contraceptive methods due to past method failure, and belief that they will not get pregnant. They also mentioned that difficulty remembering to take a pill every day, lack of motivation to go to the clinic, and male reluctance to use condoms or get a vasectomy were reasons why some couples did not use an artificial method.

Additional reasons for not using a contraceptive method included lack of knowledge of method options, perceived cost, and the fact that intercourse was unplanned. One group mentioned the teachings of the Catholic faith as a factor. Direct quotes from participants are provided in Figure 2.

Figure 2: Reasons for Non-Use of Family Planning

"I've tried a couple of different birth control methods and I haven't liked a lot of them. I have bad reactions."

"Me personally, I never have time to go to the doctor to get birth control, and I didn't have any health insurance for a period of time."

"My boyfriend thinks that it's my responsibility to find protection or get birth control. He doesn't like condoms."

"For some women, methods do not work. So they do not want to use anything."

"I [know someone] who can't remember to take the pill, so she just took herself off of it."

Participants in all the groups felt there was a need for new family planning methods in order to have more choices. They stated that the ideal method would be highly effective, natural with no hormones or side effects, non-invasive, safe, and inexpensive. Participants expressed the desire for a method that did not require daily action (so that forgetfulness would not adversely affect method use) and that only needed to be obtained once a year. Figure 3 lists direct quotes from focus group participants on this topic.

The facilitator of each focus group then told the participants about the Standard Days Method and CycleBeads and explained how the method works. Participants in all the groups thought there would be some women who would choose SDM, and some of them even mentioned that they would be interested in using it. They listed advantages of the method as the fact that it is non-hormonal and has no side effects, it can help women learn about how their bodies work, and it can involve their partners. Participants also cited other advantages to the method including that it was economical, easy to use, and reusable and long-lasting.

Figure 3: Focus group participants' opinions on a new family planning option

"Another [family planning] option is good. People can try it."

"Oh yes, we need something new. At least, I am tired of the pill."

"[An ideal method is] something without hormones, that is natural, without bad side effects."

"[I'd like something with] no side effects, weight gain, mood changes, or irregular bleeding, etc."

"I don't like the idea of something in me all the time and that I can't take out."

"An ideal method is one that works and you don't have to work too hard to keep track of it."

"I think it would be great for males to have to take on some of the responsibility as well, so that it is two people, especially when you are in a relationship."

Participants however, observed disadvantages to the method as well. For example, they acknowledged that it would not be appropriate for women with irregular menstrual cycles, and they stated that many women—particularly teens—might not be conscientious enough or have enough self-discipline to use the method correctly. Participants also indicated that some women would not have confidence in the method due to lack of understanding of the menstrual cycle and that SDM would not appeal to those seeking a highly effective method. Some representative quotes about SDM/CycleBeads from focus group participants are provided in Figure 4.

Figure 4: Focus group participants' opinions regarding SDM

"Personally, I like it a lot."
"I always wanted to do the calendar thing, but never knew how."
"I like this method because I cannot use hormones."
"I think I would worry about having unprotected sex at any point – it is nerve wracking to me."
"I am not quite convinced yet. I may need more time. I am afraid to get pregnant."
"It's natural, easy, simple. I can ask my partner, 'Honey, move the little thing for me.'" (referring to the black ring on CycleBeads)
"You can involve men. This is something visual."
"My husband will be very happy that he does not have to pull out. You really need good communication so when you tell him we are in the [fertile days] he will know what to do."
"It's a great educational tool, if anything. I never knew, none of us knew, the exact dates [when a woman is fertile]."
"My sister might like it—she's a vegetarian and rides her bike."

DISCUSSION

Overall, the needs assessment revealed that there is need for more non-hormonal options and that there is an interest in the SDM among potential clients. SDM seemed to appeal to women who wish to avoid pregnancy but do not wish to use hormones due to side effects or other reasons. At the same time, providers were open to offering it in order to expand choice for their clients and because they perceived SDM as simple to teach and as something that would help meet the needs of their clients. Their concerns about offering the method included its effectiveness, how to support correct use, cultural factors/ machismo. Clinic staff were also concerned that SDM may not be appropriate for clients who desire a highly effective method, who are unable to communicate with their partners about sex, or who cannot remember to move the ring on CycleBeads. From a systems perspective, there were no barriers to method integration that could not be resolved with minimal effort. However, procurement is likely to be a challenge in the future as the method is not on insurance formularies.

PHASE 2: INTEGRATION AND RESEARCH PHASE

At this time, SDM has been integrated into the services of all participating study clinics, and evaluation is underway. The components of the integration and evaluation phase are described below.

SDM Integration

Utilizing the results of the needs assessment, modifications were made to clinic systems to incorporate SDM. This includes billing/reporting forms, chart documentation, and protocols. No changes were required in supervision systems or clinic flow. A supply of CycleBeads was provided to each clinic, and a SDM/CycleBeads job aid was given to each staff person and placed in the counseling rooms.

The research and training centers conducted trainings for providers and counselors at each site. The trainings consisted of 2 hours on SDM/CycleBeads counseling, and 1.5-2 hours on use of educational materials and study procedures (e.g., recruiting clients into the study). Study staff conducted follow-up visits to sites throughout the year, including going to staff meetings. The information gleaned from the providers during the needs assessment enabled study staff to better tailor the trainings to their needs. For example, the training addressed certain items that came up in the needs assessment including SDM effectiveness, how to ensure proper screening of clients, and how to encourage and support correct use and male involvement. The training also addressed couple dynamics, taking into account the contextual issues that may inhibit correct use. Since FABM is not part of the counseling routine, it was stressed that SDM should be incorporated into counseling when all methods are reviewed so that clients can learn about it.

To inform potential clients of the availability of a new method—namely, the SDM—at the clinics, it was important to conduct awareness-raising activities. A sample of these activities is listed below:

- Adaptation and dissemination of posters and brochures (English and Spanish)
- Integration into ongoing outreach activities (health fairs, community talks, etc.)
- Fliers in natural food stores, yoga studios, beauty salons, coffee shops, and other women-centric establishments
- Articles in English and Spanish newspapers
- Articles in organizational newsletters
- Announcements of SDM availability on social networking sites such as Facebook

Evaluation Research

This study utilizes several methods to evaluate the effect of the introduction of the SDM by the study clinics. First, the clinics are collecting service statistics to track the number of FABM users to see if the number increases following SDM integration. Service statistics from before and after SDM integration will be analyzed on an ongoing basis.

Second, clients who choose the SDM will be invited to be interviewed via telephone by study staff. Clients who agree will be interviewed up to four times: first within two weeks of starting the method, then at three and six months, and finally at 12 months. This will enable study staff to determine client satisfaction with and correct use of the method and to assess continuation rates. Clients are being recruited into the study on a rolling basis, and these interviews are currently being conducted. Participation in the interviews is completely voluntary, and clients are able to choose the SDM without participating in the interviews.

Finally, clinic staff will be interviewed a second time six to eight months after being trained to offer the method. Through these interviews, we will learn about their experience offering the method, whether they believe their clinic should continue to offer the method, and what input they have into the production of information products to be shared during the dissemination and utilization phase that may assist other organizations to integrate the SDM into their family planning programs.

PHASE 3: DISSEMINATION AND UTILIZATION

The third year of the study will focus on dissemination and utilization of research results. This will include sharing of experiences with other organizations through conferences and meetings, development and dissemination of an SDM integration "toolkit" based on the study clinics' experiences, and potentially a video demonstrating effective SDM counseling. The specific activities and products that will be put forth during the third phase will be decided through a collaborative process involving all study partners as well as other interested organizations and stakeholders in the respective Title X regions where the study clinics are located.

CONCLUSION

According to the Strategic Approach to contraceptive introduction, the decision to offer a new method should be based on needs perceived by stakeholders, and the introduction strategy should be developed through a participatory, transparent process that focuses on client needs and quality services. Results of the needs assessment suggested that SDM would appeal to potential clients who desire a non-hormonal family planning method, and providers were amenable to offering it. Results also informed the approach to the needs assessment in terms of how systems needed to be modified, which topics should be emphasized during staff training, and what messages and channels would be most likely to reach potential clients to inform and educate them about the method. The purpose of utilizing the Strategic Approach is to increase the likelihood that quality SDM services would meet clients' needs and be sustainable and replicable within the Title X program across the country. Results of the evaluation research phase, forthcoming within the next year, will provide additional information regarding the feasibility and benefits of integrating the SDM into programs.

SOURCES CONSULTED

Arévalo, M., V. Jennings, I. Sinai. 2002. "Efficacy of a new method of family planning: the Standard Days Method." *Contraception* 65:333–338.

Bruce, J. 1990. "Fundamental elements of the quality of care: a simple framework." *Studies in Family Planning* 21:61–91.

Fajans, P., R. Simmons, L. Ghiron. 2006. "Helping public sector health systems innovate: the Strategic Approach to Strengthening Reproductive Health Policies and Programs." *American Journal of Public Health* 96:435-440.

Finer, Lawrence B. S. K. Henshaw. 2006. "Disparities in Rates of Unintended Pregnancy in the United States, 1994 and 2001." *Perspectives on Sexual and Reproductive Health* 38:90-96.

Fowler, C. I., J. Gable, J. Wang, B. Lyda-McDonald. November 2009. *Family Planning Annual Report: 2008 National Summary*. Research Triangle Park, NC: RTI International. www.hhs.gov/opa/familyplanning/tools-docs/fpar_2008_natl_summ.pdf (accessed March 10, 2010).

Gribble, J., R. Lundgren, C. Velasquez, E. Anastasi. 2008. "Being strategic about contraceptive introduction: the experience of the Standard Days Method." *Contraception* 77:147-154.

Henshaw, S. K. 1998. "Unintended pregnancy in the United States." *Family Planning Perspectives* 30:24–29, 46.

Simmons, R., P. Hall, J. Diaz, M. Diaz, P. Fajans, J. Satia. 1997. "The strategic approach to contraceptive introduction." *Studies in Family Planning* 28:79-94.

World Health Organization. 2002. *Selected practice recommendations for contraceptive use*. WHO/RHR/FCH 2nd ed. Geneva: World Health Organization.

World Health Organization Department of Reproductive Health and Research (WHO/RHR) and Johns Hopkins Bloomberg School of Public Health/Center for Communication Programs (CCP), INFO Project. 2007. *Family planning: a global handbook for providers*. Baltimore and Geneva: CCP and WHO.

8

Randomized Comparison of Two Internet-Supported Natural Family Planning Methods (Preliminary Findings)

RICHARD J. FEHRING, PHD, RN, FAAN

Professor, Director, Office of Research and Scholarship, Director, Institute for Natural Family Planning, College of Nursing, Marquette University

MARY SCHNEIDER, MSN, FNP-BC, NFPE

Assistant Director, Institute for Natural Family Planning, College of Nursing, Marquette University

ABSTRACT

The aims of this study were to determine and compare efficacy, satisfaction, ease of use, and motivation in using an internet-based method of Natural Family Planning (NFP) that utilizes either electronic hormonal fertility monitoring (EHFM) or cervical-mucus monitoring (CMM). Four hundred fifty women (mean age 30.1) and their male partners (mean age 31.9) who sought to avoid pregnancy were randomized into either an EHFM (N=228) or CMM NFP group (N=222). Both groups utilized a Web site that provided NFP instructions, an electronic charting system, and support from professional nurses. Participants were assessed for satisfaction, ease of use, and motivation in use of their respective NFP method at 1, 3, and 6 months. Unintended pregnancies were validated by pregnancy evaluations and urine tests. Correct and total pregnancy rates were determined by survival analysis. Correct and total 12 month unintended pregnancy rates for the combined participants (N=450) were 1 and

9 per 100 couple users (Std. Error = .01 and .02) respectively. The EHFM participants (N=228), however, had a typical unintended pregnancy rate of 6 (Std. Error = .03) compared to the CMM group (N=222) pregnancy rate of 13 (Std. Error = .04) per 100 users over 12 months of use. The mean satisfaction/ease of use score for the EHFM group at 6 months of use was 46.1 compared to 42.9 for the CMM group ($p < .07$). Motivation to avoid pregnancy was stronger for the CMM group compared to the EHFM group at 3 and 6 months of use (37.9 and 38.8 versus 33.7 and 33.4, $p < .01$). Although both NFP methods were highly effective methods of family planning delivered through a nurse supported Web site, at this time, the unintended pregnancy rate was lower for the EHFM group and compared well with hormonal contraception. Although acceptability of the EHFM NFP was high, motivation to avoid pregnancy with that group decreased over time.

INTRODUCTION

Studies consistently show that women want safe, effective, easy to use, and convenient methods of family planning (Arévalo1997; Severy 2001). Although Natural Family Planning (NFP) methods are free of side effects, they are often ineffective and complex to learn and use (Grimes et al. 2005). Efforts have occurred over the past 10 years to simplify the teaching and use of NFP methods and increase their efficacy. These efforts include the development of low tech calendar-based methods (Arévalo et al. 2004), simplifying instructions (Frank-Herrmann et al. 2005), and developing accurate biological markers of fertility (Guida et al. 1999).

A new high-tech electronic method to monitor fertility has recently been developed to help women determine their fertile window with ease, convenience, and accuracy (May 2001). This high-tech electronic hormonal fertility monitor (EHFM), called the ClearBlue Easy Fertility Monitor (Swiss Precision Diagnostics), measures urinary metabolites of estrogen and LH and provides the user with a daily indication of "low," "high" and "peak" fertility. A recent cohort study demonstrated that EHFM was effective when used as an aid to avoid pregnancy along with cervical mucus monitoring (CMM) as a second marker of fertility (Fehring et al. 2007) and users reported high satisfaction with the method (Severy et al. 2006). Despite this promising research, there is one task that has not yet been accomplished. There are no randomized comparison studies of EHFM NFP methods with NFP methods that utilize traditional biological markers of fertility (i.e., the Ovulation Method with cervical mucus monitoring and/or the symptom-thermal method with basal body temperature and cervical mucus monitoring combined).

Other recent efforts to increase the ease of use and convenience of NFP methods are the use of internet support for NFP instructions and automated online fertility charting (Fehring 2004; Fehring 2005; Weschler 2005). Although there have been studies to determine the knowledge base of an online hormonal contraceptive program, there have been no studies to determine the efficacy of internet-based instructions for NFP methods used to avoid pregnancy (Kaskowitz et al. 2007). Nor have there been studies to determine the efficacy and satisfaction of using an online fertility charting system for NFP purposes.

A key component in the use of NFP or any type of behavioral focused method of family planning is the motivation of both partners in the use of the method to avoid pregnancy (Sinai et al. 2006). If only one of the partners is committed to the method it will be difficult to use and the efficacy will most likely be lower. In the family planning and, in particular, the NFP community, mutual motivation has been recognized as essential for NFP efficacy (Barnett 1996; Miller, Severy and Pasta 2004; Speitzer 2006). There are, however, no recent studies investigating this aspect of the use of NFP methods.

The method of NFP called the Marquette Model utilizes the ClearBlue Easy Fertility Monitor. Developed at Marquette University's Institute for NFP, this method was further simplified to be taught in a 12-minute office session. Called, the "Marquette Light Method," it makes use of either cervical mucus or an EHFM and a calendar-based formula as a double check for the beginning and end of the fertile phase. Whether the woman user observes cervical mucus or uses the EHFM, she rates her fertility as being low, high, or peak, and utilizes the same fertility calendar-based formula for a double check. This simplified method needed to be evaluated for its efficacy.

Researchers and NFP providers at Marquette University recently developed an online system to teach couples to use NFP. The NFP Web site (http://nfp.marquette.edu) has free information on NFP, downloadable charting systems, access to protocols for special circumstances (e.g., using NFP while breastfeeding), and instructions for achieving and avoiding pregnancy. A unique aspect of the information section of the Web site is a simple one-page feature, "Quick Start Instructions," that can be read in five minutes and allows the user to begin charting and using NFP.

Couples who register on the Web site are able to access an electronic charting system and discussion forums, and they can receive consultation from professional nurse NFP teachers and an obstetrician gynecologist with expertise in the use of NFP. The online charting system also notifies the user of possible health problems, including unusual bleeding, infertility, and cycle dynamics that are out of the norm. The Marquette online NFP system is presented in both the English and Spanish languages. Neither system has been studied for its efficacy and ease of use, however. The efficacy of these systems will only be as good as the NFP method that they provide.

AIMS OF STUDY

The specific aims of this study are as follows:

1. To determine and compare the efficacy in the use of two internet-supported methods of NFP (i.e., EHFM and CMM) in aiding couples to avoid pregnancy.
2. To determine and compare the satisfaction and ease of use in the use of two internet-supported methods of NFP (i.e., EHFM and CMM) in aiding couples to avoid pregnancy.
3. To determine and compare the mutual motivation in the use of two internet-supported methods of NFP (i.e., EHFM and CMM) in aiding couples to avoid pregnancy.

METHODS

Research Design

This is a 12-month (13 cycles) prospective randomized clinical efficacy study. A minimum of 600 couples seeking to avoid pregnancy with a method of NFP and who have no known infertility problems are being sought through an online NFP web site and randomized into either a EHFM group (N=300) or a CMM only group (N=300). Any pregnancies that occur among the participants over a 12-month period are recorded and evaluated as to whether they were intended, not intended user failure, not intended system failure, or unknown.

All couple participants (men and women) are assessed as to their perceived "satisfaction" and "ease of use" with an online measurement tool at 1, 3, and 6 months of use. Mutual motivation for avoiding pregnancy is assessed before each menstrual cycle.

Sample

In order to reach a significant level of analysis for a comparison of pregnancy rates between two groups, i.e., EHFM and CMM group, a minimum of 600 women/couple participants are being sought for completion of the study. In order to achieve 80% power to detect a 10% difference in pregnancy rates between each group there needs to be a minimum of 300 couples per group. This power analysis is based on a total unintended pregnancy rate of 10% for the EHFM group and a 20% pregnancy rate for the CMM group. These rates were projected from a retrospective study that compared the CMM only method with an EHFM method (Fehring et al. 2009).

Couples who seek the Marquette online NFP services and meet the criteria for the study have the opportunity to participate in the study. All couples receive a free EHFM but those in the CMM group receive the monitor only after completing 12 months of CMM. All couples receive $10 for each menstrual cycle chart completed.

The inclusion criteria for the female participant are as follows: must be between the age of 18 and 42; have a menstrual cycle range of 21-42 days; have not used depo medroxyprogesterone acetate (DMPA) over the past 6 months; have no history of oral, patch or sub-dermal hormonal contraceptives for the past 3 months; if post breast-feeding, have experienced at least 3 cycles past weaning; have no known fertility problems; not be using medications that interfere with ovulatory function; not smoke cigarettes; and not be pregnant. The male partners of the participants are to have no known fertility problem and be between the ages of 18 and 50.

Measures

MEASUREMENT OF THE FERTILE PERIOD BY THE CLEARBLUE FERTILITY MONITOR (CBFM)

The CBFM is designed to detect the rising level of urinary estrone-3-gluconuride (E3G) and the surge in urinary LH. The CBFM is based on urinary hormonal immunoassay techniques. Product testing has shown the Clearblue monitor to be 98.8% accurate in detecting the LH surge (Unipath Diagnostics 2001). The CBFM detected the LH surge in 169 of 171 cycles from 88 women, in agreement with a quantitative radioimmunoassay for LH. Detection of urinary metabolites of urinary estradiol (E3G) has been recognized by the World Health Organization (WHO) as a reliable marker for the beginning of the fertile phase of the menstrual cycle. In a study with 90 women who used the CBFM for 1-4 cycles, in 352 cycles with an LH surge, the first day of High Fertility (i.e., the day of the first rise in E3G) was 3.01 ± 2.33 days before the LH surge (Behre et al. 2000).

The CBFM is initiated when the user pushes a button on the monitor labeled "M" on the first day of her period. The monitor then indicates which day of the cycle the user is on. The monitor requests either 10 or 20 daily urine tests per cycle. When the monitor requests a test, the user places the test strip under her urine stream for 3 seconds. The test strip is then placed in the monitor and read. The monitor will show a fertility status of "low," "high" or "peak." The user will be asked to record on the electronic NFP fertility chart her fertility status (low, high or peak) and any intercourse that occurred on a daily basis.

MEASUREMENT OF THE FERTILE PERIOD BY CERVICAL MUCUS MONITORING (CMM)

For this study, cervical mucus is self-observed and classified at three levels—low, high, and peak. Observations are based on sensations and appearance of cervical mucus. When no mucus is observed or felt, or mucus that is slightly moist and sticky, minimal, thick, white, and holds its shape, will be classified as "low" fertile mucus. Mucus that feels wetter, increases in amount, becomes thinner, cloudy and slightly stretchy will be classified as "high" fertility mucus (this mucus can be considered transitional). Any mucus that feels slippery, is abundant, thin, clear, and stretchy (like egg white) will be classified as "peak" type mucus. The peak day is the last day of peak type mucus.

Women who are in the CMM group are asked to observe for cervical mucus on a daily basis and to chart the highest level observed. They are instructed to feel for the sensation of cervical mucus (at the vulva) throughout the day and especially when voiding and before going to bed. They are also asked to observe any mucus at eye level by lifting it off a tissue and testing it between their fingers. Written, oral, and visual descriptions (pictures) of the three levels of cervical mucus were provided to the CMM users. These are standard procedures utilized in CMM NFP methods and utilized in the WHO multi-site, multi-country study of the OM (WHO 1981).

MEASUREMENT OF SATISFACTION AND EASE OF USE

Participants are asked to respond to a 10-item questionnaire on whether the online Web site was acceptable, easy to use, non-invasive, and a convenient in-home test of fertility, and whether it provides clear and objective results. The 10-item survey is a shortened form of an acceptability/ease of use questionnaire developed by Severy for evaluating an EHFM (Severy 2001). The 10 items are ranked on a scale from 1 to 7, with bipolar negative and positive adjectives. This is the same tool that was used in the prospective efficacy study of the EHFM plus CMM (Fehring et al. 2007).

MEASUREMENT OF MOTIVATION

Motivation is measured by the same system developed for the 2002 (cycle 6) *National Survey for Family Growth* (Peterson and Mosher 1999). There are two questions asked of participants (the woman and man): (1) how hard they are currently trying to not get pregnant on a scale of 0–10 (with 0 means trying hard to get pregnant and 10 means trying hard to not get pregnant); and (2) how much they want to avoid pregnancy at this time (with 0 means wanting to get pregnant and 10 means wanting to avoid pregnancy).

MARQUETTE ONLINE CHARTING SYSTEM

The Marquette University NFP online electronic charting system has designated sections for recording the results of CMM and the EHFM—as either L – low, H = high, or P = peak. The charting system provides a pop-up window for the user that illustrates the 3 levels of cervical mucus and the 3 levels provided by the fertility monitor. The charting system also has a place to record menses on a scale of 1-3 with 1 = light; 2= moderate; and 3=heavy menstrual flow and a row for recording acts of intercourse (= I). The top of the chart has room for recording intention of use (to achieve or avoid pregnancy) for each cycle. The charting automatically indicates (in light blue) the fertile phase (based on the Marquette algorithm) as the user charts. There is no guessing as to whether the day is either fertile or not.

CLASSIFICATION OF PREGNANCY

The electronic charting system automatically notifies the user of the possibility of a pregnancy when the luteal phase goes beyond 19 days. The charting system then prompts the user to take a pregnancy test and complete an online pregnancy evaluation. The online charting system also cues the woman user to a link that launches a pregnancy evaluation form on each menstrual cycle that is charted.

Two professional nurse NFP teachers evaluate all pregnancies that occur among the participants. The NFP teachers review the charting system for the days of fertility, the days of recorded intercourse, and the information on the pregnancy evaluation form. Each couple that achieves a pregnancy is asked to confirm the pregnancy with a pregnancy test kit (i.e., the ClearBlue Easy One Minute Pregnancy Test). Each pregnancy is classified (with agreement of the couple) by two professional nurse NFP teachers according to the following classification as recommended by Lamprecht and Trussell (1997): (1) pregnancies are classified as intentional only when a couple reports prior to the pregnancy cycle an intention to use the method to become pregnant; (2) all unintentional pregnancies are used in the analysis of pregnancy risk during typical use; and (3) all unintentional pregnancies occurring during cycles in which NFP rules were followed are used in the analysis of pregnancy risk during correct use.

DEMOGRAPHIC INFORMATION

Each couple (male and female participant) who enters the study completes a 21-item demographic registration form developed by Gray and Kambic (1984). The registration form asks demographic information (e.g., ethnicity, religious status), number of children, cycle history, family planning history, and intention for using NFP. The registration form automatically pops up on the NFP Web site when the couple registers.

Analysis of Evidence

All statistical analysis was carried out using significance level alpha = 0.05. In order to determine the effectiveness of the EHFM plus a fertility algorithm in aiding couples to avoid pregnancy and the CMM plus a fertility algorithm in avoiding pregnancy, cumulative pregnancy rates were calculated by (Life Table) survival analysis utilizing a 95%

confidence interval and were calculated at 3, 6, 9, and 12 months/13 cycles of use. Differences between the EHFM and the CMM group mean scores of the satisfaction/ease of use, and motivation was analyzed using independent student T-tests.

PRELIMINARY RESULTS

Although it is still rather early to start to analyze the data to meet the three aims of this study, the following are some early results.

Demographics

Table One shows a comparison of the demographics between the female participants in the monitor and mucus groups. As can been seen in the table, the mean age, number of years married, number of living children, weight, height, and age of husband/partner are similar and there are no statistical differences. In both groups the greatest percentage of participants are White and Catholic.

Table One:
Comparison of Demographics between the Monitor and Mucus group*

	Monitor group (N=228)	Mucus Group (N=222)
Mean age female	29.9 (SD=5.4)	30.3 (SD=5.3)
Mean age male	31.8 (SD=6.1)	32.1 (SD=6.1)
Mean Years Married	6.0 (SD=4.9)	6.3 (SD=5.1)
Mean # Living Children	2.1 (SD=2.0)	2.1 (SD=1.8)
Mean Weight Female	150.2 (SD=32.6)	153.6 (SD=34.7)
Mean Height Female	65.2 (SD=2.7)	65.2 (SD=2.5)
% Ethnicity Female	77% White/23% Other	84% White/20% Other
% Religion Female	81% Cath./14%Prot.	78% Cath./17%Prot.

* *There were no significant differences between the two study groups on demographic variables.*

Aim One: To determine and compare the efficacy in the use of two internet-supported methods of NFP (i.e., electronic hormonal fertility monitoring (EHFM) and traditional cervical mucus monitoring (CMM)) in aiding couples to avoid pregnancy.

Table Two:
<u>Correct Use Gross and Net Pregnancy Rates</u>: i.e., survival rates by groups per 100 women over 12 cycles of use.

<u>Gross Correct Use Pregnancy Survival Rate</u>

	Monitor (N = 227)			*Mucus (N = 219)*		
Months	reg.	Estimate	Std. Error	Preg.	Estimate	Std. Error
3	1	.989	.001	1	.988	.012
6	0	.989	.001	0	.988	.012
9	0	.989	.001	0	.988	.012
12	0	.989	.001	0	.988	.012

<u>Net Correct Use Pregnancy Survival Rate</u>

	Monitor (N = 227)			*Mucus (N = 219)*		
Months	Preg.	Estimate	Std. Error	Preg.	Estimate	Std. Error
3	0	1.00	.000	1	.988	.012
6	0	1.00	.000	0	.988	.012
9	0	1.00	.000	0	.988	.012
12	0	1.00	.000	0	.988	.012

Tables Two and Three show correct and typical use gross and net unintended pregnancy rates of the two study groups, i.e., the EHFM (monitor) and CMM (mucus) groups. The rates are based upon 1,544 cycle of use. The *gross pregnancy rate* includes all pregnancies whether it was intended or not intended. The *net pregnancy rate* is based on pregnancies that occurred when couples indicated that they intended <u>not</u> to achieve a pregnancy.

As shown in Table Two, the gross pregnancy rate per 100 women over 12 months of use in both the monitor and mucus groups is 1; however, as shown in Table Two, the net correct use unintended pregnancy rate for the monitor group is just slightly lower than the mucus group, i.e., 0 for the monitor group and 1 for the mucus group.

Table Three shows that the gross typical use pregnancy rates for the monitor group (i.e., .25) is lower for the monitor group i.e., 25 versus 16 pregnancies per 100 women over 12 months of use; however, Table Three shows there is a remarkable shift in difference in net unintended pregnancy rates between the two groups, with the monitor group

Table Three:
Typical Use Gross and Net Pregnancy Rates: i.e., survival rates by groups per 100 women over 12 cycles of use.

Gross Correct Use Pregnancy Survival Rate

	Monitor (N = 227)			*Mucus (N = 219)*		
Months	reg.	Estimate	Std. Error	Preg.	Estimate	Std. Error
3	6	.9439	.021	5	.952	.026
6	4	.900	.029	3	.899	.036
9	6	.812	.043	0	.899	.036
12	3	.752	.052	2	.839	.053

Net Correct Use Pregnancy Survival Rate

	Monitor (N = 227)			*Mucus (N = 219)*		
Months	Preg.	Estimate	Std. Error	Preg.	Estimate	Std. Error
3	4	.968	.016	1	.955	.021
6	0	.968	.016	3	.902	.036
9	2	.939	.025	0	.902	.036
12	0	.939	.025	1	.873	.045

having an unintended pregnancy rate of 6 and the mucus group 13 per 100 women over 12 months of use.

Aim Two: To determine and compare the satisfaction/ease of use in the use of two internet-supported methods of NFP (i.e., EHFM and CMM) in aiding couples to avoid pregnancy.

Ease of use and Satisfaction was measured with a 9 item questionnaire that ranked each item from 1 – 7 with 7 having better Ease of use/Satisfaction. The range of total scores is 9-63.

Table Four [next page] shows that the mean "ease of use/satisfaction" scores increase from 1 to 3 months of use in both groups. The differences in the mean scores at 6 months of use almost reach statistical significance, with the monitor group having higher scores. That said, there is not enough statistical power at this time with the study.

Aim Three: To determine and compare the mutual motivation in the use of two internet-supported methods of NFP (i.e., EHFM and CMM) in aiding couples to avoid pregnancy

Table Four:
Ease of Use/Satisfaction Mean Scores at 1, 3, and 6 months of use between Monitor and Mucus Groups

	Monitor		Mucus			
Months	N	*Mean/SD*	N	*Mean/SD.*	*t*	*Sig.*
1	135	42.0/8.6	111	40.2/ 9.6	1.57	.12
3	96	43.6/9.5	66	41.3/11.0	1.42	.16
6	66	46.1/7.2	45	42.9/11.1	1.82	.07

As shown in Table Five, mutual motivation to avoid pregnancy decreases over time for the monitor group and slightly increases for the mucus group. At three and six months of use the mucus group has statistically higher mean motivation scores.

Table Five:
Mean Motivation scores to avoid pregnancy at 1, 3, and 6 months between Monitor and Mucus Groups (female and male motivation scores combined)

		Monitor		Mucus		
Months	N	*Mean/SD*	N	*Mean/SD.*	*t*	*Sig.*
1	136	36.6/7.9	126	37.5/6.5	1.03	.31
3	101	33.7/11.9	72	37.9/4.3	2.83	.01
6	72	33.4/13.1	49	38.8/2.6	2.87	.01

DISCUSSION

Efficacy of Methods

The correct use efficacy of both the monitor and mucus group is very good, i.e., 98-100% survival rate (or a 0 – 2 unintended pregnancy rate per 100 women over 12 months of use) and compares with what is found in the literature (Trussell 2004). As predicted (hypothesized), the monitor group has a better typical use (NET) unintended pregnancy rate than the mucus group, i.e., 94% survival among the monitor group versus 87% among the mucus group. There is not, however, enough power yet to conduct a non-parametric comparison statistic. The differences in pregnancy rates between the monitor and mucus group is similar to the differences that were found in a previous cohort comparison study of the monitor plus mucus versus mucus alone as two methods of NFP (Fehring et al. 2009). The low unintended pregnancy rate (both correct and typical) are comparable to the pregnancy rates that were determined in a large European study that used mucus plus basal body temperature as a double check for the beginning and end of the fertile phase of the menstrual cycle (Frank-Herrmann et al. 2007).

Satisfaction/Ease of Use

There seems to be greater satisfaction and ease of use among the monitor group, especially as participants progress through the study. At 6 months of use, the mean difference between the groups almost reaches significance; however, there is not enough statistical power at this time to determine differences, especially because of the low response rates. The greater satisfaction might be a result of the mucus group participants dropping out (i.e., the least satisfied) and not entirely due to the use of the monitor. The increase in satisfaction over time (for couples avoiding pregnancy) is not unusual for those learning and using NFP methods. Fehring and Werner (1994) found similar results (i.e., increased satisfaction over time) with a cervical mucus only method.

Motivation

Of interest, is that the participants in the mucus group have greater motivation (at 3 and 6 months of use) to avoid pregnancy than the monitor group. This is likely due to the number of participants who enter the study intending to receive a free fertility monitor who are assigned to the monitor group, and then use the monitor to achieve a pregnancy, i.e., they intended all along to achieve a pregnancy. The participants in the mucus group have more at stake in avoiding a pregnancy and have to work hard to receive a free monitor at the end of the study. This is the first study that has prospectively measured mutual motivation in the use of NFP methods. In a previous study on the use of an electronic hormonal fertility monitor to achieve pregnancy some of the participants had a tendency to use the monitor to avoid pregnancy (Janssen and Lunsen 2000).

Practice Implications

Although this study is not completed (and will not be completed for over a year) three tentative practice implications can be identified. First, the online provision of NFP methods for both the simplified mucus method and the use of the hormonal fertility monitor are effective and efficient. Overall there is a 99% method efficacy and 95% typical efficacy with the combined results of both methods. Second, many women and couples throughout the U.S. can be reached and taught how to use NFP through the Internet and Internet-based online charting. Third, health professionals can efficiently provide health consultation and information on women's health problems, menstrual cycle questions, and related health topics through the Internet and Web- based forums. Such an online program would be one way that Title X clinics could provide NFP and women's health services.

Policy Implications

The implication the findings have on policy (so far) is that Title X Family Planning clinics (and similar type clinics) could offer NFP services through the Internet in an efficient and effective manner by use of a NFP service and support program similar to that being studied with this federal grant. In fact, the NFP services could be offered in each of the Title X regions by having a NFP Web site Internet-based NFP service and support program. These sites could be managed by 2-3 professional nurses who are familiar with NFP. The other Title X clinics in each region could be linked into the sites or the clinics could help participate in the NFP services and support by enrolling women/couples and helping to follow those couples online. A similar model could be developed for diocesan NFP programs, i.e., each diocese could have its own Internet NFP service or support system or be linked to such service sites in larger diocesan or archdiocesan programs.

Research Implications

We are just beginning to consider research implications from the preliminary findings of our study. Some speculative implications are as follows: (1) the use of an online system to enroll, randomize, survey, and maintain participants is possible and an efficient way to conduct efficacy research for NFP methods; (2) future online efficacy studies of NFP methods should consider enrolling only participants who are new to NFP—the current users of other methods of NFP have a tendency to compare their previous methods and to use them instead of the study method; (3) we would not recommend allowing participants to do retrospective charting and to make that expectation clear in the beginning of the study; (4) we would recommend use of an online system to compare other standardized methods of NFP (such as the Standard Days Method or the Two Day Method); and (5) we would recommend use of a similar online fertility awareness and educational system to determine if use of hormonal fertility charting enhances the ability to achieve pregnancy among sub-fertile women. We already have developed a proposal for such a study, i.e., to compare electronic hormonal fertility monitoring versus random acts of intercourse in helping women with sub-fertility achieve pregnancy. This proposal has been submitted to the National Institute of Nursing Research.

One problem with online systems of NFP and research is the ability to reach women/couples who do not have online access and are unable to afford such services. One way to help this might be to have online computer services available at convenient sites, like public libraries or health clinics. Another approach would be to have online charting available through cell phones and other hand held devices. We are now investigating developing such a system that could be linked to our NFP Web site.

Conclusion

Our preliminary conclusion is that the use of an online Web-based fertility education, charting, and support system to teach a method of NFP is very effective. The overall unintended pregnancy rates of the combined methods are very low. Preliminary results indicate that the use of the EHFM in an online charting system is a more effective method of NFP (when used to avoid pregnancy) than the use of CMM. There is a trend for greater satisfaction/ease of use for participants who use the EHFM for tracking fertility and for use in family planning. Motivation to avoid, however, was stronger among those using CMM to avoid pregnancy.

ACKNOWLEDGEMENT

The authors would like to recognize the invaluable medical consultation advice that Kathleen Raviele, MD, has provided and continues to provide for this federal study comparing two online-methods of NFP. In addition, commendation is given to graduate student research assistants, Teresa Roumonada and Dana Rodriguez, who have aided and continue to aid the authors in developing the data sets for this study and for helping to maintain the distribution of fertility monitors and gift cards to the many participants.

SOURCES CONSULTED

Arévalo, M. 1997. "Expanding the availability and improving delivery of natural family planning services and fertility awareness education: providers' perspectives." *Advances in Contraception* 13:275-281.

Arévalo, M., V. Jennings, M. Nikula, I. Sinai. 2004. "Efficacy of the new TwoDay Method of family planning." *Fertility and Sterility* 82:885-892.

Barnett, B. 1996. "NFP offers user-control, but requires discipline." *Contraceptive Update Network* 17:17-20.

Fehring, R. 2004. "The future of professional education in natural family planning." *Journal of Obstetrics Gynecological and Neonatal Nursing* 33:34-43.

________. 2005. "New low and high tech calendar methods of family planning." *Journal of Nurse Midwifery and Women's Health* 50:31-37.

Fehring, R., C. Werner. 1993. "Natural family planning and Catholic hospitals: A national survey." *Linacre Quarterly* 60:29-34.

Fehring, R. J., M. Schneider, K. Raviele, M. I. Barron. 2007. "Efficacy of cervical mucus observations plus electronic hormonal fertility monitoring as a method of natural family planning." *Journal of Obstetric Gynecologic and Neonatal Nursing* 36:152-60.

________. 2009. "Cohort comparison of two fertility awareness methods of family planning." *Journal of Reproductive Medicine* 54:165-170.

Frank-Herrmann, P., C. Gnoth, S. Baure, T. Strowitski, G. Freundl. 2005. "Determination of the fertile window: reproductive competence of women: European cycle databases." *Gynecology and Endocrinology* 20:305-312.

Frank-Herrmann, P., J. Heil, C. Gnoth, E. Toledo, S. Baur, C. Pyper, E. Jenetzky, T. Strowitzki, G. Fruendl. 2007. "The effectiveness of a fertility awareness based method to avoid pregnancy in relation to a couple's sexual behavior during the fertile time: a prospective longitudinal study." *Human Reproduction* 22:1310-1319.

Grimes, D. A., M. F. Gallo, V. Grigorieva, K. Nanda, K. F. Schulz. 2005. "Fertility awareness-based methods for contraception: systematic review of randomized controlled trials." *Contraception* 72:85-90.

Gray, R. H., R. Kambic. 1984. "Program evaluation and accountability." In Lanctot, C. Ed. *Natural Family Planning. Development of National Programs.* Washington, DC: International Federation for Family Life Promotion.

Guida, M., G. A.Tommaselli, S. Palomba, M. Pellicano, G. Moccia, C. DiCarlo, C. Nappi. 1999. "Efficacy of methods for determining ovulation in a natural family planning program." *Fertility and Sterility* 72:900-904.

Janssen, C. J. M., R. H. W. van Lunsen. 2000. "Profile and opinions of the female Persona user in The Netherlands." *The European Journal of Contraception and Reproductive Health Care* 5:141-146.

Kaskowitz, A. P., N. Carlson, M. Nichols, A. Edelman, J. Jensen. 2007. "Online availability of hormonal contraceptives without a health care examination: effect of knowledge and health care screening." *Contraception* 76:273-277.

Lamprecht, V., J. Trussell. 1997. "Effectiveness studies on natural methods of natural family planning." *Advances in Contraception* 13:155-165.

May, K. 2001. "Home monitoring with the ClearPlan Easy Fertility Monitor for fertility awareness." *The Journal of International Medical Research* 29 (Suppl 1):14A-20A.

Miller, W. B., L. J. Severy, D. J. Pasta. 2004. "A framework for modeling fertility motivation in couples." *Population Studies* 58:193-205.

Peterson, L. S., W. D. Mosher. 1999. "Options for measuring unintended pregnancy in cycle 6 of the National Survey of Family Growth." *Family Planning Perspectives* 31:252-253.

Severy, L. J., J. Robison, C. Findley-Klein, J. McNulty. 2006. "Acceptability of a home monitor used to aid in conception: Psychological factors and couple dynamics." *Contraception* 73:65–71.

Sinai, I., R. Lundgren, M. Arévalo, V. Jennings. 2006. "Fertility awareness-based methods of family planning: predictors of correct use." *International Family Planning Perspectives* 32:94-100.

Speizer, I. 2006. "Using strength of fertility motivation to identify family planning program strategies." *International Family Planning Perspectives* 32:185-191.

Trussell, J. 2004. "Contraceptive failure in the United States." *Contraception* 70:89-96.

UniPath Diagnostics. 2001. *Professional Information: ClearPlan Easy Fertilty Monitor.* Princeton, New Jersey: UniPath, P. C.

Weschler, T. 2005. *Taking Charge of Your Fertility.* New York, NY: Harper Collins.

World Health Organization. 1981. "A prospective multicentre trial of the ovulation method of natural family planning. II. The effectiveness phase." *Fertility and Sterility* 36:591-598.

9

Title X Client & Provider Perspectives on Natural Family Planning

Preliminary Findings

PAUL G. WHITTAKER, PHD

Associate Director of Research, Family Planning Council, Inc., Philadelphia, Adjunct Scholar, Epidemiology, University of Pennsylvania Medical School

LINDA HOCK-LONG, PHD

Director of Research, Family Planning Council

REBECCA MERKH, MS

Research Project Manager, Family Planning Council

ABSTRACT

The extent to which Title X family planning clients use, and family planning counselors and clinicians (providers) support, Natural Family Planning (NFP) strategies (here, defined as including withdrawal, Rhythm, and calendar-based methods) and fertility awareness based methods (FABM) is relatively unknown. Our mixed methods study is exploring the attitudes, beliefs, and usage/service delivery experiences of Title X clients, providers, NFP, and FABM users with regard to these methods. Provider focus groups suggest that family planning providers have mixed feelings concerning the promotion of NFP and FABM. Although they recognize that NFP and FABM methods may appeal to individuals not wishing to use hormonal contraceptives, they question whether clients possess the requisite reproductive health knowledge and skills needed to support the effective use of NFP and FABM. Providers indicate that current materials and clinic time to support client education were limited. An ongoing provider survey is collecting further data on these issues. Preliminary analysis of our survey of female Title X clients (ages 18-35) indicate that 25 (9%) of 268 clients have ever relied primarily on Rhythm/calendar or FABM methods for pregnancy prevention for more than three months. Participants generally have a low level of knowledge of their fertility, reproductive health, and specific FABM options. Future in-depth interviews are planned with women who are experienced NFP or FABM users to help to illustrate barriers/facilitators to method use and the influence of contextual factors (e.g., pregnancy intentions, partners, etc.) on use. Further analysis of provider and client survey data and a final set of provider focus groups will help identify potential strategies for integrating NFP and FABM options into current contraceptive counseling services at Title X clinics.

INTRODUCTION

Information on the extent to which women in the United States rely on natural methods of contraception such as Natural Family Planning strategies (NFP) and fertility awareness based methods (FABM) is limited. For the purposes of this study, NFP includes withdrawal, Rhythm and calendar-based methods. FABM includes methods based on basal body temperature, cervical mucus or fertility monitoring technology (please note that this is contrary to the common definition of NFP which typically includes the cervical mucus based methods, basal body temperature readings, hormonal fertility indicators and the cross check approach of the Sympto-Thermal methods).

According to the 2006 Title X Family Planning Annual Report issued by the Office of Population Affairs, less than one percent of Title X clients nationwide use fertility awareness based methods (Fowler et al. 2008). Findings from a recent Kaiser Family Foundation (2003) survey involving a national sample of adolescents and young adults suggest that reliance on NFP may be somewhat higher, as approximately one-third of the female respondents reported using withdrawal 'sometimes' or 'regularly.' A Family Planning Council (FPC) study (Whittaker et al. 2010) gives further context to the Kaiser Foundation findings and suggests that contraceptive method rates based solely on FABM may underestimate use of natural methods and potential interest in FABM options.

Many women prefer to use natural birth control methods instead of barrier or hormonal contraceptives due to such factors as religious beliefs, medical contraindications, access issues, and/or dissatisfaction with barrier and hormonal methods (Sinai et al. 2006; Stanford et al. 1998). Research suggests that NFP and FABM offer pregnancy prevention rates comparable to or better than those associated with barrier contraceptive methods. For example, according to the 2002 National Survey of Family Growth, the probability of pregnancy within the first 12 months of typical withdrawal use was 18% (Kost et al. 2008); estimates of FABM failure rates range from 2-5% for perfect use and 13-25% for typical use (Dicker et al. 1989; Jennings et al. 2004; Kambic et al. 1996). The failure rate for male condoms is estimated to be 17% (Hatcher et al. 2007).

Studies have shown that family planning providers have low levels of recommending NFP and FABM because they overestimate complexity of use and failure rates for natural methods (Gribble et al. 2008). Another provider concern is that increased availability of FABM will lead to client discontinuation of other contraceptive methods perceived to be more effective. While many national and institutional family planning policies explicitly include FABM among the method options that should be made available to clients, the full implementation of these policies is rare, due in part to provider concerns (Gribble et al. 2008).

To address critical gaps in our understanding of the determinants of NFP and FABM uptake and successful use, the Family Planning Council (FPC) of Philadelphia is conducting a mixed methods study that includes the following four aims:

1. Assess female Title X family planning clients' knowledge, attitudes, and beliefs regarding NFP and FABM and their experiences using these methods for the purpose of pregnancy prevention.

2. Explore the experiences of women who use NFP and FABM for pregnancy prevention, their attitudes and beliefs regarding these methods, and the factors that impede and/or facilitate method use.

3. Assess Title X family planning provider knowledge, attitudes, and beliefs regarding NFP and FABM options, the delivery of NFP and

FABM-related services, and the factors that impede and/or facilitate service delivery.

4. Identify potential strategies to reduce barriers to client use of NFP and FABM and the delivery of NFP and FABM-related family planning services.

METHODS

An integrated set of qualitative and quantitative data collection methods will be used in this study. Qualitative data will be obtained via provider focus groups and interviews with NFP and FABM users. We will also conduct free listing to augment discussions, which has been described as a 'bridge' technique because it uses open-ended questions to generate qualitative data, which are then analyzed quantitatively. Quantitative data will be obtained via a client Audio Computer Assisted Self-Interview (ACASI) survey and a provider survey. The Family Planning Council's IRB gave approval for the study protocol. Further IRB approval was obtained for the ACASI surveys from those participating institutions that required it.

Participants

As the Title X grantee for the Southeastern PA region (Philadelphia and the four surrounding counties), the FPC oversees a comprehensive range of family planning and reproductive health services provided through a network of 26 delegate agencies administering 75 clinical sites. Family planning clinicians and counselors (providers) across the FPC Title X network were invited to participate in focus groups at the FPC main offices in center city Philadelphia. Two focus groups were conducted at the beginning of the study and two more will take place when all other data collection has been completed. Providers were screened for eligibility when recruited and informed consent obtained at the beginning of each focus groups session. To compensate them for their time, focus group participants were given a $30 Visa gift card. We plan to have 225 providers complete the provider survey. To ensure diversity, we will aim to enroll approximately three providers from each of 75 clinics in the FPC Title X network. Providers will be given the option of completing either a web-based or paper version of the survey instrument. Instructions on how to access the web-based version of the survey were e-mailed to clinic representatives and paper copies of the provider survey instrument will be mailed to each clinic. To be eligible to participate in the study, family planning providers must: a) provide contraceptive services directly to clients, and b) have been employed by their respective agency for three or more months.

Family planning clients currently receiving services at a Title X family planning clinic in the FPC Title X network are invited to complete the ACASI survey. Approximately 400 women will be recruited to participate in this method. We will recruit clients from six clinics, administering a maximum of 70 surveys at any given clinic. A sampling strategy was selected to ensure that recruitment sites reflect the diversity of organizations (e.g., hospitals, community based clinics, Planned Parenthood affiliates) in the FPC Title X network. Study enrollment is limited to females who are 18-35 years of age, are English speaking, and are established Title X clients. In addition to flyers being posted in participating Title X clinics, research assistants (RA) approach potential participants in clinic waiting rooms. The RA provides information about the study and screens for eligibility if clients are interested in participating. Women who are eligible and agree to complete the client ACASI survey do so in a private area of the clinic after providing informed consent. To compensate them for their time, ACASI survey participants receive a $15 gift card. In the near future, qualitative interviews will be conducted with women who have used NFP or FABM for purposes of pregnancy prevention for at least three consecutive months in the past two years. We will recruit these participants from Title X clinics and via adverts and flyers throughout the FPC Title X catchment area. The interviews are estimated to last up to two hours and participants will receive a $50 Visa gift card as compensation for their time.

Procedures

PROVIDER FOCUS GROUPS

The first set of provider focus groups have been completed and are reported in this paper. They explored family planning provider knowledge, attitudes, beliefs and practices related to NFP and FABM. Focus groups also included free list exercises. A focus group facilitator (with a clinical background) followed a standard discussion guide that contained topic specific questions and probes. Information in the following areas was collected: awareness and knowledge of NFP and FABM options; advantages and disadvantages of NFP and FABM; perceptions of what others think about NFP and FABM (e.g., clients, colleagues); and factors that impede or facilitate delivery of NFP and FABM-related services. The initial focus group sessions lasted about 90 minutes. To ensure that we had a complete and accurate accounting of the focus group sessions, discussions were audio recorded.

Two additional provider focus groups will be conducted at the conclusion of the data collection period. The primary aim of these groups will be to identify potential strategies for Title X clinics to reduce client and provider-level barriers to traditional NFP and FABM uptake and successful use. To facilitate this process, we will share our prior research findings from providers, clients and NFP/FABM users at the beginning of the focus group sessions.

PROVIDER SURVEY

This activity is currently ongoing. Participants have the option of completing a web-based or paper version of the provider survey instrument. The survey includes the following domains: socio-demographics; NFP and FABM knowledge, attitudes, beliefs and practice experiences; perceived level of client experience with NFP and FABM; and perceived level of client interest in and eligibility for FABM.

CLIENT ACASI SURVEY

This activity is currently ongoing and collects information from female Title X clients in the following domains: socio-demographics (e.g., age, race, education, employment status, influence of religious beliefs on contraception use); current relationship status; fertility history; perceived pregnancy risk; pregnancy intentions; contraceptive history; fertility knowledge; NFP and FABM awareness, knowledge, attitudes, beliefs and usage experiences; and provider interactions specific to NFP and FABM use.

The survey is administered via ACASI, a software application that integrates audio and text files. The files are installed on a laptop computer, thus allowing a participant to read survey text on screen and/or listen to digitally recorded questions and corresponding response options via earphones. Purported benefits of ACASI over self-administered paper and pencil instruments and face-to-face interviews include: standardized delivery of questions; facilitated skip patterns;

increased likelihood of accurate responses to sensitive questions; decreased likelihood of socially desirable responses; and increased privacy and confidentiality. In light of the aural and graphic options ACASI provides, it is well-suited for individuals with low literacy and/or limited computer skills.

The research assistant (RA) orients participants to the computer, explains that they can listen to the questions using earphones and/or view them on the computer screen, and stresses the importance of completing all questions and providing accurate responses. At the same time, she explains that participants can choose to skip any question they do not wish to answer. An external mouse is used to select yes/no and multiple choice/Likert scale responses and the keyboard is used to enter textual responses, (e.g., age, zip code, explanations when the 'other' category is selected). The RA ensures that the computer is positioned such that no one other than the participant can view the screen during survey administration and remains within hearing distance should the participant need assistance as she completes the survey. The survey takes a maximum of 45 minutes to complete.

INTERVIEWS WITH NFP/FABM USERS

Qualitative interviews will be conducted with women who have a history of using NFP or FABM for pregnancy prevention. Interviews will be used to explore key behavioral, normative, and control beliefs related to NFP and FABM, as well as individual-, social-, and environmental-level influences on usage experiences. Domains will include: childbearing desires/pregnancy intentions; contraceptive beliefs, attitudes and history; individual, social, and environmental factors influencing NFP and FABM uptake and use; perceived advantages/disadvantages and barriers/facilitators of NFP and FABM use; and perceived efficacy in using NFP and FABM. To ensure the interviews approximate a natural conversation, participants will be encouraged to share their experiences in their own words. The interviews will be audio recorded.

DATA ANALYSIS

Screening, demographic and survey data are analyzed using SPSS 16.0. For the client ACASI surveys, individual responses are saved to a data file and uploaded to the ACASI data base. The survey data is then imported into SPSS. For the provider survey, frequency distributions can be generated directly from the web-based survey software. Completed provider surveys on paper will be entered manually into a database and merged with the web-based responses.

Notes on the proceedings of the focus groups were written up and were cross-checked with the audio recordings. The interviews will be transcribed verbatim, coded using Atlas.ti software and summarized. The team meets regularly to discuss themes and patterns emerging from the data and, after all relevant data have been reviewed, reaches consensus regarding key themes and findings.

RESULTS

Initial Provider Focus Groups

Two focus groups were held, one with 5 participants and another with 4 participants. Eight participants worked at a hospital-based family planning clinic and one worked at a federally qualified health center. Five participants were counselors/health educators, two were clinicians, one was an administrator, and one played both clinical and administrative roles. Four had been working in the family planning field for more than 20 years, one for 15 years, one for 8 years, and three for three or fewer years. Six participants self-identified as Caucasian and three as African-American. Participant age ranged from 28 to 59 years, with a mean of 43.

It was perceived as common for clients to report misinformation or myths about hormonal contraceptives. Providers indicated that some clients don't want to use hormonal contraception because of side effects and difficulty with adherence to regimens, other clients believe they can't get pregnant (and so don't use reliable contraception), while some clients are worried hormonal contraception will make them infertile and/or they may wait too long if they decide they want to get pregnant. Providers agreed that two of the NFP methods, Rhythm and calendar-based methods, and FABM can be very effective when used correctly and consistently (though there was no consensus on the effectiveness of withdrawal). Providers did not recall receiving any specific, in-depth training on natural methods and said they would be interested in having such training. According to providers, many clients have limited knowledge about the length of their menstrual cycle and when their fertile period is, which indicates a need for education in these areas if natural methods are promoted. Potential *advantages* of NFP and FABM cited by providers were that they: have no side effects, have little or no cost, are always available, can be used when conditions prevent hormonal method use, facilitate women knowing more about (and being more comfortable with) their bodies, encourage positive communication between partners, facilitate deeper intimacy, accommodate cultural/religious beliefs, and allow for changes in pregnancy intentions. Potential *disadvantages* of NFP and FABM cited by providers were as follows, that they: require time (that wasn't available) to provide adequate patient education, and entail a high level of knowledge and attentiveness, are difficult to use, suffer from improper use and non-compliance, require a regular menstrual cycle, a 'regular' lifestyle and partner cooperation, entail planning for fertile periods. Providers expressed some discomfort in condoning condom non-use in communities with high STD rates. While some providers expressed reservations about clients using natural methods, all would educate a client about a natural method if he or she specifically asked about it.

Provider Survey

The survey was launched in May 2010. Preliminary results are provided for the 50 providers who completed the survey as of 6/23/10. Some questions use a Likert scale. For example, "How *effective* are FABM?" uses a 4 point scale: 1 = "not at all," 2 = "not very," 3 = "somewhat," 4 = "very." The question, "How often do I ask clients if they use an FABM?" also uses a 4 point scale: 1 = "never," 2 = "rarely," 3 = "usually," 4 = "always." Responses to these and similar questions are shown in Table 1 below.

When asked if they had ever received training on Rhythm/calendar or FABM, 58% and 43% (respectively) indicated they had. According to providers, the main *advantages* of offering natural methods are an opportunity to educate clients (53% Rhythm/calendar, 66% FABM) and no side effects/health risks (55% Rhythm/calendar, 42% FABM). The main *challenges* of offering natural methods are clients won't understand correct use (57% Rhythm/calendar, 61% FABM) and clients would not be able to abstain/use condoms during their fertile period (67% Rhythm/calendar, 37% FABM). Providers considered that the clients most appropriate for natural methods would be those who are very motivated, organized and willing to abstain (27% Rhythm/

calendar, 38% FABM) and those having regular cycles and who are "in touch" with their body (29% Rhythm/calendar, 28% FABM).

Client ACASI Survey

Surveys have been conducted with clients at five clinics thus far. As of 6/8/10, results were available for 250 clients. Clients have been recruited from three hospitals and two community health centers. Four clinics are in Philadelphia and one is in Chester, PA. More than 90% of all clients at these five clinics have incomes below 125% of the 2009 federal poverty level.

DEMOGRAPHICS

Clients' median age is 24 (range 18-35), 92% are Black and 6% Hispanic. Sixty-nine percent had an established religious affiliation (33% Protestant, 13% Christian, 13% Muslim, 10% Catholic). Forty-five percent said religious/spiritual beliefs have 'some' or 'a lot' of influence on their contraceptive decisions.

Table 1 Provider Survey – responses from fifty participants.

Provider survey questions	Withdrawal	Rhythm/ Calendar	FAM
	% marking 'somewhat/very'		
Method considered effective	58	80	90
Clients' interest in method	-	33	13
Comfort with client using method	34	73	53
How hard is it for the client to use method?	96	85	89
	% marking 'usually/always'		
How often I ask client about method	44	24	15
If client asks about method, I recommend an alternative	75	33	19
If client asks about method, I describe it	42	61	49
If client asks about method, I give written info	4	38	44

RELATIONSHIP AND REPRODUCTIVE FACTORS

Sixty-three percent of clients were in a serious relationship, 33% were cohabiting and 13% were married. In the past six months, 8% had no sexual partner, 59% had one, 27% had two to four, and 6% had five or more partners. Primary contraceptive methods currently being used were: hormonal (50%), condom (31%), withdrawal (14%), Rhythm/calendar (3%) and no method (24%). Seventy percent said preventing pregnancy now was "important" or "very important."

Sixty percent described their menstrual cycles as "regular" over the past year. Thirty-one percent indicated their usual cycle having '26-32' days, 34% '25 or fewer' days, and 32% indicated they 'don't know.' Thirty-one percent knew when in the menstrual cycle is the fertile time (i.e., two weeks before her period starts) and 51% estimated their one-month likelihood of getting pregnant if not using contraception as 'likely' or 'very likely.' Eighteen percent knew the clinically accepted likelihood (85%) of an average woman getting pregnant if she doesn't use contraception for one year. Providers were reported as being the most common source of reproductive health information, followed by adult family members, sex education classes, TV/magazines/movies, friends and the Internet.

WITHDRAWAL, RHYTHM/CALENDAR (R/C), FERTILITY AWARENESS BASED METHODS (FABM)

A series of questions asked about these natural methods for pregnancy prevention. Fifty percent said withdrawal is not effective while 45% said it is common. Twenty-five percent considered R/C and FABM as not effective and 15% said they are common. More than eighty percent said that providers never asked or talked to them about these methods. About 74% had never heard of or knew nothing about FABM and three common methods of assessing fertility (basal body temperature, cervical mucus and fertile monitoring technology). The proportion that had *ever* used withdrawal, R/C or FABM as their primary contraceptive method was 39%, 13% and 9% respectively and for *at least three months* was 22%, 5% and 4 % respectively. Of those who ever used these methods, 40-60% told their provider, 54-66% felt comfortable doing so and 61-67% said it would be helpful if providers gave them information on these methods.

Some questions use a Likert scale. For example, "How *confident* were you in your ability to use FABM the right way?" uses a 5 point scale where 1 = "not at all" and 5 = "very." Responses to these and similar questions are shown in Table 2 below.

CONCLUSIONS

Provider Focus Groups and Survey

Few participants recalled specific training on NFP or FABM but would be interested in this. Providers agreed that Rhythm/calendar and FABM can be very effective when used correctly. Providers cited various advantages that NFP and FABM had over other methods, including: no side effects, ease of availability, little or no cost, improved partner communication, and accommodation of certain religious/cultural beliefs. Providers had reservations, however, about their clients using NFP or FABM due to their perception of clients' limited knowledge about their menstrual cycles and fertility, the anticipated difficulty of using these methods correctly, and the limited time and materials available to educate clients about correct method use. In addition, some providers were hesitant to condone condom non-use due to the high STD rates among the population they serve. Despite their reservations, providers agreed they would educate a client about NFP or FABM if the client asked them to do so.

Client ACASI Survey

Only a minority of clients had suitable cycle and fertility knowledge to be candidates for Rhythm, calendar-based methods and FABM. Clients were not generally aware of FABM options. Those who had used any of the natural methods were interested in having further discussions with providers about them. Of those using NFP or FABM for more than three months, a substantial proportion indicated difficulty with correct use and worry about getting pregnant when using the method. A majority of R/C and FABM users, however, also indicated satisfaction with these methods as contraception. Future analysis on the complete dataset will explore reasons for use, barriers, and the involvement of partners. These factors will also be given greater context by our qualitative interviews with experienced NFP and FABM users.

Table 2. Client Survey – responses from NFP users (for at least three months).

ACASI questions	% marking 4 or 5 on a scale with 5 being highest rating	
	Withdrawal	R/C &FAM
	n=60	n=25
Confidence in ability to use method correctly	55	56
Difficulty using method every time	29	36
Used method correctly >half/all time	59	44
How likely to get pregnant using this method	42	32
How worried about pregnancy using this method	45	44
Satisfaction with the method	38	68

Implications

The primary aim of the two additional provider focus groups at the conclusion of the data collection period will be to identify potential strategies for Title X clinics to reduce client and provider-level barriers to traditional NFP and FABM uptake and successful use. To facilitate this process, we will share our findings from providers, clients and NFP/FABM users at the beginning of the focus group sessions. Findings from our study have the potential to be relevant to a range of settings providing reproductive health services.

SOURCES CONSULTED

Dicker, D., T. Wachsman, D. Feldberg. 1989. "The vaginal contraception diaphragm and the condom: An evaluation and comparison of two barrier methods with the rhythm method." *Contraception* 40:497-503.

Fowler, C. I., J. Gable, J. Wang. 2008. *Family planning annual report: 2006 national summary*. Research Triangle Park: RTI International.

Gribble, J. N., R. I. Lundgren, C. Velasquez, E. E. Anastasi. 2008. "Being strategic about contraceptive introduction: The experience of the Standard Days Method." *Contraception* 77: 147-154.

Hatcher, R. A., J. Trussell, A. L. Nelson, W. Cates, F. H. Stewart, D. Kowal. 2007. *Contraceptive Technology: Nineteenth Revised Edition.* New York: Ardent Media.

Jennings, V. H., M. Arévalo, D. Kowal. 2004. "Fertility awareness-based methods." In R. A. Hatcher, et al. Eds. *Contraceptive Technology*, pp. 317-329. New York: Ardent Media, Inc.

Kaiser Family Foundation. 2003. *National survey of adolescents and young adults: Sexual Health knowledge, attitudes and experiences.* www.kff.org/youthhivstds/3218-index.cfm (accessed June 5, 2011).

Kambic, R. T. ,V. Lamprecht. 1996. "Calendar rhythm method efficacy: A review." *Advances in Contraception* 12:123-128.

Kost, K., S. Singh, B. Vaughan, J. Trussell, A. Bankole. 2008. "Estimates of contraceptive failure from the 2002 National Survey of Family Growth." *Contraception* 77:10-21.

Sinai, I., R. Lundgren, M. Arévalo, V. Jennings. 2006. "Fertility awareness-based methods of family planning: Predictors of correct use." *Perspectives on Sexual and Reproductive Health* 32: 94-100.

Stanford, J. B., J. C. Lemaire, P. B. Thurman. 1998. "Women's interest in natural family planning." *Journal of Family Practice* 46:65-71.

Whittaker, P. G., R. D. Merkh, D. Henry-Moss, L. Hock-Long. 2010. "Withdrawal attitudes and experiences: a qualitative perspective among young urban adults." *Perspectives on Sexual and Reproductive Health* 42:102-109.

PANEL IV

STATUS OF NFP: HOW MANY, WHO, WHY?

10

Status of NFP in the U.S. & Developing Countries

A review of data from the National Survey of Family Growth & the Demographic & Health Surveys

IRIT SINAI, PHD

Senior Research Officer, Institute for Reproductive Health, Georgetown University

VICTORIA JENNINGS, PHD

Director, Institute for Reproductive Health, Georgetown University

ABSTRACT

Large standardized surveys that are periodically collected in most countries, such as the Demographic and Health Surveys (DHS) in developing countries and the National Survey of Family Growth (NSFG) in the United States of America, can provide rich data about the health of the population, including their use of family planning. In this study we explore the suitability of these data as currently collected to measure the prevalence of Natural Family Planning (NFP) use, and attempt to measure it. We also show that the questions, probes, and procedures used for data collection cannot accurately measure NFP use, but that NFP prevalence is uniformly low. Finally we conclude that those interested in promoting NFP use should advocate for more accurate representation in these surveys of NFP methods, as well as collect and publish statistics of NFP users. In addition, the reasons why NFP methods are not used by more couples should be explored.

INTRODUCTION

Most countries periodically collect data using large nationally representative surveys about a variety of health and demographic indicators. These surveys, which are designed to provide the government with important information that can be used to make development policy decisions, is then made publically available, and is routinely used by stakeholders, health program managers, and researchers.

In the United States the National Survey of Family Growth (NSFG) serves this purpose. The NSFG gathers information on family life, marriage and divorce, pregnancy, infertility, use of family planning methods, and men's and women's health. The data are collected by the Centers for Disease Control and Prevention (CDC), and are used by the U.S. Department of Health and Human Services and others to plan health services and health education programs, and to do statistical studies of families, fertility, and health. Rounds 1-6 of the NSFG were collected in 1973, 1976, 1982, 1988, 1995, and 2002. The latest round of data collection, round 7, was continuous in the years 2006-2010, where data were collected 48 weeks of every year for four years. In each year, a nationally representative sample of men and women age 15-44 in 33 areas was interviewed. By the end of the four years of interviewing, in June 2010, over 22,600 interviews had been completed in 110 areas (CDC 2010).

In most developing countries, nationally representative health data are collected through the Demographic and Health Surveys (DHS), about every five years. Sample sizes are large (usually between 5,000 and 30,000 households). In all households, women age 15-49 are interviewed. In many countries men from a sub-sample of households are also interviewed. There are three core questionnaires in DHS surveys: A Household Questionnaire, a Women's Questionnaire, and a Male Questionnaire. There are also several standardized modules for countries with interest in additional topics. The data are collected by the appropriate ministry of each country with technical assistance of the Measure DHS project, which is funded by the United States Agency for International Development (USAID). Since 1984 over

240 DHS surveys have been undertaken in over 85 countries. DHS has earned a worldwide reputation for collecting and disseminating accurate, nationally representative data on fertility, family planning, maternal and child health, gender, HIV/AIDS, malaria, and nutrition (Measure DHS 2010).

This paper reviews the status of Natural Family Planning (NFP) use in the United States and in developing countries using NSFG and DHS data. NFP methods provide women with guidelines to determine the days each cycle when they are most likely to become pregnant (the fertile window). Couples use this information to avoid or achieve pregnancy. The umbrella term NFP consists of several methods with many variations. Using some methods involves monitoring the biological symptoms of fertility and ovulation, while other methods require monitoring cycle days. NFP methods are available in many parts of the world. Some, like the Standard Days Method®, are provided at the community level as well as in family planning and health facilities, while others, such as the Billings Ovulation Method (BOM) and the Sympto-Thermal Method (STM) are usually offered by non-profit volunteer organizations. These programs and providers can benefit from information about the prevalence of method use. This paper examines the data available on NFP use in the NSFG and DHS data, reviews the challenges of using these data to determine prevalence of use, and studies some trends the data demonstrate.

NFP IN DEVELOPING COUNTRIES

The broadest definition of NFP is a group of methods in which a couple wishing to avoid pregnancy abstains from sexual intercourse on the days their method identifies as potentially fertile, based on the identification of certain signs or symptoms of fertility or on specific cycle days. The key words are 'their method identifies.' This definition encompasses a variety of algorithms, or rules, that identify the fertile window. The Billings Ovulation Method (BOM) and the TwoDay Method®, for example, use the presence of cervical secretions to determine the days in the cycle a woman is most likely to become pregnant. Standard Days Method users, on the other hand, determine their fertile window by considering the day of the menstrual cycle the woman is on. However, not all 'methods' that women can use provide correct information. Some forms of periodic abstinence that have never been tested, and in fact are not very effective, are highly prevalent in some settings (Arévalo 1997). In the DHS these so called methods usually are referred to as the Rhythm Method. Rhythm Method users often learn to use their 'method' from friends, relatives, or others in the community. Yet Rhythm fits the broad definition of NFP. This presents a challenge when gathering data about NFP use.

The DHS questionnaire includes questions about women's knowledge of the fertile time. The respondent is first asked: "From one menstrual period to the next, are there certain days when a woman is more likely to become pregnant?" If she answers in the affirmative, she is then asked: "Is this time just before her period begins, during her period, right after her period has ended, or halfway between two periods?" Figure 1 shows the percent of women who had ever used Rhythm, and the percent of them who recognized that a woman is most likely to conceive halfway between two periods, in selected countries, randomly selected from the list of all developing countries for which the information is available. The figure in parenthesis next to each country name represents the year in which the latest DHS was undertaken in that country. Each column shows the percent of women in each country who said they have ever used the Rhythm Method. The upper section of the column represents the percent of ever Rhythm users,

Figure 1. Percent of women who know that a woman is fertile halfway between two periods, from those who had ever used the Rhythm method (DHS data, selected countries)

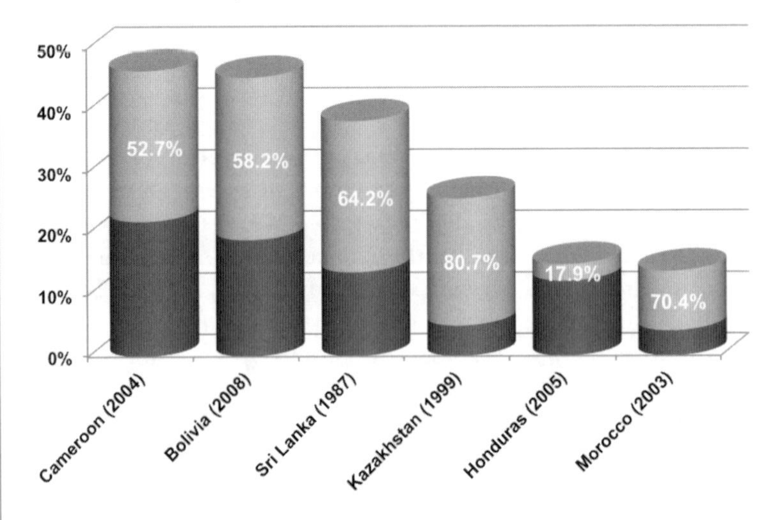

who demonstrate basic fertility awareness. Clearly, many women who had ever used some variation of the Rhythm Method used a rule that does not actually work.

Half-way between two periods, which is the best option women can choose as they respond to the second question, is not exactly accurate. Some modern NFP methods have more complex rules. For example, the Billings Ovulation method (BOM) instructs women to also abstain every other day until their mucus pattern begins. Therefore real NFP users could be confused by the question. Figure 2 shows the distribution of answers to the second question in Kenya. Again, the country was randomly selected from a list of all DHS studies. The figure shows that the most prevalent response is 'right after her period has ended,' which is incorrect. Clearly, many Rhythm users use incorrect rules.

These figures suggest that the DHS may not be an appropriate source of information about the prevalence of NFP use, because Rhythm, which is measured in all countries, includes also ineffective rules, and not only NFP. People who are less familiar with NFP perceive Rhythm users to be users of NFP. Since many Rhythm users use ineffective rules, many get pregnant while using their version of it. As a result, NFP is often incorrectly perceived as being an ineffective family planning method.

Figure 2. Responses to the question about when in the cycle a woman could become pregnant (DHS, Kenya, 2008)

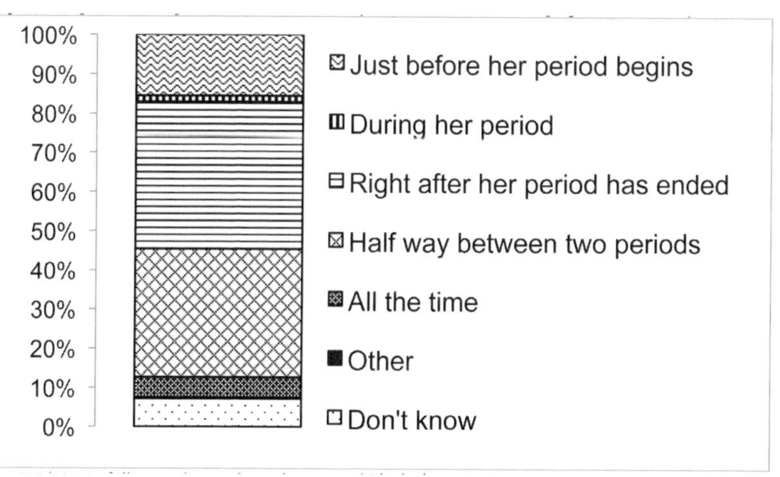

n = 756 (13.5% of all respondents – those who ever used Rhythm)

Table 1. Ever use of Rhythm by continent (DHS, most recent downloadable data, 71 countries)

	Minimum	Maximum	Mean
Africa (38 countries)	Egypt (2008) 0.9%	Congo Brazzaville (2005) 85.4%	15.3%
Asia (14 countries)	Nepal (2006) 4.5%	Sri Lanka (1987) 38.2%	14.5%
Europe (5 countries)	Turkey (2003) 8.4%	Ukraine (2007) 40.5%	19.7%
America (14 countries)	Nicaragua (2001) 9.5%	Bolivia (2003) 45.3%	19.6%

With this in mind, we can review the percent of DHS respondents who have ever used the Rhythm Method. This is shown in Table 1. The figures were drawn from the most recent DHS Studies for which data are available online (71 countries). We downloaded these data to calculate indicators. The data show considerable variation between countries, however the figure for 89% of the countries was less than 30%. Given that many of these Rhythm users were not actual NFP users, the actual rate for ever use of NFP is probably significantly lower.

A similar pattern emerges when we review current use of Rhythm. Means per continent shown in Table 2 are probably lower than actual Rhythm use, because of the way interviewers are trained to code

Table 2. Current use of Rhythm by continent (DHS, most recent downloadable data, 71 countries)

	Mean
Africa (38 countries)	4.1%
Asia (14 countries)	4.0%
Europe (5 countries)	3.8%
America (14 countries)	5.5%

responses. When a respondent lists more than one method as her current family planning method, interviewers are instructed to code it as if she uses the more effective method only. While NFP methods instruct users to abstain from sex during the fertile days, it is a fact that some users choose to use a condom on their fertile days from time to time. Because of the reputation of Rhythm as being ineffective, if a woman says she uses it with condoms, she is counted as a condom user, not a Rhythm user. This practice results in underreporting of Rhythm users. These figures, again, include NFP users, as well as users of other periodic abstinence rules that may not be very effective.

While in most developing countries Rhythm is the only NFP method listed in the DHS, there are some exceptions. As the Standard Days Method becomes available in more countries, it is increasingly included in the DHS as a method separate form Rhythm. Table 3 is drawn from recent surveys that include Standard Days Method use. Considering that the method was available in these countries for no more than 1-2 years at the time the surveys were conducted, and was available only in pilot sites, these results are encouraging.

Table 3. Standard Days Method use in recent DHS surveys

Country	Ever use	Currently using
Benin (2006)	0.3%	0.1%
Bolivia (2008)	1.4%	0.2%
Madagascar (2008)	0.2%	<0.1%
Peru (2004-08)	0.2%	<0.1%
Philippines (2008)	0.4%	0.1%
Rwanda (2007-08)	1.9%	0.5%

The Philippines is the only country in which NFP methods other than the Standard Days Method are listed separately. Figure 3 shows the list of NFP methods in the Philippines questionnaire, and the prompt associated with each. While these prompts may not be completely accurate descriptions of the methods (for example, the Sympto-Thermal Method is not just a combination of the other methods), these can clearly better identify NFP users. Table 4 shows the percentage of Filipino respondents who have used NFP, from the 2008 DHS.

Table 4. NFP use in the Philippines (DHS, 2008)

Method	Ever use	Currently using
Mucus	1.1%	0.1%
BBT	0.6%	<0.1%
Symptothermal	0.2%	<0.1%
Standard Days Method	0.4%	0.1%
Rhythm	19.5%	6.2%

NFP IN THE UNITED STATES

The NSFG includes the following questions:

"Have you ever used Rhythm or safe period by calendar to prevent pregnancy?"

and

"Have you ever used Natural Family Planning or safe period by temperature or cervical mucus test to prevent pregnancy?"

In the survey report, CDC statisticians interpreted the first question as "Periodic abstinence—calendar rhythm," and the second as "Periodic abstinence—Natural Family Planning." While these questions are more specific than that DHS question, they still do not provide a good description of NFP methods. Therefore these questions may result in some underreporting. However, as Table 5 shows, few women report using NFP. Even if there was no underreporting, the figures would still be low.

Table 5. NFP use in the United States (NSFG, 2008)

Method	Ever use	Currently using
Periodic abstinence – calendar rhythm	19.4%	0.5%
Periodic abstinence – natural family planning	4.6%	0.1%

Figure 3. DHS prompts for NFP in the Philippines

MUCUS, BILLINGS, OVULATION. Women can monitor the cervical mucus to determine the days of the month they are most likely to get pregnant.

BASAL BODY TEMPERATURE. Women can monitor the body temperature to determine the days of the month they are most likely to get pregnant.

SYMPTOTHERMAL. It is a combination of Basal Body Temperature and Mucus, Billings, Ovulation Method.

STANDARD DAYS METHOD. This method uses a beaded necklace on which each bead represents the days of a woman's cycle. The necklace would help determine the days when the woman is likely to get pregnant.

CALENDAR OR RHYTHM OR PERIODIC ABSTINENCE. Every month that a woman is sexually active she can avoid pregnancy by not having sexual intercourse on the days of the month she is most likely to get pregnant.

DISCUSSION

Our findings highlight several difficulties in collecting information about the prevalence of NFP use worldwide from existing data sources. Inappropriate questions and misguided interviewer training result in under-reporting of NFP users. Yet even accounting for this, the number of NFP users in the world is small, considering the effort of dedicated providers everywhere to provide NFP methods. When researchers include NFP users in the Rhythm category it results in the misconception that NFP methods are not effective. This is so because so many women who report that they are Rhythm users have no understanding of their fertility.

It is important that those interested in promoting NFP advocate for including NFP methods in DHS surveys. The Standard Days

Method is included in more and more DHS surveys as the method becomes available in these countries because developers of the questionnaires are willing to include methods they believe will be identified by a statistically significant number of respondents. There are strong NFP programs in many countries, and these programs should promote the inclusion of NFP methods, separate from Rhythm, in the surveys of their respective countries, as has been accomplished in the Philippines.

It is very important that definitions and probes in these surveys are accurate. The relevant question in the DHS is too broad; the question in the NSFG is more specific, yet not sufficiently accurate. Probes given in the DHS to respondents who do not spontaneously say that they have heard of the method can be misleading, and need to be corrected.

But advocacy efforts to improve questions and probes take time. It may be years before DHS and NSFG surveys can provide accurate information about the prevalence of NFP use. In the meantime, programs that provide NFP should be encouraged to collect service statistics and publish their results. The Standard Days Method is often offered in public health facilities, which routinely collect service statistics. Nonetheless, there is some under-reporting, as Standard Days Method users who request condoms to use on the fertile days are often incorrectly classified as condoms users. For example, we know that during the period from July 2008 through June 2010, about 5,400 women in Guatemala received counseling in the Standard Days Method in public facilities, and started using the method. We also know from the manufacturer of CycleBeads® (a string of color-coded beads that helps Standard Days Method users keep track of their fertile days), that over 10,115 were sold in Guatemala in the same period. While some of these were distributed for training and advocacy purposes, this figure can still be informative regarding expected demand for the method. With respect to other NFP methods, there are many small NFP programs that do not collect data at all. For most of those that do, any information they collect regarding the number of users is not aggregated or published.

We encourage programs to collect and aggregate data, keeping in mind the definition of a 'user.' We need to ensure that the definition used is the same definition of users that is utilized elsewhere. It is not 'users' that should be aggregated, but 'new users,' as we can never assume that everyone who starts using the method continues to do so.

Therefore, programs need to devise a recording system, where couples who learn to use the method are tallied. They should only be recorded as they start using the method, and should be counted as new users.

At the same time, we need to think creatively about generating more demand for NFP methods. We know that these methods can meet the needs of many couples, and studies have shown that a significant proportion of people are interested in learning more about them (Stanford et al. 1998; FHI 2010). What is it that keeps more people from using them? Is it the message we give them about the methods? Is it how, where, or by whom the methods are being provided? Is it the methods themselves? What other barriers exist, such as attitudes toward NFP on the part of health providers, program managers, and policy makers? We need to study what it is that keeps more couples from using NFP in various settings, so that we know what we need to address.

SOURCES CONSULTED

Arévalo, M. 1997. "Expanding the availability and improving delivery of natural family planning services and fertility awareness education: providers' perspectives." *Advances in Contraception* 13: 275-281.

Centers for Disease Control and Prevention (CDC). 2010. *About the National Survey of Family Growth*, available online at www.cdc.gov/nchs/nsfg/about_nsfg.htm (Accessed May 22, 2011).

Family Health International (FHI). 2010. Progress in Family Planning. Mobile technology: Text messages for better reproductive health. Available online at www.fhi.org/en/Research/Projects/Progress/GTL/mobile_tech.htm#formative_research (Accessed May 22, 2011).

Measure DHS. 2010. *Demographic and Health Surveys*, available online at www.measuredhs.com/aboutdhs/ (Accessed May 22, 2011).

Stanford, J. B., J. C. Lemaire, P. B. Thurman. 1998. "Women's interest in natural family planning." *Journal of Family Practice* 46: 65-71

11

Trends in NFP Services in the Catholic Dioceses of the United States

An Overview of Data from the National Survey of Diocesan NFP Programs (Profile)

REV. ROBERT R. CANNON, MA, MED, MTH, JCL

Consultant, NFP Program, United States Conference of Catholic Bishops

ABSTRACT

The Catholic Church has developed a variety of educational and support programs for engaged and married couples. Among these are diocesan programs of Natural Family Planning (NFP). In the United States, it is possible to determine trends in these Church sponsored NFP services based on the *Annual National Diocesan NFP Survey* (commonly called the *Profile*). The Natural Family Planning Program of the United States Conference of Catholic Bishops (USCCB) conducts the survey and produces the *Profile*.

The *Profile* provides a wealth of information on diocesan NFP educational support services. The data gathered in this survey identify the strengths and weaknesses of diocesan NFP ministry both locally and nationally. It is an important pastoral tool for directing the development of national resources to help facilitate the growth of NFP ministry in the U.S. Catholic dioceses.

This paper discusses the following trends. The majority of Catholic dioceses have a designated NFP coordinator. Most dioceses have NFP education included in their programs of marriage preparation. All major NFP providers are represented in the dioceses. Despite these strengths, NFP ministry continues to be fragile due to poor funding and other limited resources.

BACKGROUND

The Catholic Church has a beautiful and rich theological understanding of human sexuality (including human fertility), marriage, conjugal love and responsible parenthood, the value of children and the good of the family. Catholic belief regarding human sexuality is rooted in Sacred Scripture and Catholic Tradition. Conference speakers have delved into many of these Church teachings through the fine theological papers presented. This paper complements and builds upon those presentations from a programmatic perspective. It looks at the concrete institutional strengths and weaknesses of Natural Family Planning Ministry efforts in the Catholic dioceses within the United States.

The Catholic Church has developed a variety of educational and spiritual programs for engaged and married couples. Among the support programs for marriage are diocesan programs of Natural Family Planning (NFP). In the United States, it is possible to gain insights from trends in these Church sponsored NFP services based on the *Annual National Diocesan NFP Survey* (commonly called the *Profile*). The Natural Family Planning Program of the United States Conference of Catholic Bishops (USCCB) conducts the survey and produces the *Profile*.

The *Profile* was the idea of the late Bishop James McHugh. It was Bishop McHugh who designed and first directed the USCCB's NFP Program (NFPP). He saw the necessity of gathering specific information on each diocesan NFP program in order to provide better support to dioceses and to offer specific guidance to dioceses with particular pastoral circumstances. At the same time, Bishop McHugh understood that the data gathered by the *Profile* would enable the staff of the NFP Program to recognized national patterns of strengths and weaknesses and thus be better equipped to guide the dioceses in their NFP efforts. Similarly, Bishop McHugh thought that the insights gained from the *Profile* would prove useful to his fellow bishops, who have the ultimate pastoral responsibility for NFP services in their own dioceses.

The *Profile's* design is focused on programmatic information. Its foundation is rooted in an earlier five-year nationwide study of diocesan NFP programs and couples who used NFP between 1988 and 1992. A debt of gratitude is owed to Robert Kambic, MSH, for this foundational and original NFP research (see Kambic and Notare 1994). Building upon the work of Kambic, the current NFP *Profile* survey questionnaire is divided into four areas:

1. General information (name of diocesan NFP coordinator, address, etc.)
2. Program management (how the ministry is structured, which department it falls under, number of teachers, NFP schools that train the teachers, etc.)
3. Budget (all funding sources)
4. Program service (what the program provides to the local church, NFP methods represented, introductory programs, NFP presence in marriage preparation programs, NFP classes, etc.)

The *Profile* provides a wealth of information on diocesan NFP services. The data gathered in this survey identifies the strengths and weaknesses of diocesan NFP ministry both locally and nationally. It is an important instrument for directing the development of national resources that facilitate the growth of NFP ministry in the U.S. Catholic dioceses. In anthropological terms, the *Profile* serves as a type of "ecclesiastical" ethnographic study. It examines the concrete efforts by the Catholic Church to assist the faithful, especially those who are preparing for marriage and those already married, to live Church teaching on human sexuality, marriage, conjugal love, and responsible parenthood.

The variety of diocesan NFP ministry efforts affects the precision of the data reported in the *Profile*. For example, the survey does not have strict control of many of the variables of similar sociological research. The USCCB's NFPP staff cannot require all diocesan NFP coordinators to consistently participate in the survey. The NFPP staff can only "invite" participation. The number of dioceses that participate in the survey changes from year to year. Some diocesan NFP coordinators fail to meet the survey deadline. Staffing changes or other administrative glitches result in dioceses not participating in the survey. Each year, the NFPP staff urges all diocesan NFP coordinators to complete the survey. Due to these efforts, about half of the diocesan NFP coordinators consistently submit their questionnaires.

In addition to the diocesan coordinator who submits the data to the national NFP office, the accessibility of precise numerical information available varies not only from diocese to diocese but even within a diocesan NFP program from year to year. In some dioceses for example, NFP teachers who are not officially affiliated with a particular diocese but who work within the geographic area of the diocese, may or may not submit their data on clients taught in a given year. The local NFP coordinator can only invite these NFP teachers to participate in the survey. They cannot require them to submit their data. This variable obviously affects the total number of clients taught in a diocese. Similarly, inconsistent diocesan infrastructure is visible when calculating diocesan NFP budgets. Although the majority of dioceses establish a fee scale, some dioceses encourage their NFP teachers to charge their own fees for NFP classes. Other teachers follow a fee scale suggested by national NFP providers. Still others dioceses allow a national provider to be the sole agent to charge fees for NFP classes in a diocese.

Despite these survey reporting limitations, the design of the *Profile*'s questions reduce much of this respondent variability from year to year in order to reveal broad trends over time. The analysis of the cumulative data creates a picture, albeit, an imprecise one, of NFP activity in dioceses across the United States. When these annual snapshots are compared, a fairly clear picture of NFP diocesan ministry emerges.

As a survey, the *Profile* is not designed to answer NFP methodological questions, examine consistency of client use, critique individual providers, evaluate teacher competency, or answer the myriad of other such questions. The main intent of the *Profile* is to gather specific concrete information on how NFP ministry operates within the diocesan structure and delivers NFP services.

When the diocesan data is tabulated and examined, the *Diocesan Natural Family Planning Ministry National Profile Report* is generated. The *Profile* report serves as an educational tool for bishops and diocesan NFP coordinators. The *Profile* report allows bishops and their respective coordinators to compare their own diocesan NFP ministry efforts with that of the larger Church (for past reports see www.old.usccb.org/prolife/issues/nfp/surveyarchives.shtml).

What does the *Profile* reveal about Roman Catholic sponsored NFP services in the United States? This analysis covers the years 2000 to 2009. Four sections of the *Profile* will be discussed: (1) Program management; (2) Program budget; (3) Program service; and (4) Interpolation of the data and reflection on some anecdotal comments by respondents.

PROGRAM MANAGEMENT

Most dioceses have a person who serves as the designated NFP coordinator responsible for NFP ministry. This is a significant improvement from the 1980s and 1990s. For most diocesan NFP coordinators this responsibility is only one of many jobs. For example, typically the marriage and family life director is responsible for NFP ministry. That same person may also be responsible for youth ministry, respect life activities, or other ministries as well. Nevertheless, it is significant that there is an NFP contact person in most dioceses. As a group, they represent an ecclesial network for giving and receiving NFP information and servicing from the USCCB Natural Family Planning Program. Almost all NFP coordinators are trained in an NFP methodology. This is a significant improvement. For many years, this was not true.

The bulk of NFP ministry provided in dioceses is done by committed lay men and women who volunteer their time as teachers to support NFP. Without this cadre of laity, most NFP diocesan programs would collapse without their generous sacrifices. The motivation for these teachers is the truth of Catholic teaching on conjugal love and responsible parenthood. They are the unsung heroes of NFP ministry.

A variety of organizations train diocesan NFP teachers. These include: Billings Ovulation Method Association (BOMA), Couple to Couple League (CCL), Northwest Family Services, Creighton Model Fertility*Care*™, Family of the Americas Foundation, Marquette University Institute for NFP (Marquette Model), smaller diocesan programs (e.g., Dioceses of Cleveland, Phoenix, and Archdiocese of Boston), and non-diocesan programs (e.g., Southern Star NFP, etc.).

Although it may seem insignificant, about half of diocesan NFP programs are asked by their supervisors to prepare an annual diocesan report on NFP ministry. The symbolic implication is obvious. If the diocesan NFP coordinator is not asked to prepare a report on NFP activities, it may imply a lack of concern about this pastoral area of Church life, indicate a poor system of internal accountability or both possibilities.

PROGRAM BUDGET

All dioceses are under financial constraints. Funding correlates with diocesan priorities. The funding of diocesan NFP programs is and remains, in most dioceses, problematic at best. Across the United States, diocesan NFP programs have remained underfunded. Only a handful of diocesan NFP programs are well funded. As mentioned previously, if not for lay volunteer teachers most dioceses would have no NFP program. The majority of the budgets are so small that NFP efforts do not warrant a line item within diocesan departmental budgets.

Over half of all diocesan NFP programs receive less than $10,000 annually. Only a handful of dioceses spent more than $50,000 annually. In these instances, the bulk of the funds are used to pay the salary for a full-time diocesan NFP coordinator. To supplant the shortfall in diocesan funding, many NFP programs rely on fees for materials used in introductory sessions, tuition for a full course of NFP instruction, donations from seminars to various groups, free use of facilities for NFP instruction, and donations from various organizations, such as the Knights of Columbus.

PROGRAM SERVICE

From 2000 to 2009, the number of dioceses that included NFP as a component of their marriage preparation guidelines grew significantly. In almost all dioceses, a presentation on NFP is required. But with closer scrutiny, the length of time of the NFP presentations varies greatly. Typical NFP presentations last between fifteen minutes to an hour. Ideally, the hope is that couples will be inspired to take a full course of NFP instruction.

Today, one third of dioceses require an introduction to NFP. This is a huge improvement in conveying the beauty of NFP in relation to conjugal love and married life. There are seven dioceses that require a full course of NFP as part of their marriage preparation programs (for a report see, www.old.usccb.org/prolife/issues/nfp/report_requiring_%20NFP_%2008.pdf). Both the Sympto-Thermal Method and the Cervical Mucus Method are taught in most dioceses. The diversity of methods allows users to choose the method that best serves their needs. As mentioned previously, teachers have been trained by a variety of organization such as BOMA, CCL, Creighton Model Fertility*Care*™, and smaller diocesan/regional programs.

INTERPOLATION OF THE DATA

At the conclusion of the first decade of the 21st century, when viewed nationally, NFP programs fluctuate from robust to anemic. Some dioceses have very strong educational programs that integrate NFP into all educational efforts treating human sexuality, marriage, and family life. Through hard work and dedication, some dioceses have made tremendous strides improving the quality of their NFP programs in order to meet the USCCB's *Standards for Diocesan NFP Ministry*. But, as one diocese improves its NFP program, another diocese experiences a retraction in its NFP program, either through teacher loss (individuals moving out of diocese), budget cuts, and or diocesan restructuring (over the last few years departments of marriage and family life have been reduced or merged with other departments). Despite the richness that NFP adds to the Church's teaching on human sexuality and conjugal life in a practical way, one has to conclude that NFP remains a fragile pastoral program in the majority of dioceses.

Even though the majority of dioceses include NFP in their marriage preparation guidelines, in reality, most newly married couples fail to take full advantage of Natural Family Planning in their conjugal life. This observation is strongly suggested when the total number of marriages is compared with the total number of individuals that took a class/instruction in NFP (see Cannon 2009, question 22). In a culture where the twofold meaning of the conjugal act (unitive and procreative) has been severed by a contraceptive dominated mentality, much more must be done to inspire couples to fully understand the call "to embrace and reverence God's vision of human sexuality" (Committee for Pro-Life Activities 1993).

Each year, respondents are asked to offer their personal observations on what is needed to promote the use of NFP. A few remarks appear with regular frequency. There is a hunger for bishops to support NFP efforts as a ministry within their respective dioceses. Where there is identifiable support by the local bishop, lay volunteers work tirelessly to enrich couples about God's design of the human body and the nature of genuine spousal love. In our highly pragmatic culture, dollars speak louder than words. When scrutinizing the funding levels of NFP programs nationally, the funding is paltry, almost scandalous. But again, the cry of NFP providers and teachers is rarely for huge dollars to be directed to NFP efforts. The plea is for those charged with

Church teaching to publicly, institutionally and educationally promote the efficacy of NFP as a morally sound approach to cooperating with the love and life-giving plan of God in marriage.

CONCLUSION

Occasionally articles are published comparing various populations on contraceptive use. They typically reveal that Catholic couples use contraception at the same rates as the general public. This is not surprising given the overwhelming acceptance of contraception as a modern means to manage human fertility. What most people do not realize is that acceptance of contraception is also indicative of a devaluation of the awe inspiring power of procreation. In fact, due to the preoccupation with sex for pleasure and as an end in itself, the current American culture is fostering a greatly impoverished and even false understanding of the nature of sexual intercourse. In this scheme, marriage itself is devalued.

To fight against this diminished approach to human sexuality, the Catholic Church must invest in providing reasonable support for its members to learn how to live the mystery and beauty of marital sexuality (in the Church this is also referred to as "marital chastity"). Otherwise, the power of the Church's moral authority will continue to be dismissed as irrelevant and viewed as vacuous for modern life. It is often said by NFP teachers that NFP is a *hidden treasure* of the Church. If the national picture of NFP efforts drawn by the *Profile* over the last 10 years is any indication, an independent observer can certainly come to this same conclusion.

On a personal note, the heart-felt motivation that led me to offer my professional expertise to the USCCB's NFP Program in developing and analyzing the *Profile* from its inception was the result of a counseling session years ago that I had with a wonderful young married couple. The couple had three small children. The last pregnancy was problematic. The wife's gynecologist told her that another pregnancy would most likely be life threatening. He recommended a tubal ligation for her or a vasectomy for her husband. The couple decided to use a less drastic means. She went on a birth control regimen. On a marriage retreat the couple heard about NFP for the first time as a practical and reasonable method to steward their shared fertility. Inspired and motivated from what they heard, they asked me where they could go to learn about NFP. To my chagrin, the only teacher in the diocese was a two-hour drive away. Eventually, they took a correspondence course and had many long distance telephone calls to learn how to use NFP correctly. The desire of this couple to be faithful to Church teaching given the limited resources available at the time, led me to do what I can in this area of Church life.

Finally, and regardless of the diocese, when examining any NFP program, the most important pastoral question is summed up with this simple "yes" or "no" question: Can Catholic couples who wish to be faithful to Church teaching on conjugal love and responsible parenthood readily get the NFP support they need? The answer to this basic question will determine how to best plan support for local diocesan NFP ministry (Cannon 2009).

SOURCES CONSULTED

Cannon, Robert R. 2009. *Diocesan Natural Family Planning Ministry, National 2009 Profile Report.* Washington, DC: NFP Program, United States Conference of Catholic Bishops www.old.usccb.org/prolife/issues/nfp/09profile.pdf; accessed June 13, 2011.

Committee for Pro-Life Activities, 1993. *Human Sexuality from God's Perspective,* Humanae Vitae *25 Years Later*. Washington, DC: United States Conference of Catholic Bishops.

Kambic, Robert T., Theresa Notare. 1994. "Roman Catholic Church-sponsored natural family planning services in the United States." *Advances in Contraception* 10:85-92.

12

Scaling-Up Natural Family Planning

Models & Results from Five Countries

REBECKA I. LUNDGREN, MPH

Deputy Director, Director of Research, Institute for Reproductive Health, School of Medicine, Georgetown University

with

KATHERINE LAVOIE CAIN, MPH

Independent Consultant

ABSTRACT

Natural Family Planning (NFP) provides couples with an effective and safe approach for managing their fertility. Despite the many benefits of NFP and the persistent efforts of many NFP organizations and teachers, NFP services are not widely available in the United States, and the number of couples using them is very small. NFP groups invest considerable commitment and effort in providing services, yet these efforts have not yet resulted in a significant numbers of NFP users.

The promotion and practice of NFP can be aided by the implementation of a "scale-up" strategy. Core elements of a scale-up strategy include the NFP method's credibility, both its method effectiveness and the overall quality of the program through which the NFP method is taught; its relative advantage (benefits); ease to teach; and its ability to be evaluated.

This article discusses all the core elements of scale-up strategy and recommends how they can be helpful to NFP information dissemination and client use.

INTRODUCTION

Natural Family Planning (NFP) provides couples with an effective and safe approach for managing their fertility. Couples choose a natural method for a variety of reasons—religious beliefs, health concerns, the desire to work together as a couple to plan a family, or simply to understand the signs and symptoms of their combined fertility. Fertility awareness, the basis of NFP, increases both women's and men's knowledge of their reproductive potential and enhances self-reliance. Despite the efforts of many individuals and organizations to develop an array of methods and to streamline and improve approaches for teaching couples to use them, NFP services are not widely available in the United States, and the number of couples using them is very small. NFP groups invest considerable commitment and effort in providing services, yet these efforts have not yet resulted in a significant numbers of NFP users.

On a global level, hundreds of pilot and experimental projects—many successful—have been launched in developing countries aimed at improving access to high quality reproductive health services, including NFP. The influence of these small-scale interventions, however, has largely remained confined to original target areas, thus limiting their overall impact. Little systematic attention has been paid to how benefits achieved in pilot projects can be expanded to serve more people, and significant gaps remain in understanding the processes by which innovations are implemented and sustained.

Without a better grasp of how scale-up happens, promising reproductive health interventions—such as NFP—cannot realize their full potential. Increasingly policy makers, practitioners, and researchers agree that we face a formidable gap between health innovations and their delivery to communities around the world. Realizing the need for a quantitative, scientific framework to guide health-care scale-up, researchers in health, engineering, and business are building interest in implementation science. Unlike routine applied research, implementation science creates generalized knowledge that can be applied across settings and contexts to answer central questions about scale-up (Madon 2007; Fixsen 2005).

Reproductive health researchers and their counterparts in a range of other areas of public health are concerned why "evidence-based best practices" are rarely incorporated—that is, scaled-up into "standard practices." Serious gaps exist in understanding the processes by which innovations are implemented and sustained. As part of the Fertility Awareness-Based Methods (FABM) Project, Georgetown University's Institute for Reproductive Health (IRH) is scaling up a new family planning innovation, Standard Days Method® (SDM), and studying the process along the way. SDM is a natural method of family planning based on a woman's menstrual cycle. Appropriate for women who have most menstrual cycles between 26 and 32 days long, the method identifies days 8 through 19 as the fertile days. A woman can use Cycle Beads®, a color-coded string of beads, to help track the days of her menstrual cycle and see which days she is most likely to get pregnant. Field experience and results from clinical trials show that this method is effective, low cost and particularly useful for expanding contraceptive prevalence and addresses the family planning needs of many couples. It appeals primarily to those who are new to family planning or who are concerned about side-effects with other modern methods of family planning (Arévalo et al. 2001; Gribble et al. 2008).

The purpose of studying the scale-up process is to identify factors that facilitate or constrain sustainable scale-up of innovations with an emphasis on those that can be manipulated by program managers. This endeavor will examine the extent to which SDM scale-up was achieved as well as the facilitators and barriers to this process. IRH is conducting a five-year prospective, multi-site comparative study of the process and outcomes of scaling up SDM in five countries, drawing upon the ExpandNet/World Health Organization (WHO) scale-up model. The ExpandNet/WHO model grounded development of a feasible yet rigorous methodology and facilitated operationalization of the scale-up concept.

Once an innovation has been tested and proven on a small scale, the question naturally becomes how to expand it to achieve maximum benefit. In order to address this question, this paper examines the notion of scaling up, drawing from diffusion of innovation theory and considering examples from IRH's five-year prospective case study of scaling up SDM in the Democratic Republic of Congo (DRC), Guatemala, India, Mali and Rwanda.

WHAT IS SCALE-UP?

Scaling up is defined as, "deliberate efforts to increase the impact of health service innovations successfully tested in pilot or experimental projects so as to benefit more people and to foster policy and program development on a lasting basis" (Simmons et al. 2007). Notably, this definition includes several key concepts. Most importantly, scale-up rarely happens spontaneously. Deliberate, planned, strategic action must be taken to achieve it. With scale-up, we are trying to reach more people with an innovation, in order to maximize its impact. Using this definition, the innovation being scaled up has already been tested successfully on a small scale. Finally, inherent in the concept of scale-up is sustainability. It is an ineffective use of resources to scale something up today that is forgotten about tomorrow.

Thinking about scaling up NFP, we must consider some key questions. First, what exactly should be scaled up? With regard to NFP, is it the rules or guidelines of a particular method? Are there particular teaching or tracking tools and/or a systematic way of teaching the method that must also be scaled up? Alternatively, do we want to scale-up a way of life or an expression of faith? These questions are worth considering, as the answers will guide scale-up efforts. But even before addressing these issues, we must start with the question of why we want to scale-up NFP. Is scale-up important to our program? We each define scale-up according to our particular vision and mission. What does scale-up mean to us? Whom are we trying to reach? To what end? This is something each of us and our programs must decide for ourselves. Making these goals and assumptions explicit will facilitate the task of scaling up, and are even essential to the starting point of deciding whether or not to scale-up.

Finally, how do we define successful NFP scale-up? This is another question best answered by thoughtful reflection. Each program must determine its own definition of scale-up. Here are a few questions to consider:

- How many people use NFP now?
- To what extent is NFP available at the national, sub-national and organizational levels?
- What is the capacity of providers to offer NFP?

HOW DO WE SCALE-UP?

Once we have asked ourselves these questions and are confident we know what we are scaling up, why we want to do it, and what success means to us, we need to consider the best way to actually do it. In contrast to the spontaneous diffusion of innovations, scaling up is a social, political, and institutional process that engages multiple actors, interest groups and organizations. Currently, the scale-up literature focuses primarily on the attributes of the innovation, patterns of innovation/technology adoption, and use of opinion leaders. Much less has been written on the process of scaling up itself (Simmons et al. 2007; Greenhalgh 2004). The dearth of literature on the scale-up process may, in part, be due to the considerable challenges inherent in this type of research including the complex interpretive process underlying adoption, pervasive pro-innovation bias on the part of researchers, and the need to incorporate several research methodologies to gather information on both process and impact.

Scaling up must be strategically planned because it will not happen automatically, even when the merits of the pilot program become known to stakeholders. During the process of studying the scaling up of SDM into family planning programs, IRH has found that successful scale-ups call for careful planning, a systems approach, and evidence-based practices. These are core principles of the ExpandNet/WHO model of scaling up that IRH has adopted. This model emphasizes partnering with other organizations, involving stakeholders, working

Figure 1. The ExpandNet framework for scaling up

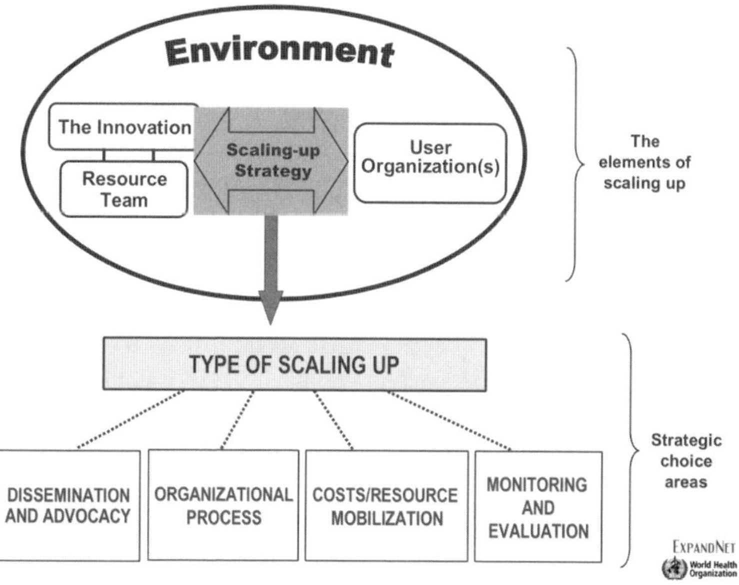

with different cadres of providers, and supporting scale-up through research, monitoring, and evaluation. The ExpandNet/WHO framework is based on a review of literature from the fields of family planning, health and development, from the diffusion of innovations and research utilization, and from the management and policy sciences (ExpandNet 2004).

Figure 1 provides an overview of the framework, representing the system that must be kept in mind when planning and managing the process of scaling up. The centerpiece is the scaling-up strategy, that is, the means by which successfully-tested innovations are communicated, transferred, or otherwise promoted and managed. An effective scaling-up strategy must be congruent with the elements which surround it—the innovation, the user organization expected to implement the innovation on a large scale, the resource team which supports the process, and the larger social, economic and institutional environment in which scale-up takes place—so as to maximize the potential for success. At the same time, a set of strategic choices must be made related to the types of scaling up, dissemination and advocacy, the organizational processes to be used, resource mobilization and monitoring and evaluation. Institutionalization and expansion are the two most critical areas for successful scale-up. Institutionalization refers to ways of anchoring the innovation in policies, regulations, norms, budgets, logistics and management information systems, etc, so that the innovation and its processes will naturally be perpetuated in the host program/agency. Expansion is the process of replicating an innovation in different geographic sites or serving larger or different population groups (Simmons et al. 2007; ExpandNet 2009). Careful adaptation of the innovation to the needs of new sites is at the heart of successful scale-up. In turn, knowing what to adapt—and what needs to be changed when the scale-up is underway—depends on a systems-based approach to research, monitoring and evaluation. A systems approach is necessary because the environment in which scale-up occurs goes beyond the programs that serve clients. It includes the larger service delivery system and its many components (e.g., training, supervision, reporting, procurement), in addition to the socio-cultural and economic characteristics of families and communities. The environment also includes the influence of media, the role of opinion leaders and the policy climate upon which approvals and financing depend.

DIFFUSION OF INNOVATIONS THEORY

Relevant to, yet distinct from, scale-up theory is literature on diffusion of innovations which examines how, why, and at what rate new ideas and technologies are spread. According to this theory, made famous by Evert Rogers, a new idea is adopted very slowly by individuals until it hits a "tipping point"—where the rate of adopting an innovation speeds up and then levels off, as depicted in Figure 2 (Rogers 1995). This concept is discussed in Malcolm Gladwell's book, *The Tipping Point*, which describes how a small number of people who adopt an idea or habit can grow into a critical mass and affect great change.

The community of NFP researchers and practitioners has developed an impressive number of innovations over the decades since the Billings Ovulation Method was developed. These include the Marquette and Creighton models, a "double check" approach to the Sympto-Thermal Method and internet applications for teaching and learning NFP, along with SDM and the TwoDay Method. According to diffusion theory, the degree to which these innovations spread depends on a set of factors, such as: (1) characteristics of the innovation;

Figure 2: Diffusion of Innovation: Rate of Adoption

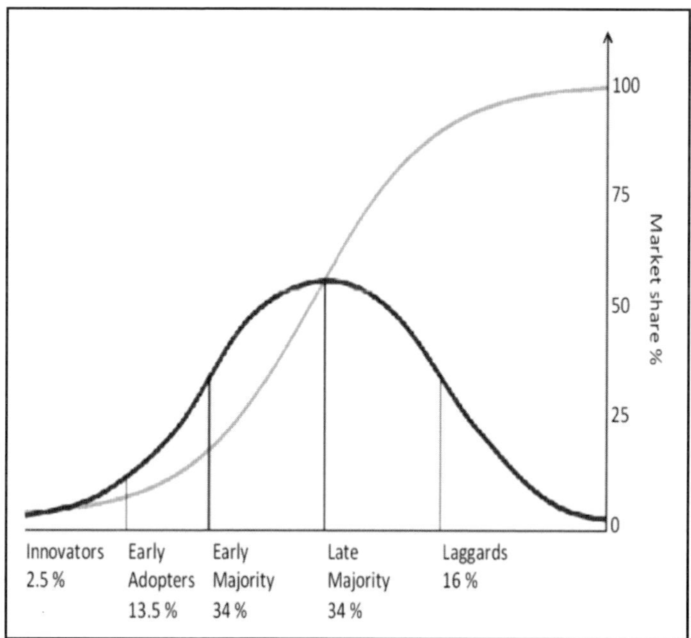

(2) access, availability and quality of services; (3) attitudes of opinion leaders (medical/academic); and (4) communication strategies (Greenhalgh 2004; Rogers 1995). Some innovations spread quickly, even if they are not beneficial. Innovations which are low cost, consistent with prevailing beliefs and practices, and easy to adopt are likely to spread quickly through social networks.

SCALING UP AS A SCIENCE AND AN ART

While it is useful to consider how information diffuses, we cannot rely on important health interventions to spread randomly, in fact, they do not. We must more deeply understand the scale-up process and take concrete actions to achieve broad impact. Whereas diffusion of innovations can be passive, scale-up efforts are proactive. Other ways to characterize scale-up include:

- Interactive, overlapping phases require differing inputs and approaches.
- Multi-level, multi-dimensional, multi-partner. Wide geographical scale-up requires involvement and collaboration at the national, state, and local level. A wide range of groups must be involved, and in fact, partnerships are key. Groups to consider include government, professional schools, influential non-profit organizations, and the private sector.
- A non-linear, long-term process. In the process of scale-up, it is common to experience a combination of victories and setbacks. For example, advocacy efforts to gain the support of a key political figure can become irrelevant if and when that figure is transferred to an area outside your scale-up area. Government changes happen. We take victories where we can.

Managing the scale-up process involves sensitivity to trends and the ability to think fast and seize opportunities that arise. For this reason, scale-up is not only a science, but an art.

EXPANDNET/WHO FRAMEWORK

While the above concepts apply to scale-up efforts in general, the ExpandNet/WHO framework for scale-up is based on several key principles that are not graphically depicted in the framework yet serve as a guidepost for all key decision making regarding the scale-up process (see ExpandNet 2009). They are:

1) *Systems approach.*

   This framework takes into account all the components of the health system, from health centers, to health information systems, to the health workforce, and more. However, it also looks at the broader system in which scale-up takes place, including political processes, social norms and values, and key systems such as education, government, and finance.

2) *Focus on access, rights, participation, quality, and equity.*

   This principle is critical in that we keep in mind the entire reason we are working to scale-up in the first place: to benefit people. Quality services are essential. Equity can refer to gender, class, caste, ethnicity, socioeconomic status, and more. A key component in terms of rights related to family planning is that of informed choice; a woman should be well informed of her options and freely choose what will best suit her needs. In order to ensure that values are upheld and community needs are being met, participation of both governments and individuals is required.

3) *Strive for sustainability.*

   Scaling up is one thing; scaling up sustainable services is another. When you strive for sustainability, you must consider how the innovation will last in the long term. If you simply train providers, what will happen after staff turnover takes place? This is just one example how you must build in sustainability into your scale-up plans. Scale-up requires considerable financial investment. In order for this investment to pay dividends in the long term, you must build in sustainability.

4) *Guided by evidence.*

   To scale something up, you should be confident that it works and is beneficial enough to make it worth the effort. Only a proven innovation should be scaled up, and the process by which it is integrated should also be based on what has been shown to work, to the extent possible. The scale-up phase follows the research and development phase and the pilot/introduction phase.

TYPES OF SCALE-UP TO ENSURE SUSTAINABILITY

Scaling up is often associated with the "roll out" of a tested innovation to new sites or populations. Such expansion will not be sustainable, however, unless it is accompanied by a process of anchoring the innovation in policies, regulations, norms, or training curricula or through other national or sub-national institutional mechanisms. The ExpandNet model defines the concepts of vertical scale-up and horizontal scale-up. Both are important and necessary. By vertical scale-up, we are referring to integration from the political, policy, institutional and legal perspective. This includes getting the method into relevant norms and guidelines in addition to garnering political support for the method. In essence, these are key activities that "sanction" expansion. Horizontal scale-up is also referred to as replication or geographic expansion. With horizontal scale-up, the innovation is available through a wider geographic area, reaching more people.

Vertical and horizontal scale-up complement each other. Without vertical scale-up, you do not have the official sanctioning of the innovation and the "go ahead" for people to take it on. However, vertical scale-up in itself will not mean that the method automatically becomes integrated into services guided by those policies and guidelines. For example, Title X legislation specifically requires grantees to include NFP in their programming. While some give lip-service to doing so, in fact NFP is rarely available through Title X programs. At the end of the day, we want impact on a large scale. So, while vertical scale-up, i.e. institutionalization, provides a strong foundation for scale-up, we must take action to extend the reach geographically to bring greater benefit.

It is important to ensure that the scale-up process not be viewed as simply the integration of NFP into norms, plus provider training. So what are the steps required to achieve scale-up? Our experience with the FABM Project has revealed that it is important to consider both systems and services integration, tasks that can only be achieved with political support and technical leadership. Systems integration includes ensuring that the innovation in question is included in norms and procedures, training curricula, supervision systems, health information systems, procurement and distribution mechanisms, and budget lines. At the same time, the innovation must be included in services through provider training, availability of supplies, supportive supervision and information, education, and communication (IEC) efforts. For example, SDM is included in the four key family planning guidance documents put forth by the WHO, including the Medical Eligibility Criteria for Contraceptive Use, the Decision-making Tool for Family Planning Clients and Providers, and Family Planning: A Global Handbook for Providers. While the inclusion of SDM in these documents has been critical, it alone does not assure that the method is actually offered in programs around the world.

SCALING UP CASE STUDY—JHARKHAND

The case study of the FABM Project's scale-up activities in Jharkhand—a state in north east India—provides an example of how the ExpandNet/WHO model can be useful when scaling up NFP. Jharkhand is a relatively new state formed in 2002. It has a population of 27 million, with more than 90% living in rural areas. State wide, the literacy rate is only 54%. In terms of health indicators, the total fertility rate is 3.3, and contraceptive prevalence is 36%, with 8% of women using a spacing method (IIPS, Macro 2007). In India, female sterilization has long been the backbone of the official family planning program.

Figure 4. Components of Expandnet/WHO Framework

"CORRECT"

The innovation refers to the health service interventions that are being scaled up, or to other new practices such as community or school based interventions that are being introduced. Attributes of a successful innovation can be summarized in the acronym,

Credible
Observable
Relevant
Relative Advantage
Easy to install
Compatible
Testable

Prior to the decision to scale-up SDM, IRH and the Ministry of Health (MOH) conducted a pilot project in Jharkhand to introduce SDM in limited areas of one district. Since 2007, under the FABM Project, IRH has been working to expand family planning options by scaling up access to SDM with a focus on public sector programs in the state of Jharkhand. IRH has a memorandum of understanding with the state government through which the government is committing funds to SDM scale-up, in addition to considerable in-kind support.

The remaining of this article will examine SDM scale-up in Jharkhand through the lens of the ExpandNet model.

The Innovation

It is useful to apply the "CORRECT" acronym (see box above) to the innovation you are seeking to scale-up to identify any areas of concern which will need to be addressed during scale-up. Credibility of the innovation is critical to scale-up. IRH continually shares evidence on the efficacy of SDM, but provider attitudes tend to be more influenced by personal experience, or even lack of experience in offering the method. The use of CycleBeads as a mnemonic device contributes to the scalability of SDM by providing concrete, observable evidence of NFP introduction, something less evident with other fertility awareness-based methods. In the case of SDM, policy makers and users in Jharkhand recognize that it is relevant given the high use of ineffective, traditional methods, and presents a relative advantage to methods frequently relied upon, such as periodic abstinence or withdrawal. With regards to the ease of SDM introduction, there are differing opinions. While introducing the SDM does not require any special equipment or clinical training, good quality services do require strong counseling centered on women's needs—not a strength of the health system in Jharkhand. While users find SDM compatible with existing abstinence practices, it is not compatible with the India family planning program's traditional emphasis on permanent methods. Prior operations research on SDM in India has demonstrated that it is testable, and evaluation efforts continue during the scale-up process.

Although SDM is at the core, the innovation which is being scaled up in India is a comprehensive package consisting of CycleBeads, the accompanying low-literacy Hindi insert, simple provider training and job aids, awareness raising and efforts to engage men in SDM use. As stated earlier, according to the definition of scale-up, innovations must first be tested before they are expanded. SDM is an evidence based practice, successfully tested in a pilot-project in Jharkhand in addition to other areas of India and worldwide. Nevertheless, scaling-up conditions are often different than pilot project conditions. In a pilot project, researchers and programmers are typically able to devote more resources to a concentrated area. Such intensity is often not possible during scale-up, and therefore, the innovation may need to be adapted to scale-up conditions. For example, as IRH and partners started planning the scale-up process, we realized that the training curriculum used during the pilot in Jharkhand needed to be condensed to fit into the amount of time available for training. Also, it was necessary to revise materials for lower-literacy providers and clients. Therefore, we adapted the materials and evaluated their use in part of the state prior to further expansion.

Scaling up is an ongoing process of developing and testing approaches to facilitate expansion, ownership and sustainability. Community radio broadcasts and social marketing of CycleBeads were not part of the pilot project in Jharkhand but were introduced during the scale-up phase as promising strategies to expand access to SDM. These new initiatives were piloted to ensure that they were appropriate and effective.

Resource Team

Scaling up differs from routine program implementation; it requires more attention than established services. The resource team is a dedicated team that plans and supports the scale-up of innovations tested in pilot projects. The resource team will usually include multiple organizations which enhances its credibility and effectiveness. A multi-organizational team will be more effective at leveraging resources for scale-up and maintaining consistency in messaging across organizations. Their involvement creates a sense of ownership among the organizations that will have to sustain implementation of the innovation and contributes their valuable knowledge and skills to the process of scaling up.

It can be challenging, however, to form such a team, given the nature of funding which encourages vertical programming and institutional competition for limited resources. In Jharkhand, the resource team is primarily composed of IRH and the MOH, although the MOH is not capable of managing scale-up on its own at this point and relies on the technical support of IRH. Other TA groups are involved to a limited extent, participating in periodic partner meetings, offering input, and integrating NFP into their own initiatives. Ideally, more partners would be actively involved in the resource team, though Jharkhand being a relatively new state lacks family planning institutions and organizations.

User organization

In the ExpandNet framework, the user organization refers to the institutions or organizations that seek to adopt and implement the innovation. The Government of Jharkhand, encompassing the MOH as well as other government departments that oversee social welfare initiatives (and maintain a cadre of community health workers), is the primary user organization as we strive to integrate SDM into public sector health facilities and programs in scale-up districts. During the scale-up process, the goal is for some members of the user organization(s) to become part of the resource team. Therefore, we are working to build the capacity of the MOH not only to offer the method as part of public sector services, but also to serve as a resource organization to other groups who wish to include SDM in their program.

Benefits to working with the Government of Jharkhand include the fact that the government brings significant financial resources to the table and has committed funding to provider training and production of IEC materials. Since the government is by far the biggest health providing organization in the state, its inclusion is essential. One of the challenges to working with the government, however, is the need for intensive coordination at all levels of the state system, including the block, district and central levels. In addition, some elements of the health program are controlled by the national government, so coordination and advocacy in Delhi is necessary also.

Environment

The environment, including social, political, and other factors, has a major effect on scaling up. The environment in Jharkhand is very dynamic and requires persistence and flexibility. The state government changed twice in 2009/2010, requiring doubled efforts to create a common vision, and commitment to on-going SDM integration efforts. Likewise, provider turnover requires that incoming staff be continually trained in SDM counseling. While turnover affects other services as well, it is particularly an issue for an "innovation" that is not already well established.

In order to respond to frequent changes in governments and government officials, advocacy efforts are intensive and ongoing. Decisions and resource commitments obtained after months of negotiation can be reversed overnight when personnel changes. In addition, although the environment in Jharkhand is supportive of SDM, it is highly influenced by the central level government, which does not see SDM as contributing to their long term goals. Furthermore, because Jharkhand is a new state, key institutions and capacity have not yet been established. For example, there is no state institute for health training that can take on the function of SDM training although many of the health providers and program managers are inexperienced and require substantial capacity building. In addition, family planning, especially birth spacing methods, is not a priority of the health system at this time, which means that resources and political commitment for SDM integration are limited, as they are for all family planning initiatives.

There are advantages to working in a new state, however. The piloting and roll out of new systems can provide opportunities for integration and scale-up. For example, over the last few years, Jharkhand has been involved in identifying and training a large cadre of new community level providers (over 60,000). IRH is working closely with the government to include SDM in their responsibilities and training. Finally, other environmental factors such as natural disasters and political unrest significantly influence the pace of scale-up. There is an ongoing separatist Maoist movement in Jharkhand that limits our ability to mobilize in particular areas, causing last minute cancellations of trainings and meetings.

Strategy/Approaches

The scaling up strategy designates the means by which the innovation is communicated, disseminated, transferred or otherwise promoted. In Jharkhand, for example, we are working with the MOH to scale up SDM in phases. We started in three districts and have added more districts each year. We are currently working in twelve districts, which represent half of the districts in the state. To build capacity within the MOH, we utilize a cascade training approach, training outstanding MOH providers as master trainers who then train other MOH staff at the district level. We have also worked with the MOH to develop a supportive supervision strategy and a quality assurance strategy that includes regular provider knowledge checks and client follow up. We have also provided assistance to the MOH in developing and disseminating provider job aids and client materials, and ensuring that CycleBeads reach service delivery sites.

In Jharkhand and in other areas of India, we are testing new strategies to teach health workers how to offer SDM as well as to inform the public about the method. The need to reach large numbers of people with limited resources has led to the development of innovative strategies including the use of satellite teaching, distance learning, e-learning (on line), mobile health technologies and paper images of CycleBeads as tear-outs in women's magazines.

Monitoring and Evaluation

Why measure? One reason for measurement is that it is required for reporting purposes. This is important to maintain a flow of resources for scaling up. However, there are more important reasons for measurement, namely, to improve the program and maximize the impact of the innovation. Monitoring the scale-up process is more complex than measuring routine reporting indicators; in fact, it is not possible to manage scale-up using only routine reporting indicators. It is important to monitor key sub/systems processes/outcomes. Measurement

Figure 5

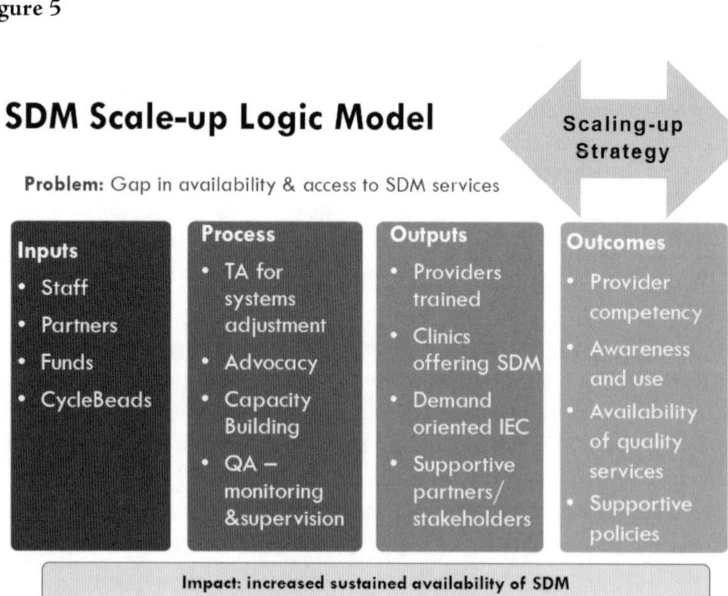

for scale-up is further complicated by the fact that at different stages of scaling up (i.e., as we reach certain milestones in the process), we will need different kinds of information about the functioning of the system. Early on, as we are refining the innovation, we may need more types of information, such as verification that the refinements made to the innovation achieve the desired effects. As the innovation goes to scale, we will need to monitor expansion and institutionalization. As the innovation becomes established, routine performance monitoring of process and outcomes is needed.

A logic model is a useful tool for monitoring and evaluation of scale-up. In the logic model above (Figure 5), the inputs, or resources, invested into scaling up SDM in Jharkhand include IRH's staff, partners (the most important being the MOH in this case) funds, and CycleBeads. The processes describe the role of IRH staff in scale-up, which include providing technical assistance for integrating SDM into training and health management systems, advocating for appropriate inclusion of SDM, building the capacity of providers and health systems to offer the method and conducting quality assurance through supportive supervision. Outputs are the activities undertaken through the scale-up process, such as training providers; offering SDM in clinics, engaging in IEC activities to generate awareness and demand for SDM, and building support for the method among partners and stakeholders. Outcomes show the expected changes or benefits that will result from scaling up SDM: more competent providers, greater awareness of SDM and increased use of the method, availability of quality services and inclusion into norms and policies. The impact of successful scale-up of SDM in Jharkhand will be the sustained availability of SDM through the government health system in the state.

While the MOH is greatly contributing to SDM scale-up efforts now, our goal is for the process to continue even after the institution providing technical assistance has left the picture. Therefore, the process must become fully entrenched into the service delivery system so as to protect against inevitable provider and MOH leadership turnover. At the same time, MOH personnel must become fully invested in including SDM in their program and take on ownership of the scale-up process.

To monitor expansion and institutionalization, IRH has developed monitoring indicators and end-of-project benchmarks. Establishing the benchmarks was a lengthy process, involving discussion with partners coupled with a realistic appraisal of what could actually be accomplished. With these benchmarks, we are able to track progress over time. IRH monitors the scaling up process through benchmark tables that are updated quarterly (see Table 1 below). Goals are adjusted annually, and the resource team adjusts its work plan as needed. The table below summarizes the extent of SDM access and institutionalization in Jharkhand achieved so far. These tables are based on the ExpandNet framework and are organized by horizontal and vertical scaling up indicators. Examples of horizontal scale-up indicators include:

- Proportion of service delivery points (SDPs) that include SDM as part of the method mix
- Estimated number of individuals trained to counsel clients in SDM (IRH-supported).
- Some examples of vertical scale-up indicators are:
- SDM included in essential or key policies, norms, guidelines, and protocols
- Presence of public or private training organizations that include SDM in pre-service training and/or continuing education.

The benchmark tables include indicators to track progress on activities associated with all elements of the ExpandNet framework. For example, an environment indicator tracks whether SDM is included in essential policies, norms, guidelines, and protocols. To gauge status of scaling up within user organizations, IRH tracks the number of public or private training organizations that include SDM in pre-service training, in service, and/or continuing education. To track success of the scaling up strategy, for example, IRH monitors the inclusion of SDM in IEC activities, materials and mass media, such as posters, street theater, radio spots, and flyers. Finally, service statistics are periodically aggregated from the respective national health information systems to monitor changes in demand for SDM compared to other FP methods available in-country.

In Jharkhand, data collection has included service statistics, household surveys, facility assessments, in-depth provider/stakeholder interviews, Most Significant Change (MSC) story collection and process tracking. The ExpandNet model grounded development of our methodology and facilitated operationalization of the scale-up concept through ten critical indicators of scale-up and developed a simple annual process to monitor benchmarks. In the course of integrating

SDM into 12 districts in Jharkhand, the India team, including IRH and the MOH, has learned how to utilize routinely gathered monitoring information to evaluate progress and adapt the scaling-up intervention. Data from training programs, MOH service statistics, application of a Knowledge Improvement Tool (KIT) to assess provider competency, and client follow-up data are regularly collected and analyzed at the district level. Results are shared monthly and quarterly with MOH officials at the district and state level.

Table 1. Monitoring Performance Benchmarks

Monitoring Performance Benchmarks – India, Jharkhand

Selected Indicators	(as of 6/10)
VERTICAL	
No. of resource organizations	3 of 8
SDM included in key policies, norms, protocols	2 of 2
SDM in pre-service training	In process
Commodities in logistics & procurement systems	Partially
SDM in IEC materials	6 of 9
SDM in HMIS	In process
FAM in surveys (DHS)	No
Funds leveraged for FAM	$360,000
HORIZONTAL	
Proportion of SDPs with FAM in method mix	38%
Providers trained	5,700 of 15,000

CONCLUSIONS: SCALING UP CONSIDERATIONS FOR NFP PROGRAMS

IRH has found the ExpandNet framework to be an invaluable tool in helping us to strategize and plan for sustainable scale-up. The framework has a great deal to offer, and our experience with SDM in Jharkhand is just one example of how it can be applied. NFP groups, whether in the U.S. or abroad, may find the framework useful as well. Table 2 below presents some questions related to scale-up process and outcome which may be useful to consider during the expansion process.

Process	
Resource team	Do user organizations assume the roles, responsibilities and ownership of the resource team during scale-up process?
Advocacy & dissemination	What strategies work best? What is the role of NFP champions?
Organizational choices	Is NFP offered in a variety of settings (e.g. faith based, private, public)?
Outcomes	
Clients	What is the experience of couples with NFP when scaled-up? (Knowledge, attitudes and use)
Service provision	Is NFP offered correctly?
System integration	To what extent has NFP been integrated into training, IEC, procurement and distribution, and HMIS? Is it included in norms, protocols and guidelines?
Resource mobilization	What is the level of resources dedicated to NFP?

Successful scale-up calls for careful planning, a systems approach, and evidence-based practices. Based on its experiences thus far, IRH has learned a number of important lessons regarding NFP scale-up.

- Replicate the essential features of the successful pilot when scaling up: these include careful planning based on research, adopting a systems approach, partnering with relevant organizations, involving diverse stakeholders, working with different cadres of providers, and communicating needed data to policymakers.
- Assessments prior to and throughout the process of scaling up are critical to identify needed adjustments and course corrections in the new sites, maintain momentum and accountability, and build strategic planning skills among stakeholders.
- To best evaluate outcomes, it is important to understand the characteristics of the healthcare delivery system and

operationally define indicators for access to the new FP method and its integration into the health system.

- Research, monitoring and evaluation are crucial to successful scale-up. Involving multiple partners increases their commitment and builds their research skills.
- Balancing research and programmatic needs is important as is producing relevant, timely data for stakeholders with diverse needs.
- Additional resources (i.e. financing, human resources, and time) are needed for scaling up an innovation as compared to the resources needed for routine service provision. These scale-up resources are often overlooked by donors and participating organizations alike.

SOURCES CONSULTED

Arévalo, M. et al. 2001. "Efficacy of a new method of family planning: the Standard Days Method.®" *Contraception* 65: 333-338.

ExpandNet, World Health Organization. 2009. *Practical guidance for scaling up health service innovations*. Geneva: World Health Organization.

Fixsen, D., S. F. Naoom, K. A. Blasé et al. 2005. *Implementation Research: A Synthesis of the Literature*. University of South Florida, Louis de la Parte Florida Mental Health Institute, The National Implementation Research Network (FMHI Publication #231).

Greenhalgh, T., G. Robert, F. MacFarlane, P. Bete, O. Kyriakidou. 2004. "Diffusion of innovation in service organizations, systematic review and recommendation." *Milbank Quarterly* 82: 281-629.

Gribble, J. et al. 2008. "Being strategic about contraceptive introduction: the experience of the Standard Days Method.®" *Contraception* 77: 147-154.

International Institute for Population Sciences (IIPS) and Macro International. 2007. *National Family Health Survey (NFHS-3), 2005–06*. India: Volume I. Mumbai: IIPS.

Madon, T. et al. 2007. "Implementation Science." *Science Magazine* (December 14 2007) 318: 1728-1729.

Rogers, E. M. 1995. *Diffusion of innovations*. 4th ed. New York: Free Press.

Simmons, R., P. Fajans, L. Ghiron. Eds. 2007. *Scaling up health service delivery: from pilot innovations to policies and programmes*. Geneva: World Health Organization.

PART II

Faith & Culture

13

An Anthropology of Love: Caritas in Veritate

MARY SHIVANANDAN, STD

Professor of Theology, John Paul II Institute for Studies on Marriage and the Family at The Catholic University of America, Washington, DC

ABSTRACT

This paper examines the interconnection between philosophical and theological ideas on love, marriage, and the human person and scientific discoveries of human fertility. The Catholic Church holds that there can be no contradiction between reason and faith because God is the author of both revealed truth and the truths discovered by human reason in the created world. While faulty theories of biology have distorted the truth of the human person and marriage in the past, the new more complete discoveries of human fertility have brought new insights into the nature of man and woman, procreation, and the bond of spousal and maternal love. Three philosopher/theologians have been at the forefront of developing a theology to meet the challenges of new discoveries of human fertility in the 20th century, which for the first time enable couples to consciously achieve or avoid pregnancy. Dietrich von Hildebrand, influenced by the phenomenology of Edmund Husserl, analyzes marital love in the light of new thinking on the subjectivity of the person. It is not enough to view conjugal sex simply from its procreative end. It has an intrinsic human value from the fulfillment it brings, which in the case of wedded love he calls *supervalue response*. The intensity of the sex act, which is always in danger of overwhelming the spiritual dimensions of the person, finds its fulfillment in a total mutual self-surrender of the whole of life in the sight of God. Karol Wojtyla/John Paul II continues the emphasis on total mutual self gift in marriage, developing what is called the *logic of the gift* from God's creation of the world out of love and man and woman's imaging of the mutual self-giving of the divine Persons in the Trinity. He finds in the body itself "anticipated signs of the gift." Pope Benedict XVI proposes for the first time that the Church's teaching on human life and love has a pivotal role to play in society and human development not least because it brings to the public square the concept of the human person as fundamentally ordered to relation and not simply an autonomous individual, with consequences for all human activity.

INTRODUCTION

The first part of this paper will consider the unity of faith and science, showing how the Catholic Church holds that there can be no contradiction between them. It will go on to show how different scientific theories influence philosophical and theological accounts of the human person, procreation, gender, and vice versa. The newer, more complete discoveries in the 20th century, by challenging traditional scientific, philosophical, and theological interpretations of marriage and procreation, have contributed to a great development in the theology of marriage. The second part of the paper will briefly outline the theological anthropologies of three philosopher/theologians at the forefront of these new developments.

THE UNITY OF SCIENCE AND FAITH

In the modern era, science and faith are often perceived as opposed to one another. The scientific community recalls the Church's condemnation of Galileo and theologians are troubled by what they call "scientific universalism" or the tendency of contemporary science to absolutize the scientific method to the exclusion of other methods of accessing truth. Pope Benedict XVI describes this as considering only "the kind of certainty resulting from the interplay of mathematical and empirical elements. … By its very nature it excludes the question of God, making it appear an unscientific or pre-scientific question" (Benedict XVI 2006, "Faith, Reason and the University," no. 5). This dichotomy was not always the case. In an earlier era, science and faith worked hand in hand in search of truth. A major reason for this happy collaboration was that science (*scientia*) referred to everything constituting rational thought, not only facts about nature and its internal laws, but deductive judgments of philosophy and theological reason. It implied a study of the respective nature of actual beings according to the formal object of the specific science. The formal object of theology is God, of philosophy Being, and of the physical sciences the phenomena of nature (Aquinas 1945, *S.T.*, Q. 1:1). In this view, scientific reasoning arrives at truth from the conformity of its reasoning to the object under consideration (*adaequatio intellectus et rei*).[1] The certitude claimed is that of scientific judgment, which is based on its agreement with other judgments and on the facts themselves. Scientific judgments or the judgments of reason apply as much to the practice of philosophy and theology as to the physical sciences. The trend in the modern era to exclude from the domain of science all but observed phenomena, has driven a wedge between truths acquired by the modern scientific method and by faith. There is no room for a God who reveals objective truths about himself and the world.

Thomas Aquinas

At the beginning of his monumental *Summa Theologica* on the nature of God, man, and the cosmos, Thomas Aquinas explains why revelation is necessary. Although many truths even about God himself can be discovered from creation through reason, these truths would be known only by a few after a long time and with the admixture of many errors (Aquinas 1945, *S.T.*, Q1:1). Secondly, men and women have an eternal destiny, which can only be known through revelation. The *Summa Theologica* is itself a masterly integration of the truths of Aristotelian science and philosophy with Christian faith. In fact that was Thomas's great work, according to Pope Benedict. He was not afraid to encounter the pre-Christian culture of Aristotle with its "radical rationality." He created a synthesis, showing how they belonged together. "What seemed to be reason incompatible with faith was not reason, and what seemed to be faith was not faith, in so far as it was opposed to true rationality" (Benedict XVI 2010, "General Audience," no. 2). Pope Benedict XVI credits Aquinas especially with showing the natural harmony between Christian faith and reason and bringing about the rapprochement between biblical faith and Greek philosophical inquiry. He considers this integration to be of "decisive importance not only from the standpoint of the history of religions, but also from that of world history" (Benedict XVI 2006, "Faith, Reason and the University," no. 3). There can be no contradiction between faith and reason, since the author of creation and revelation is one and the same God.

The Church has continued to take this position even when it was challenged by the rise of Cartesian dualism and the explosion of scientific discoveries in the 19th and 20th centuries. Both the First and Second Vatican Councils have reaffirmed the compatibility between reason and faith.. For example, the First Vatican Council states:

> The same holy mother, the Church, holds and teaches that God, the source and end of all things, can be known with certainty from the consideration of created things by the natural power of human reason: ever since the creation of the world, his invisible nature has been perceived in the things that have been made. It was, however, pleasing to his wisdom and goodness to reveal himself and the eternal laws of his will to the human race by another, and that a supernatural way ... it is, indeed, thanks to this divine revelation, that those matters concerning God which are not of themselves beyond the scope of human reason, can, even in the present state of the human race, be known by everyone without difficulty, with firm certitude and with no intermingling of error. It is not because of this that one must hold revelation to be absolutely necessary; the reason is that God directed human beings to a supernatural end, that is a sharing in the good things of God that utterly surpasses the understanding of the human mind. (*Dogmatic Constitution on the Catholic Faith*, nos. 13-15; the Second Vatican Council fathers echo this statement in *Dei Verbum*, no. 6)

JOHN PAUL II AND KNOWLEDGE AS ENCOUNTER

Above all, their unity was taken up by John Paul II in his encyclical, *Fides et Ratio* (*Faith and Reason*, hereafter FR), where he states that the "unity of truth is a fundamental premise of human reasoning, as the principle of noncontradiction makes clear. Revelation renders this unity certain, showing that the God of creation is also the God of Salvation History" (FR, nos. 34 and 9). In explaining the reasonableness of faith, John Paul II points out that more truths are simply believed than acquired by personal verification. This is as true in the field of science as of faith. "In believing we entrust ourselves to the knowledge acquired by other people" (FR, no. 31). Therefore, all knowledge involves an interpersonal relationship, entrusting oneself to another. The truths of faith and reason both meet in the human person and depend on his capacity both to know and to entrust himself to another.

In his interpretation of the text of Genesis, which gives a theological account of the creation of man, it is significant that John Paul II begins with the text, "'It is not good that man [male] 'should be alone; I want to make him a help similar to himself'" (Gen 2:18). The starting point is one directly concerned with relationship or the lack thereof (John Paul II 2006, *Man and Woman*, no. 5:2). It is within the context of relationship that man comes to knowledge of himself and the world. Knowledge comes through an encounter with objective reality, whether the cosmos, himself or another human being. Angelo Scola has developed most fully the nature of knowledge as encounter (Scola 2005, pp. 224-227). He has coined the term "symbolic ontology" to capture the fact that being cannot be grasped directly by man. It does not mean that man cannot touch the real itself through intuition but the real communicates itself in a sign to form concepts. This encounter constitutes an event. Man must choose it in freedom, but the thing always remains other. This otherness or difference allows for relationship and encounter. Sexual difference is a primary form of otherness. John Paul II emphasizes that knowledge comes by way of experience, our ordinary human experiences. The appeal to experience is fundamental because man is a body. He goes so far as to say that "our experience is in some way a legitimate means for theological interpretation" (John Paul II 2006, *Man and Woman*, no. 4: 4, 5 and fn. 8). Although faith and science are two distinct disciplines, they meet in the human person and his experience.

John Paul II summarizes his argument as follows. It is the nature of the human person to seek truth, not just partial truths from empirical or scientific evidence or the true good in individual acts of decision-making. The person looks for an ultimate truth that would explain the meaning of life. The search can only end in "reaching the absolute," as the ancient philosophers concluded. But the search for truth also needs trust and friendship, which was well accepted by these philosophers. Therefore, there is both "a search for truth and a search for a person to whom they might entrust themselves." Christian faith offers Jesus Christ, both true God and true man. Through the order of grace Christ offers participation in divine mysteries and coherent knowledge of the Triune God. Through his humanity, the goodness of the order of creation is confirmed. There can be no contradiction between the order of faith and the order of reason, both of which are united in the person of Christ. In entrusting themselves to the person of Jesus, believers find a *fullness* of truth not available to reason alone (FR, no. 33).

Especially important in the Genesis text is the use of the verb "know" for conjugal relations. It means first of all that the biblical text raises the level of the conjugal act from the merely biological to the personal. Secondly, in the biblical understanding of "know" there are two aspects, intentionality and the reality of the union in one flesh. Both the husband and the wife know each other reciprocally and by doing so discover the depths of their own specific "I." Each is known as an "*unrepeatable feminine or masculine 'I'*" (John Paul II 2006, *Man and Woman*, no. 20:5). This reciprocal knowledge, he says, "establishes a kind of personal archetype of human bodiliness and sexuality" (John Paul II 2006, no. 21:1). He goes on to say that

> the 'man' who for the first time 'knows' the woman, his wife, in the act of conjugal union is in fact the same one who—in giving names, that is, also, by 'knowing'—differentiated himself from the whole world of living beings or *animalia*, thus affirming himself as a person and a subject (John Paul II 2006, *Man and Woman*, no. 21:1).

Canadian philosopher, Kenneth Schmitz has brought out well the relational dimension of knowledge not just of one human being to another but of things in themselves in a metaphysics of being. "Knowledge," he says, "is precisely the relation in and through which we come to know things as they are in their own being" (Schmitz 2008, p. 11). By being intelligible to man, things are rendered explicit in themselves. This makes them available for a relationship in which they retain their own integrity. In giving themselves they also affirm their identity (Schmitz 2008, p. 11). According to David Schindler, "Knowing at root is but the distinctly cognitive manner of participating in the relations of love and beauty implicit in an ontology of creation" (Schindler 1999, p. 527). He proposes that "knowledge is first and foremost a matter of relation, the order of which is disclosed in the creation of all things by and in the triune God revealed in Jesus Christ" (Schindler 1999, p. 527). In love the subject discovers the self in relation first to the Other who gives himself together with the gift of the world. The relationship with God is primary. Therefore there is a priority of the 'objective' as already given as a gift of God and the world. "What this means," says Schindler, "is that knowledge takes its first and most basic order from within relation or relationship defined by love and beauty, which originates in submission of the self to the other (God and all others in God)" (Schindler 1999, p. 527).

It is clear then from these fundamental biblical texts that: the search for truth about God, the world and man himself takes place only in interpersonal relationship; and through the conjugal act, man comes to the truth about himself and his creation in love. The search for truth by science and faith cannot be separated because they both meet in the human person who is a unity of body and soul. Furthermore the human person is made for love, especially the fundamental love between man and woman in marriage. Both science and faith are necessary for an anthropology of love.

INTERACTION BETWEEN SCIENTIFIC THEORIES OF REPRODUCTION AND PHILOSOPHY/THEOLOGY

In the past, inadequate and/or incorrect scientific explanations of biological facts have contributed to faulty interpretations of the nature of the human person, fertility, and gender, with detrimental effects on both theology and philosophy. In its turn theology has continually reflected on scientific discoveries and theories, keeping in mind the dignity of the human person and marriage. Before the 18th century, when modern scientific methods were applied to the study of biology, two theories predominated on the process of conception in the human being.

Aristotle & Aquinas

Aristotle hypothesized from his study of animals and his philosophic theory of potency and act that the male provided the seed and the female the matter. It was from the male that the new human being took its soul or form, while the female only provided the matter. Furthermore, the only way a female could be conceived was if there were some defect in the male seed/form, so in essence the female was a defective male (McLaren 1984, p. 16; see also Allen 1997, pp. 95-102). It is not hard to imagine what effect this may have on the philosophic understanding of masculinity and femininity. Aquinas struggled to make this congruent with revealed truth on the equal dignity of man and woman as image of God. His commentary on the Letter to the Ephesians is a good illustration of difficulties in interpreting the biblical text in light of the sex polarity inherited from Aristotle (see Aquinas 1966, pp. 216-217).

Hippocrates & Galen

The other theory put forth by Hippocrates and taken up by Galen in the 2nd century AD was that both the man and the woman provided the seed. Furthermore, in order for conception to take place sexual pleasure was necessary to provide the stimulus to activate the process. Since both shared in the process and sexual pleasure was necessary for both, it resulted in a greater equality between the sexes, at least in this one area, in marriage (McLaren 1984, pp. 17, 18-20).[2] The effects of this theory are evident in the way marriage was lived among Protestants (Puritans included) and among Catholic moralists, who regarded procreation as the end of marriage. The view that Puritan couples expected to enjoy friendship, affection and sexual pleasure within marriage is confirmed by secular historians John D'Emilio and Estelle B. Freedman (see D'Emilio and Freedman 1989, p. 16). It must be noted that Aquinas, following Aristotle's *Ethics* had legitimated sexual pleasure in marriage in a more explicit way than St. Augustine, so that the Council of Trent in 1546 declared that concupiscence was the "germ" of sin but not in itself sinful (Gardella 1985, p. 13). The American bishop Francis Patrick Kenrick in his discussion of desire in his *Theologiae Moralis* wrote: "There are some more severe philosophers who reject all enjoyment, but, as St. Thomas [Aquinas] said, they counsel badly." He also argued that consent to passion resulting from a good act, was itself another good act (Gardella 1985, p. 12). This belies conventional wisdom that an appreciation for sexual pleasure in marriage originated in the 18th century. The opposite may, in fact, be more accurate with regard to the role of woman and sexual pleasure.

Modern Theories of Conception

A change came at the beginning of the 19th century when medical science applied the new experimental methods to embryology. Both the role of the sperm and the ovum in conception were discovered, along with the fact that sexual pleasure in the female was not necessary for conception (McLaren 1984, pp. 23, 26, 27). This discovery, when coupled with cultural forces of the time, led to the unforeseen consequence of assigning a passive role to the female. As one historian commented, "the medical literature depicts a change from the sexually active woman of the seventeenth century to the passionless creature of the nineteenth" (McLaren 1984, p. 27).

From these examples it can be seen how scientific theories of human conception interact with philosophical and theological concepts of the nature of man and woman and marriage. Not surprisingly, new discoveries in the 20th century, especially of the reproductive hormones in fertility, had equally profound effects on philosophical and theological concepts of love and marriage. It is noteworthy here how many of the medical researchers, such as Doctors John and Evelyn Billings, were motivated by their Catholic faith. John Billings, a neurologist, was asked to assist married couples coming for instruction in fertility regulation at a Catholic Marriage Guidance Center in Melbourne, Australia in 1953. Together with his wife, Evelyn, he devoted the rest of his medical career to developing the Ovulation Method of Natural Family Planning (Shivanandan 1999, pp. 279-280). Because so much attention has been paid to the Church's opposition to contraception, little attention has been given outside the Church to the challenges posed by these new discoveries to the theology of marriage within the Church.

For the first time in history, with the development of the natural methods of family planning, couples are able to monitor their fertility accurately and make a conscious decision whether to conceive a child or not through periodic abstinence. New questions arose: "Is this legitimate? What now are the respective roles of love and procreation in marriage?" One of the first manuals published on the Rhythm Method devoted Part III to the ethical aspects. It begins with the questions: "Is it wrong to take advantage of the rhythm of sterility and fertility, to practice a natural method of birth control? What does the Pope say?" Out of forty pages dealing with ethics, only six refer to the illicitness of contraception. The rest are all concerned with the licitness of Rhythm (Latz 1932, pp. 110-151). To this day heated debates continue on these very issues.

As a result, the 20th century has seen the greatest development of the theology of marriage since the high Middle Ages and that is thanks, in part, to the new and more accurate understanding of fertility achieved by modern science. Three philosopher/theologians have been at the forefront of grappling with these challenges and for the remainder of this article I shall outline the key contribution of each.

AN ENRICHED ANTHROPOLOGY OF LOVE

Dietrich von Hildebrand

Dietrich von Hildebrand, a German Catholic philosopher, brought to bear the phenomenological method of Edmund Husserl and Max Scheler to an investigation of love and marriage. His first book on the subject, with the seemingly paradoxical title, *In Defense of Purity*, was published in English in 1931. It was not, in his own words, a defense of purity and virginity "against his detractors" but a study of what constitutes "the complete virtue of purity" (von Hildebrand 1970, p. v). The decisive factor for purity, whether in virginity or marriage, is the person. In other words, without understanding the nature of the person and love, neither Christian marriage nor virginity can be understood.

THE NATURE OF PURITY

Von Hildebrand begins by distinguishing between the sexual appetites and other appetites of the body such as eating and drinking. These appetites remain on the surface, whereas sexual desire reaches to man's deepest being and overflows into the psychological and spiritual spheres. Here the body and soul meet in a singular fashion. His purpose is to argue for the significance of conjugal sex beyond its biological end of procreation. As a phenomenologist he takes into account the *experience* of physical sex as providing a fullness of completion. It has a significance for man *as such*, not just as the propagator of the species. Such an attitude was challenging to the Catholic theologians and canonists in the 1920s. Equally challenging to sexologists such as Havelock Ellis[3] was his contention that only in wedded love between a man and a woman is the meaning of sex as intimate mutual self-donation and self-revelation to be truly found (von Hildebrand 1970, p. 12).

He is emphatic that the love between a man and a woman is not a sublimation of the sex instinct. Love can be understood without any reference to sex. Wedded love itself does not depend on the physical aspect. What distinguishes it from other forms of love is the particular completion between the man and the woman that takes place in the conjugal act. Wedded sex can only be understood from above;

otherwise the ultimate significance is lost (von Hildebrand 1970, pp. 7, 9-10). Von Hildebrand notes intrinsic dangers to marital love stemming from the intensity of the sex act itself. It is as it were the "awakening of corporeal nature." The spirit is exposed to being "swamped" by the convulsive nature of the sex act, tending to drag it into the domain of the body. There are two senses in which the person can be carried away and lose possession of himself, one in spite of himself and the other by deliberately throwing himself away in the heat of the moment. To do so in the sex act without a corresponding giving away of oneself in the spiritual sphere is to risk flinging away one's very existence. There needs to be a more powerful spiritual experience, fully anchored in God, which sanctions the flinging away of self, and which paradoxically ends in finding oneself. This legitimation occurs in marriage (von Hildebrand 1970, pp. 61-65).

There are two attitudes that essentially belong to wedded love, first the desire to "share in the *being* of the other, not just in his or her life and thoughts" (von Hildebrand 1970, p. 67) and secondly the surrender of oneself to the other for the whole of life, a giving over that must take place in the sight of God. Only such love can transform the conjugal act into one that is truly pure. "Wedded love alone," says von Hildebrand, "holds ... the key, which by realizing it, can unlock the significance of sex as an experience and reveal to the person its true positive aspect" von Hildebrand 1970, pp. 68, 69).

Published in German in 1927, von Hildebrand's *In Defense of Purity* had a profound effect on Pope Pius XI, at a time when the Church was faced with widespread advocacy of contraception in the name of marital love. When the worldwide gathering of Anglican bishops met in England at Lambeth Palace in 1930 and endorsed the limited use of contraception in marriage, Pius XI issued a papal encyclical. The encyclical, *Casti Connubii*, reaffirmed the Church's ban on the use of contraception in marriage for any reason. This encyclical was binding on all Roman Catholics. While the language of the encyclical was traditional in style, referring to marriage as a contract rather than a covenant, there is one paragraph, which confounded many in the Church since it advanced what was referred to as a "personalist" view of marriage.

> This mutual inward molding of husband and wife, this determined effort to perfect each other, can in a very real sense, as the Roman Catechism teaches, be said to be the chief reason and purpose of

> matrimony provided matrimony be looked at not in the restricted sense as instituted for the proper conception and education of the child, but more widely as the blending of life as a whole and the mutual interchange and sharing thereof (*Casti Connubii*, no. 14).

This paragraph was left out of the translation copyrighted in 1951 by the National Catholic Welfare Association of the United States (now the United States Conference of Catholic Bishops) perhaps to forestall any interpretation that procreation was no longer considered the primary end of marriage (Shivanandan1999, p. 199, fn76). *Casti Connubii* was first published in German as *Die Ehe*. Dietrich von Hildebrand draws attention to this paragraph in a book for the general public he later wrote on marriage, which was published in English in 1942. In the preface to the English edition, von Hildebrand notes how his ideas brought about an increased stress on the role of love in Christian marriage in Italy and France in the years between the wars (von Hildebrand 1991, pp. vi, vii).

PERSONALISM AND MARITAL LOVE

In all his writings on ethics and marriage, von Hildebrand contrasted the philosophy of personalism, which emphasizes the spiritual nature of man in a unity of body and soul, with biological materialism, which views man as simply a superior animal. The notion of "subjectivity" (or *Eigenleben*) is central to von Hildebrand's ethics of personalism. The interest in the objective good for persons is not the whole of the moral life. The subjective element, affirming the value in the objective good is necessary. Such an affirmation is called a value response. Von Hildebrand discerns three kinds of value: the subjectively satisfying; the objectively good in itself; and the objectively good for the person or the beneficial good (von Hildebrand 2009, p. xvii).[4] It is the nature of the person to transcend himself in seeking the value or good in an object. Von Hildebrand further distinguishes two kinds of persons, those who bend to themselves what is merely subjectively satisfying in the object, and those who live by value response. A value is revealed as value precisely through its capacity to give delight. It can be both objectively good in itself and a beneficial good for me. Love is a "super-value response" because in love each becomes objectively good, a delight, for the other. The lover wills to be the source of happiness for the beloved and also to receive from her his deepest happiness. What constitutes love as super-value response is the lover's self-giving. In a relationship that is merely subjectively satisfying, the person bends the other to his own benefit without giving himself in return (von Hildebrand 2009, pp. xvi, xxiv, xxv). This articulation of love as super-value response enabled von Hildebrand to give full value to the reciprocal self-giving at the heart of marriage, expressed in ecstatic sexual union, while at the same time, distinguishing it from what is merely subjectively satisfying, the pursuit of sex for its own sake.

John Paul II & the Logic of the Gift

While von Hildebrand wished to stress the spiritual dimension of the conjugal union, raising it to the level of the person from the merely biological, John Paul II sought to discover how the body, far from being a hindrance to the spiritual, has the capacity in itself for expressing love. In fact it is specifically designed to express love. He approached the subject of conjugal love from both metaphysics (philosophy) and later, revelation (theology). His treatise, *Love and Responsibility*, was published in Poland in 1960 and translated into English in 1981. In a remarkable statement, he writes, "The sexual urge is something even more basic than the psychological and physiological attributes of man and woman in themselves, though it does not manifest itself or function without them" (Wojtyla 1993, p. 49). It follows from the contingent nature of the person, who needs another for completion and at the same time wishes to share his riches with another. In other words, it has a spiritual source and is more strongly linked to the spiritual nature of the person than the biological.

PHILOSOPHIC ANALYSIS

Common language makes the distinction between an object, even a living object as *some/thing* and a person who is *some/one*. To treat a person, *some/one*, as some thing is to treat him as less than human. Wojtyla cites the categorical imperative of German philosopher, Immanuel Kant, "Act always in such a way that the other person is the end not merely the instrument of your action." Wojtyla expands the axiom further by saying that in any action between persons the other must always be treated as a personal subject and not merely as an object. He notes that this lies at the basis of all human freedoms (Wojtyla 1993, pp. 27, 28). It is especially important in the sexual relation, where the other is in one sense an object of the sexual urge. What raises the action to the level of persons is love, which receives the other as gift.

"But how does a person enjoy sexual relations without using the other person?" Karol Wojtyla examined this dilemma in his philosophical treatise, *The Acting Person.* He distinguished between what merely happens in man and what he chooses to do. Hunger, thirst, and sexual desire are what happen in man. It is the task of the person to integrate what happens in him into a human act, an act that ensures the primacy of the spiritual nature of man, his reason and well-being over the physical and emotional drives. In the sexual sphere this obviously means not suppressing the sexual urge, which is a good in itself, and oriented to the survival of the species, but channeling it to express love (Wojtyla 1993, p. 123). As experience teaches, chastity or self-mastery over the sexual urge comes only after much effort. It is both motivated by love and enables love. Here is the great strength of periodic abstinence in Natural Family Planning as it facilitates self-mastery.

Love is in essence the affirmation of the value of the person. In order truly to give herself in the sexual relation, the woman, especially, needs to value herself as a person and also value the man as a person, because the paradox of erotic love is that the person wishes to surrender his very being to the other. Only if the sexual relation is an expression of a unification through the total mutual gift of self in *marriage,* will the lover not lose himself but gain himself in a new way. Indeed by going outside himself (ecstasy) each finds a fuller existence in the other (Wojtyla 1993, p. 129, cf., pp. 125, 126).

THEOLOGICAL ANALYSIS

The future Pope John Paul II discovered the truth about love, especially erotic love and its relationship to self-gift, by reason. He turns to revelation for the full understanding of what theologically is described as the *logic of the gift.* The first verse of the Bible reveals God as creator of the universe out of nothing: "In the beginning, God created the heavens and the earth" (Gen. 1:1). Canadian philosopher Kenneth Schmitz points out that reason alone could not postulate creation out of nothing as it is beyond human experience and comprehension (Schmitz 1982, p. 13). Creation is a freely willed gift of the Creator, who does not have to create. He creates out of the desire to share his goodness (*bonum diffusum sui*). Subsequent biblical verses tell how man is made in God's image and is called to a one-flesh union with the woman. Love is both the motive of creation and its *raison d'etre*. As the highest point of creation, man and woman are ultimately called to share in the mutual self-giving love of the three divine Persons in the Trinity.

Only if man and woman are equal as persons but different can they find fulfillment and happiness in mutual self-giving. It is the body in its masculinity and femininity that reveals both the similarity and difference and the call to communion. The body itself is nuptial or spousal. It speaks a language of which it is not the author. It speaks the language of fidelity and total self-giving in marriage and the language of deception outside of marriage. In the Old Testament the language of the body provides the key analogy for the fidelity or infidelity of God's people. In the New Testament, the love of Christ for the Church is compared to the love of the bridegroom for the bride. The husband is admonished to give himself up for his wife as Christ gives himself up for the Church (Eph 5:26) .(John Paul II 2006, *Man and Woman*, no. 92).

THE BODY ORIENTED TO SELF-GIFT

In his encyclical, *Veritatis Splendor*, John Paul II speaks of finding "anticipated signs, the expression and the promise of the gift of self" in the body (*Veritatis Splendor*, no. 48). In commenting on the different bodily constitution of man and woman, he says "we know in fact today that it is different even in the deepest bio-physical determinants" (John Paul II 2006, *Man and Woman*, no. 21). Science has unveiled the difference. It reveals the equal but different roles of the male and the female in creating new life, with the woman's cervical mucus guiding, protecting and nourishing the sperm; it shows the part hormones play in bonding between the man and the woman in sexual union and between mother and child during nursing. Feminist author, Emily Martin, who has made a study of medical textbooks on human reproduction, is troubled by the trend of pushing back the boundaries of the body to the cellular level so that no matter what the intentions of the couple, within their bodies a "cellular 'bride' (or *femme fatale*) and a cellular 'groom' (or her victim) make a cellular baby" (Shivanandan 2000, p. 172). John Paul II, far from being troubled by such an interpretation of human love and procreation, goes so far as to declare, "In the whole perspective of his own history, man will not fail to confer a nuptial meaning on his own body." In spite of many distortions, "it will always remain the deepest level, which demands to be revealed in all its simplicity and purity, and to be shown in its whole truth, as a sign of the 'image of God'" (John Paul II 2006, *Man and Woman* , no. 15).

Pope Benedict & Caritas in Veritate

Pope Benedict, in his turn, has boldly taken up the theological and philosophical reflections on human and divine love of both von Hildebrand and John Paul II.

EROS AND AGAPE

At the beginning of the first encyclical of his pontificate, *Deus Caritas Est* (*God is Love*; hereafter DCE), he reiterates what John Paul II had already affirmed, the unity of *eros* and *agape* in the conjugal embrace. They must be united because "it is neither the spirit alone, not the body alone, that loves; it is man, the person, a unified creature composed of body and soul" (DCE, no. 5). *Eros* is often referred to as ascending love since it arises in the body and moves toward possession of the beloved while *agape* is called descending love, which is of divine origin and seeks the good of the beloved (DCE, no. 7).

As von Hildebrand pointed out, *eros* as sexual desire can either elicit a subjectively satisfying response in the lover or move to a true value response of the person through love (*caritas*). Pope Benedict sees them as seamlessly united in both human and divine love. What is more, *eros* has its place not only in man's ecstatic love of God but in God's love of each person. The total self-gift of Christ on the cross is the supreme example of the unity of *eros* and *agape* in divine love (DCE, nos. 10, 12). "In this the love of God was made manifest among us, that God sent his only Son into the world, so that we might live through him" (1 Jn 4: 9).

HUMANAE VITAE AND INTEGRAL HUMAN DEVELOPMENT

Pope Benedict's first encyclical is not primarily about the love between a man and a woman, but the love of God and neighbor as it pertains to justice and charity in the Church's social mission. What was surprising in it is the analysis of the two kinds of love, *eros* and *agape* and their intimate relationship in both human and divine love, as a prelude to the practical aspects of Christian charity in the world. What is unexpected about the encyclical, *Caritas in Veritate* (*Charity in Truth*; hereafter CIV), yet follows logically from *Deus Caritas Est*, is the proposal for the first time that the Church's teaching in *Humanae Vitae* (*Of Human Life*) is essential to true human development (CIV, no.28). Secular development agencies have generally viewed the Church's insistence on openness to life as a perverse block to development, viewing development primarily as material prosperity, without concern for man's spiritual life.

The Church has always insisted on the promotion of "the whole man," not partial aspects such as material needs. If development excludes God, it cannot encompass the value of the whole person (CIV, no. 18). Pope Benedict proposes that *Humanae Vitae,* by marking the strong links between life ethics and social ethics, ushers in a "new area of Magisterial teaching" (CIV, no. 15). In the encyclical *Humanae Vitae* (hereafter HV) Pope Paul VI speaks of an "integral vision of man and his vocation," one that includes both "his natural and supernatural vocation (HV, no. 7). Pope Benedict applies this concept to society and speaks of integral human development in his encyclical *Caritas in Veritate*. Responsible procreation has a particular contribution to make to integral development, especially through its promotion of the "beauty of marriage and family, institutions which "correspond to the deepest needs and dignity of the person" (CIV, no. 44). The person received as gift and called to communion is above all lived out in the family.

In the chapter of the encyclical on "*Fraternity, Economic Development and Civil Society,*" Pope Benedict defines the meaning of charity in truth (*caritas in veritate*) as placing man before "the astonishing experience of gift." The truth of the human being is that he is gift and made for gift. First and foremost the human being receives his being from an "Other" as a fruit of God's gratuitous love. In the same way the truth of ourselves is given to us. "Truth, like love, 'is neither planned not willed, but somehow imposes itself upon human beings" (CIV, no. 34). In an echo of von Hildebrand, Pope Benedict speaks of the superabundant nature of gift. It overflows in communion. In fact the logic of fraternity can and must overflow into normal economic and political activity, not instead of, but together with it (CIV, nos. 36, 37). Attitudes of gratuitousness cannot be legislated. Such attitudes are developed in the family through the reciprocal gift of self. Pope Benedict affirms John Paul II's emphasis on the human being as fundamentally relational. A philosophical understanding of interpersonal relations greatly aids their personal development. The person does not mature except in relation to others and God. Christian revelation confirms reason in providing the example of the interpersonal relations in the Trinity, where the community does not annihilate the individuality of each divine Person. It is the same way in the family (CIV, nos. 53, 54, 55).

John Paul II has cited both the family and the state as the place where the greatest abuses can occur because every person is born into a family and into a state. It is imperative that in both societies the dignity of the person be upheld. At the dawn of modern democracy, political theorists such as John Locke proposed the contract as the primary bond linking individuals to the state. The contract is not grounded in the relational notion of the human person but in the autonomous individual and his rights. For Locke every society is formed by voluntary contract and can be dissolved by the consent of its members whether it has fulfilled or perverted its purpose. Even in the case of marriage, Locke did not rule out the separation of husband and wife whether the children had reached maturity or not (Yolton 1977, p. 238).

As we have seen in the 20th century, this notion of contract has spread from the larger entity of the state to the family in a more radical way, so that, with the new reproductive technologies especially, it is not nature or even nurture that unites family members but arbitrarily chosen relations through contracts. In *Caritas in Veritate* Pope Benedict seeks to reverse the order and to extend the covenantal relations in the family, predicated on the person as a freely willed gift called to communion, to the larger society. Principles of justice and equality in difference lie at the core of the family as well as society. This article does not allow space for elaborating on how Pope Benedict develops this concept. Suffice to say that it is through the quality of mercy that a relational concept of the human person would be extended from the family into society.

Conclusion

The Church & Reproductive Science

By opposing contraception and various reproductive technologies, is the Church opposed to all technological developments in human fertility? By no means! The modern methods of Natural Family Planning are based on the latest scientific discoveries and the Church welcomes new research, such as that on adult stem cells, which bring great promise of healing. Pope Benedict affirms:

> True progress does not arise primarily from doing. Progress is first an intelligence capable of thinking in a technical way and perceiving clearly the human meaning of a human action, in the perspective of the significance of the person viewed in the totality of his being.[6]

Far from being opposed to technology, the pope calls it a "profoundly human reality, linked to the autonomy and freedom of man" (CIV, no. 69). Technology "touches the heart of the vocation of human labor" because it enables man to exercise dominion over matter and to improve the conditions of life. It is in a sense "a response to God's command to till and to keep the land (cf. Gen 2:15)" (CIV, no. 69). The painstaking labor of scientific research, which discovered the secrets of human fertility, made possible this very conference, yet technology is not enough. It needs to be set in the context of the person in the fullness of who he is and his call to communion. It needs *caritas in veritate,* that is, charity in truth.

END NOTES

1. An excellent contemporary discussion of the traditional holistic view of science can be found in "Bishop Lafitte's address to the White Mass, www.zenit.org/article-28849?1=English, ZE10040301-2010-04-03; accessed May 2011.
2. Galen, however, was less supportive of breastfeeding, believing that "carnal copulation troubleth the blood, and so by consequence the milk," a view which may have influenced husbands to send their infants to wet nurses (see Hardyment 1983, p. 4).
3. Havelock Ellis was at the forefront of the sexual revolution. He authored six volumes entitled *Studies in the Psychology of Sex* (published between 1897 and 1910) in which he attacked almost every aspect of the Judeo-Christian heritage on marriage and sexuality. He questioned marriage as an institution, holding that it stifled passion. He approved of cohabitation before marriage, masturbation and even homosexual behavior. (See D'Emilio and Freedman 1989, p. 224.) In his highly popular book *The Dance of Life,* he advocated an aesthetic morality that adhered to no rules, concluding: "In so far as we can infuse it [morality] with the spirit and method of art, we have transformed morality into something beyond morality; it has become the complete embodiment of the Dance of Life." (Ellis 1923, p. 270.)
4. This summary is taken from the introductory study by John Henry Crosby. In discussion of von Hildebrand's treatment of conjugal sexuality, it is important to state that it does not preclude the concept of original sin. As John Paul II later would say, sin originates in the heart with the

imperfection of self-gift. Any expression of genital sex outside marriage is by its very nature defective in total self-gift.

5. In a study of Natural Family Planning manuals of instruction, both secular and Catholic, words such as harmony, gift, and union predominate. Martin sees the aggressive and hostile words used to describe the same facts in secular medical textbooks, as reflecting a contemporary culture hostile to women and their bodies (see Shivanandan 2000, pp. 170-182).

6. *Etenim vera progressio non ex faciendo potissimum oritur. Profectus principium est intellectus, technicam artem cogitandi percipiendique plane humanum sensum humanae actionis capax, in conspectu significationis personae, quae tota in sua essentia suscipitur.* The translation given in this paper is that of the author and replaces the one in the official translation, which does not seem to the author to capture the full significance of the Latin text: "The key to human development is a mind capable of thinking in technological terms and grasping the fully human meaning of human activities within the context of the holistic meaning of the individual's being." For example, "*humanae actionis*" or human action has a particular meaning in Thomistic philosophy in reference to action that is specifically human as opposed to animal and the translator has lost the significance of the concept of person by translating it "individual." "Person" has the implication of transcendence that the word "individual" does not possess.

SOURCES CONSULTED

Allen, Prudence. 1997. *The Concept of Woman: The Aristotelian Revolution, 750 B.C. to A.D. 1250.* Grand Rapids, MI: William B. Eerdmans Publishing Co.

Aquinas, Thomas. 1966. *Commentary on St. Paul's Epistle to the Ephesians.* Aquinas Scripture Series. Albany, NY: Magi Books.

Benedict XVI. 2005. *Deus Caritas Est* (*God is Love*). Papal encyclical. *Origins* 35(33): 541-560.

———. 2006. "Faith, Reason and the University: Memories and Reflections." Lecture, University of Regensburg, Germany, September 12, 2006. The Holy See online. www.vatican.va/holy_father/benedict_xvi/speeches/2006/september/documents/hf_ben-xvi_spe_20060912_university-regensburg_en.html; accessed May 2011.

———. 2009. *Caritas in Veritate* (*Charity in Truth*). Papal encyclical. Washington, DC:

United States Conference of Catholic Bishops.

———. 2010. "General Audience: Saint Thomas Aquinas." General Audience, Vatican City,

June 2, 2010. The Holy See online. www.vatican.va/holy_father/benedict_xvi/audiences/2010/documents/hf_ben-xvi_aud_20100602_en.html; accessed May 2011.

D'Emilio, J. and E. B. Freedman. 1988. *Intimate Matters: A History of Sexuality in America*. New York: Harper and Row Publishers.

Ellis, Havelock. 1923. *The Dance of Life*. New York: Grosset and Dunlap.

First Vatican Council. 1869-1870. *Dogmatic Constitution on the Catholic Faith*, Ch. 4 "On Faith and Reason" and Canon 4. EWTN. www.ewtn.com/library/councils/vi.htm; accessed July 2010.

Flannery, O.P., Austin. Ed. 2004. *Vatican Council II,Tthe Conciliar and Post Conciliar Documents*. Northport, New York: Costello Publishing Company.

Gardella, P. 1985. *Innocent Ecstasy: How Christianity Gave America an Ethic of Sexual Pleasure*. New York: Oxford University Press.

Hardyment, Christina. 1983. *Dream Babies: Three Centuries of Good Advice on Child Care*. New York: Harper and Row Publishers.

John Paul II. 1993. *Veritatis Splendor* (*The Splendor of Truth*). Boston: St. Paul Books and Media; see also, *Origins* 23 (18).

———. 1998. *Fides et Ratio* (*Faith and* Reason). Papal encyclical. *Origins* 28 (19).

———. 2006. *Man and Woman He Created Them: A Theology of the Body*. Boston: Pauline Books and Media.

Latz, L. J. 1934. *The Rhythm of Sterility and Fertility in Women*. Chicago: Latz Foundation.

McLaren, A. 1984. *Reproductive Rituals: The Perception of Fertility in England from the Sixteenth to the Nineteenth Century*. New York: Methuen.

Paul VI. 1973. *Humanae Vitae* (*Of Human Life*). Papal encyclical. In *Good News for Married Love*. Collegeville, MN: The Liturgical Press, 33-78; see also Holy See online, www.vatican.va/holy_father/paul_vi/encyclicals/documents/hf_p-vi_enc_25071968_humanae-vitae_en.html; accessed May 2011.

Pegis, A. C., Ed. 1945. *Basic Writings of Saint Thomas Aquinas*. New York: Random House.

Pius XI. 1930. *Casti Connubii* (*Encyclical Letter of Pope Pius XI on Christian Marriage*). Boston: St. Paul Books and Media; see also Holy See online, www.vatican.va/holy_father/pius_xi/encyclicals/documents/hf_p-xi_enc_31121930_casti-connubii_en.html; accessed May 2011.

Schindler, D. L. 1999. "God and the End of Intelligence: Knowledge as Relationship." *Communio* 26 (3 Fall): 511-540.

Schmitz, K. L. 1982. *The Gift: Creation*. Milwaukee: Marquette University Press.

———. 2008. "*Human Nature and Human Culture.*" *A Common Morality for the Global Age: In gratitude for what we have been given*. Washington, DC: Catholic University of America, Center for Law and Culture, unpublished paper.

Scola, A. 2005. *The Nuptial Mystery*. Grand Rapids MI: William B. Eerdmans Publishing Co.

Shivanandan, M. 1999. *Crossing the Threshold of Love: A New Vision of Marriage*. Edinburgh: T&T Clarke.

———. 2000. "Body Narratives: Language of Truth?" *Logos* 3: 166-193.

von Hildebrand, D. 1970. *In Defense of Purity*. Chicago: Franciscan Herald Press.

———. 1991. *Marriage: the Mystery of Faithful Love*. Manchester, NH: Sophia Institute Press.

———. 2009. *The Nature of Love*. South Bend, IN: St. Augustine's Press.

Wojtyla, K. 1979. *The Acting Person*. Dordrecht, Holland: Reidel.

———. 1993. *Love and Responsibility*. San Francisco: Ignatius Press.

PANEL I

CO-CREATING WITH THE CREATOR

14

Biblical Reflections on Co-Creating with the Redeemer

WILLIAM S. KURZ, SJ, PHD

Professor, Department of Theology, Marquette University
with

ANNE CARPENTER

With gratitude for Anne Carpenter's research and editorial assistance

ABSTRACT

The Bible does not explicitly answer questions about co-creating with God and discerning whether to try to have children. In consulting Scripture regarding contemporary concerns, one needs to go beyond historical exegesis. Reading Scripture as God's Word requires seeking what God, the divine author of all of Scripture, is currently saying in the biblical passages under study.

The primary foundation for biblical teaching about marriage and family is Genesis, especially concerning God's original intention in creating marriage (Gen 1-2). Humans are created in the image of God as male and female, and marriage is the two becoming one flesh.

Most of Scripture treats adjustments that were made *after* marriage and family were gravely wounded by human rebellion against the Creator's plan (Gen 3).

The Book of Ruth demonstrates the broader familial contexts and purposes of marriage beyond the couple. The Song of Songs is a powerful poem celebrating the passion, emotion, and love in courtship and marriage. The prophet Hosea portrays the relation of God to his people as that of the covenant between husband and bride, on which the New Testament Letter to the Ephesians builds, in comparing Christian marriage to the mystery or sacrament of Christ's marriage covenant with his bride, the Church. Sayings of Jesus make obvious that after death there will be no more purpose for marriage and procreation in our immortal resurrected bodies. St. Paul develops the meaning of celibacy from these eschatological sayings of Jesus, and discusses a topic closely related to the topics in this conference: temporary sexual abstinence in marriage (see 1 Cor 7).

The more synthetic section on "theology of the body" and magisterial summaries of biblical teaching is structured by the topics introduced in Vatican II's *Gaudium et Spes*: how marriage is ordained toward begetting and educating children; warnings against lust toward one's spouse as supporting communion of persons of equal dignity in marriage; openness to life and Jesus' welcoming of children; co-creating and receptivity to God's gift of life in marriage; and discernment about bringing new life into the world. Specific answers will require the cooperation of theologians and others, as is manifested in the schedule of papers in this conference.

INTRODUCTION

The particular topic of married couples co-creating with God is obviously not explicitly taken up in Scripture. In previous writings, I discussed how one can find biblical guidance for contemporary questions that may not always be expressly treated in biblical texts written two thousand and more years ago (Kurz 2003; Kurz 2004; Kurz 2001). Rather than seeking biblical proof texts or focusing on explicitly legal and ethical passages that relate to sexuality, let us try a more inclusive approach to consulting the entire canon of Scripture for its overall "worldview" on how the complete Bible describes the place of humans as male and female in the world and before their Creator God.

Searching the Scriptures for guidance about contemporary topics requires going beyond historical critical exegeses of particular texts in their original meanings, as much as is possible (e.g., Hahn and Flaherty 2007). For example, this investigation will begin with the classic biblical introduction to the Bible's worldview, the Genesis creation texts, especially those relating to the creation of man and woman and to human rebellion from divine limits in Genesis 1-3. Although critics have long noted that Genesis 1-3 combine two independent accounts of creation, our analysis follows the example of both ancient Jews and Christians, who searched the two accounts together as they are now canonically merged into a single presentation of God's creation of the universe and of humans. Indeed, more recent popes, imitating *Gaudium et Spes* (hereafter GS), treat these two creation accounts as a united, authoritative canonical source in discussing sexuality, marriage, and family. Though the texts are not strung together as if they were identical, they are frequently placed into context together (see for example, GS, no. 50; *Mulieris Dignitatem* [MD], no. 6; Benedict XVI 2006b, *Sunday Angelus*).

As explained in the articles mentioned above, guides to finding the message of Scripture's divine author are the steps recommended in Vatican II's dogmatic constitution on divine revelation, *Dei Verbum* (DV, no. 12 § 4). To make them even more available, they are repeated in the *Catechism of the Catholic Church* (CCC 1997, nos. 111-114). Because we believe Scripture is divinely inspired, for correct interpretation, "Sacred Scripture must be read and interpreted in the light of the same Spirit by whom it was written" (CCC 1997, no. 111; DV, no. 12; Pius XII 1943, *Divino Afflante Spiritu* [DAS]). Both Vatican II and the *Catechism* then outline a simple three-step process for so interpreting Scripture in the light of the Holy Spirit.

The *Catechism* repeats the three practical steps recommended in *Dei Verbum*: "1. Be especially attentive 'to the content and unity of the whole Scripture'" (CCC 1997, no. 112). Christians interpret Scripture by other parts of both Old and New Testaments, because God is the ultimate author of the entire Bible and he does not contradict himself. "2. Read the Scripture within the 'living tradition of the whole Church'" (CCC 1997, no. 113). Catholics read the Bible as earlier Catholics have interpreted it and lived it through the centuries, for the same Spirit that inspired Scripture has continued to inspire and guide the Church to this day. "3. Be attentive to the analogy of faith.

By 'analogy of faith' we mean the coherence of truths of faith among themselves and within the whole plan of revelation" (CCC 1997, no. 114). For example, believers seeking biblical guidance about relationships among men, women, marriage, and family can understand and relate what the Bible says about these relationships to their own personal experience of these realities and as they are taught and lived in the Church or by relatives or acquaintances from their own or other times and cultures. These approaches provide a good entry into theological interpretation of Scripture for those who are not specialists in biblical studies.[1]

SACRED SCRIPTURE RELATING TO MARRIAGE AND FAMILY

"In the Beginning"— Genesis on God's Original Intention for Man & Woman

The foundational creation texts from Genesis 1-3 have been frequently discussed—more recently and famously by Pope John Paul II in his "Theology of the Body" homilies on Genesis and other scriptures (John Paul II 2006, *Man and Woman*). Still, a summary here of the main teachings of the creation accounts about God, the world, humanity, and the interrelationships among them can provide a necessary foundation for more particular biblical insights concerning marriage and parenthood. These accounts contribute to a "biblical worldview" that can ground and provide a context for biblical considerations of marriage and having children.[2]

CREATION OF MAN IN THE IMAGE OF GOD AS MALE & FEMALE

The Genesis creation account narrates God's ordering of the world and creation of various material life-forms, from vegetation to water creatures and birds, whom God commanded, "Be fruitful and multiply and fill the waters in the seas, and let birds multiply on the earth" (Gen 1:22, *RSV*). After these early steps in God's creating and ordering the world, including the sexual propagation of animals, Genesis comments, "And God saw that it was good" (Gen 1:25; compare 1:4, 10, 12, 18, 21). But after creating humans as male and female in his image and likeness, God exclaimed even more forcefully, "And God saw everything that he had made, and behold, it was *very good*" (Gen 1:31, emphasis mine). The fact that Genesis describes God creating everything (including both animal and human sexuality) as *good*, and the human male and female as *very good*, is quite important for discussion about the meaning of human sexuality, marriage, and parenthood. It precludes negative attitudes toward human sexuality and marriage. God created our sexuality as good.

The Bible emphasizes the importance of human creation by presenting God as first pausing to consult with himself about creating man. "Then God said: 'Let us make man in our image, after our likeness'" (Gen 1:26a). In the meditations of later Old Testament authors, Second Temple writers, and rabbis, the only living God may have originally been imagined as here addressing his angelic heavenly court. However, almost from the beginning of Christianity, New Testament and Patristic authors understood that the plural "Let us make" prefigured an inner-Trinitarian council among Father, Son, and Holy Spirit. For both Jews and Christians, God's preparatory consultation invests God's creation of humans with great solemnity.

Absolutely foundational in both Jewish and especially Christian meditations on Gen 1:26 is that God made "man in our image, after our likeness." That humans are in the image of God is our principle distinction from the animals that God had created before us. There is a scholarly consensus that it is precisely because humans are "in our image" that they are placed in authority over sub-human material creation as God's image, representative, and steward.[3] Many of the Church Fathers who reflected on this verse have concluded that even after human rebellion and alienation from God and the undermining of human authority over nature as a result of the primeval sin in Genesis 3, humans retain the image of God. However, by sin we have lost our likeness to God, which will have to be restored by repentance and holiness of life (Louth 2007).

Jewish and Christian reflections on how humans are in God's image have tended to focus on human endowment with intellect and will. Like God and unlike animals, we have an intellect by which we can know God as our Creator, and we have a will by which we can either return or reject the love that God first offers to us (Williams 2007).

HUMAN AUTHORITY OVER NATURE AS GOD'S IMAGE

Because humans are in the image of God and God's representatives or stewards, God places them in the "garden" of the earth to tend to the plants and animals it contains. As "in our image," God orders, "let them have dominion over the fish of the sea, and over the birds of the air, and over the cattle, and over all the earth, and over every creeping thing that creeps upon the earth" Gen 1:26b). Humans have God's delegated authority over animals and nature, but God, the one who created animals and nature "as good," remains their sole owner.

God's commission of humans to exercise dominion over and to tend animals and plants and, by extension, the whole earth and all of God's material nature as God's "garden," is based on the human capacity, unlike animals, to plan and make decisions using their intellect and will. For example, God's gift to the human couple of "every plant yielding seed which is upon the face of all the earth, and every tree with seed in its fruit" to "have them for food" (Gen 1:29), implies human understanding and decisions about how to plant and tend the seeds until the grown plants bear fruit.

Likewise, Genesis 2 shows Adam making decisions in naming the animals (Gen 2:19), and presumably in taking care of them. Thus in Genesis 4, Cain will have agricultural produce from which to offer God "an offering of the fruit of the ground," and Abel can offer the "firstlings of his flock" (Gen 4:3, 4). The fact that Scripture presumes that humans make decisions about tending animals and plants provides a biblical foundation for further considering the human role in making decisions about their own fertility and sexuality.

What have been vigorously debated, at least since the1960s, have been the extent and limits of human decisions and control over their fertility and sexuality. Do humans have complete domination over their fertility? Or, like human dominion over everything else in nature, is their dominion over their sexuality limited by God in any way? Humans are manifestly only God's stewards responsible for making decisions about other aspects of nature. Therefore, although humans have broad authority to develop nature (e.g., by breeding mules from horses and donkeys), they are not owners of nature who can dominate (and pollute) nature in any way that they might wish.

It seems reasonable to suppose that human dominion over their own bodies and sexuality is similarly a stewardship, in which they are responsible to God. This is presumed in non-sexual contemporary cultural contexts in which people are exhorted to be responsible for how they treat their bodies, in order to preserve their health. Abuse of one's body by smoking, overeating and drinking, and controlled substances is commonly considered wrong and a "lack of respect" for one's body (which believers hold is given by the Creator).

Dominion over nature will play an important role in twentieth-century debates about dominion over our sexuality through artificial, chemical, or mechanical contraception, or by fertility procedures, as *in vitro* fertilization (IVF). Genesis already makes clear that human dominion over nature is not the dominion of God, but only *a delegated dominion* that must respect the limits that God places on it. For example, the first creation account narrates limits for both animals and humans, who were given only plants to eat, not other animals (which only occurred after the fall and the flood, Gen 9:3-4). In respect to the sexual begetting of children, Eve's remark makes clear our human dependence on God. After Adam and Eve had sinned and were banished from Eden, "Adam knew Eve his wife, and she conceived and bore Cain, saying, "I have gotten a man with the help of the LORD" (Gen 4:1). Humans can only beget children "with the help of the LORD." Therefore, childbearing is not an action autonomous from God, but it is under the Lord's authority.

IN THE IMAGE OF GOD HE CREATED HIM; MALE & FEMALE HE CREATED THEM. (GEN 1:27)

The climax of this first creation account is the creation of man: "So God created man in his own image, in the image of God he created him; male and female he created them" (Gen 1:27). This verse clearly refers to "man" (Hebrew *ha adam*, LXX *ton anthrōpon*) as a genus of being. It shifts to the plural to indicate that this genus of "man" exists as plural and differentiated: "in the image of God he created him; *male and female* he created *them*" (1:27b, emphasis mine). Unlike more philosophical reflections on God's image that focus on an individual human as possessing the spiritual powers of intellect and will, this verse clearly emphasizes that "man" is in God's image not only as a solitary individual but as a sexually differentiated but united couple—as "male and female." This will lead to two kinds of reflections in Christian biblical interpretation. One is on humans in community imaging the Trinity of Divine Persons. The second is on the united (married) male and female *couple* as the human image of God, not just as individual humans (Scola 2005, pp. 42-52).

The blessing that God gives to this human couple becomes also the primeval human commission in creation as originally intended by

God. This commission lays the biblical foundation for all discussions of human sexuality, marriage, and having children. It adds to this human mission to multiply the human race a commission to do the work of tending for God's nature (Gen 1:28).

For an original human couple to spread over the entire earth and tame it, they had to "be fruitful and multiply, and fill the earth and subdue it." Therefore, the more basic human commission is to populate this planet earth. The related and consequent commission is to tend to the earth, as Adam and Eve had tended to plants (and presumably to animals, whom they named) in Eden. This is an intriguing reversal of the attitude of many married couples today, for whom their work and careers are more important than having and raising children. Genesis reveals no conflict in God's creative plan between human population growth, human work with nature, and human respect for earth's ecology.

MARRIAGE & FAMILY RELATIONSHIPS MARRED AFTER HUMAN REBELLION

Human rebellion against the limits God set for them in his original plan of creation, however, significantly damaged God's original intentions for human marriage and family. In place of the "very good" married "two-in-one-flesh" relationship planned by God and attained by mutual and complete self-giving, selfishness and power grabbing invaded the husband-wife interrelationship. Almost of necessity, God's perfect plan gave way to some harsh realities of the fallen condition of marriage and family. A brief summary exposition of Genesis 3 can trace how this came about.

In Genesis 3, God's plan was soon challenged by the tempter, portrayed as a wily serpent, but later in Scripture identified as the devil or Satan (Wis 2:24; John 8:44; Rev 12:9). He challenged the woman about the limits that God placed on what trees they could eat from in Eden. When she exaggerated God's warning not to eat from the one tree in the middle of the garden, "neither shall you touch it" (Gen 3:3), under pain of dying, the devil contradicted God. "But the serpent said to the woman, 'You will not die. For God knows that when you eat of it your eyes will be opened, and you will be like God, knowing good and evil'" (Gen 3:4-5). She put more faith in the affirmation of the serpent than that of God. She and her husband became discontented with God's permission to eat from all but this one tree, for the devil was tempting them to resist any divine limits, to "be like God, knowing good and evil" (v 5).

The human desire to "be like God" can be called the primeval and underlying temptation, from which flows all others. Humans were rejecting any divine limits over their freedom (having to say "No" to any choice). A similar insistence on the autonomy to decide for oneself what is good and evil in sexual behavior is at the very heart of the modern sexual revolution (Kurz 2003).

The consequence of the human couple's disobedience to God's command was immediate and catastrophic. It severely damaged their sexuality, their marriage, and their relationships not only with God but with each other. "Then the eyes of both were opened, and they knew that they were naked" (Gen 3:7). In their new shame at their bodies they tried to cover themselves with fig leaves, no longer completely open to each other. When they heard God approaching, "the man and his wife hid themselves from the presence of the LORD God among the trees of the garden" (v 8b). Their former friendship with God was replaced by terror at his approach.

When God asked Adam why he was hiding, he answered, "I was afraid, because I was naked; and I hid myself" (v 10b). God immediately designated the heart of the problem as their disobedience. "Who told you that you were naked? Have you eaten of the tree of which I commanded you not to eat?" (v11). Instead of admitting his guilt, the man blames the woman "whom thou gavest to be with me" (implicitly blaming also God, v 12); in turn, she also refuses to take personal responsibility and blames the serpent (v 13). The close friendship between God and humans has been fractured and replaced by human fear of and alienation from God.

God's curse of the serpent also included a promise of future salvation through the seed of the woman. Both Jewish and Christian readers interpreted this as prophesying a messianic figure who would save humans from the devil. "I will put enmity between you and the woman, and between your seed and her seed; he shall bruise your head, and you shall bruise his heel" (Gen 3:15). This is also a promise to heal and exalt marriage, in contrast to its wounding after the Fall (cf., Eph 5).

The "punishments" pronounced on both man and woman signaled a clear end to the paradisiacal conditions of Eden. No longer were husband and wife acting as "two in one flesh" joined together by God, but the relationship between women and men became perverted to historical conditions quite unjust to women. Regarding the human commission to "increase and multiply and fill the earth" (Gen 1:28), woman's motherly role of bearing children will cost her great suffering. Her relationship with her husband will be degraded from mutual and self-giving love between equals to one of lust and domination (Gen 3:16). This passage has become a classic explanation for the contention between the sexes, which throughout human history (and still today) has been filled with lust, power, domination, abuse, resentment, and hatred.[4]

The second human commission, to "fill the earth and subdue it; and have dominion over the fish of the sea and over the birds of the air and over every living thing that moves upon the earth" (Gen 1:28b), will likewise become quite onerous, as expressed in Adam's punishment: "cursed is the ground because of you; in toil you shall eat of it all the days of your life; thorns and thistles it shall bring forth to you" (Gen 3:17-19). Because humans challenged the dominion of God over them, sub-human nature will similarly rebel against dominion of humans over it. Instead of fruit (as in Eden) the earth will produce "thorns and thistles." As the woman will suffer a great deal in her maternal duties, the man will find his efforts to grow food similarly burdensome. God's plan for human love, marriage, family, and work has been deeply wounded.

The Book of Ruth

The Book of Ruth provides complementary insights into God's divine plan for marriage and having children within his more inclusive plan to save and reconcile humans to himself. The presumed cultural background to the account of Ruth and her mother-in-law Naomi is the Israelite law about a close relative providing heirs to the widow of a dead husband in order to preserve and pass on the family inheritance and property.[5] Not only did the Israelite Naomi's husband die in Moab, but the two sons he left her both also died childless, despite their marriages to Moabite women, Orpah and Ruth.

In effect, Naomi found herself thus abandoned without living heirs to inherit her and her husband's property in Israel and to provide for Naomi in her old age. Naomi, in despair of ever having heirs in Israel, urged her two Moabite daughters-in-law to provide for themselves by seeking new husbands among their Moabite countrymen (Ruth 1:13).

However, the Moabite widow Ruth's fidelity to her Israelite mother-in-law, Naomi, leads Ruth to return to Israel with Naomi and to seek to provide an heir to Naomi and her dead son through marrying a close relative to Naomi and her son, who can fulfill the Old Testament obligation of providing an heir for Naomi and for Ruth's dead husband, Naomi's dead son. Their situation makes clear how critically important marriage and having children are for the perpetuation of a family into future generations and for the preservation of the family's ancestral property. God rewarded Ruth's fidelity to Naomi by caring for Ruth through Boaz, a close relative of her dead husband, who married Ruth and raised up children for her dead husband and for Naomi her mother-in-law. In addition, Ruth's exemplary fidelity to her deceased husband and to Naomi her mother-in-law played an important role in God's more general plan of salvation for Israel. Through her son by Boaz, Obed, Ruth became an ancestress of King David and ultimately of the Messiah and Savior Jesus.[6]

The Song of Songs

The Song of Songs reminds believers of the emotional, romantic, even passionate aspects of married love. It focuses on the unitive aspects of the marriage act, whereas many other Old Testament treatments of marriage put more emphasis on procreation in marriage. Although contemporary culture tends to overdo the romantic and unitive aspects of human sexuality to the neglect of its procreative purposes, within the ancient biblical perspective, the Song of Songs provides an important canonical biblical balance toward the second principal purpose of the marriage act, the unitive.

From very early times, the Song of Songs is interpreted both by Old Testament and later Jewish writers as a symbol of God's spousal love for his people. The Fathers of the Church also explicated this romantic poetry as symbolizing Christ's spousal love for the Church, his Body. The most explicit celebrations of married human sexual love and romance in Scripture become quasi-sacramental signs for the deeply loving covenant union between God and his "Chosen People" and between Christ and his Church.

The Prophets Hosea and Isaiah

The prophets, especially Hosea, frequently compare God's love for his people to a husband's love for his bride (see also *Deus Caritas Est*

[DCE], no. 9). This comparison is a forerunner of the very important New Testament comparison of married love to the love of Christ to his bride, which will transform, elevate, and ennoble the natural beauty and significance of marriage into the supernatural mystery of marriage as a sacrament. Throughout the Old Testament, especially in the prophets, the analogy between human spouses with God and his people deepens insight into the relationship of human married love to God's love for his people that will be further developed in the New Testament.

In Hosea 1, God's offer and human rejection of God's love are portrayed in the living example of marriage to a prostitute who committed adultery with other gods. After God's punishment of his adulterous people, he promises (Hosea 2:14-23) to forgive and restore her, referring to her time in the desert when she was faithful, before going after the pagan god Baal in the promised land: "And in that day, says the LORD, you will call me, 'My husband,' and no longer will you call me, 'My Ba`al.' For I will remove the names of the Ba`als from her mouth, and they shall be mentioned by name no more" (Hos 2:16-17).

Though much less frequently than Hosea, Isaiah, too, compares God's relationship with his people to marriage. Thus, Isaiah 62:5b prophesies: "and as the bridegroom rejoices over the bride, so shall your God rejoice over you." In the Old Testament, however, marriage is not just a matter of a closed husband-wife relationship. Marriage, as seen in the Book of Ruth, is meant to bless also extended families and to participate in God's blessing of all people. Thus, the canonical Book of Isaiah has a very strong universalist theme. God's special love for his people is meant to bless not only his chosen people but all nations.

This is vividly portrayed in God's vocation to his Servant, "It is too light a thing that you should be my servant to raise up the tribes of Jacob and to restore the preserved of Israel; I will give you as a light to the nations, that my salvation may reach to the end of the earth" (Is 49:6). Thus, the Old Testament analogy of God's love with married love has a universalist aspect that directly prepares for the New Testament comparison of Jesus as Bridegroom loving his bride the Church for the salvation of all nations. Isaiah's servant theme is applied in the New Testament not only to Jesus (who is called "a light for revelation to the Gentiles, and for glory to thy people Israel," Luke 2:32), but also to Sts. Paul and Barnabas ("For so the Lord has commanded us, saying, 'I have set you to be a light for the Gentiles, that you may bring salvation to the uttermost parts of the earth,'" Acts 13:47).

NEW TESTAMENT TEXTS IMPORTANT FOR MARRIAGE AND FAMILY

Ephesians 5:21-33

Ephesians reveals an even deeper meaning to the natural covenant of marriage, in which "the two shall become one flesh" (Eph 5:31). Already Jesus in his ministry had made clear that "in the beginning" the husband and wife were to become two in one flesh, joined by God and not to be separated by men (Matt 19:6 and parallels). Because of this divine joining of husband and wife in God's original plan for marriage, Jesus had forbidden divorce and remarriage, despite concessions in the Law due to the people's "hardness of [their] hearts" (Matt 19:8).

The author of Ephesians explores this "two in one" union even further. "'For this reason a man shall leave his father and mother and be joined to his wife, and the two shall become one flesh.' This mystery is a profound one, and I am saying that it refers to Christ and the church" (Eph 5:31-32). Paul is referring to human marriage as a mystery from of old whose meaning is newly revealed in Christ. The natural and divinely instituted covenant of marriage that unites husband and wife is now understood to reveal a new covenant of marriage between Christ and his bridal Church. As Pope John Paul II, interprets it,

> The covenant proper to spouses "explains" the spousal character of the union of Christ with the Church, and in its turn this union, as a "great sacrament", determines the sacramentality of marriage as a holy covenant between the two spouses, man and woman (MD, no. 23 §34).

In other words, this physical "two in one" covenanted union of marriage from the creation of the world now carries in Christ an even more profound meaning. Human marriage is now comprehended as a profound mystery that reveals the marital union of Christ and his Church. As created by God "in the beginning," marriage, as God's "two in one" union of husband and wife, was not to be sundered by humans. Now that this same marriage union symbolizes the union of Christ and his Church, it takes on additional qualities from how Christ relates to his Church.

Not only that: the husband in Christian marriage is to relate to his wife as Jesus acted toward his Church. "Husbands, love your wives, as Christ loved the church and gave himself up for her" (Eph 5:25). Husbands are to sacrifice themselves for their wives as Christ gave up his life on the cross for his Church. Compare John 15:13, "Greater love has no man than this, that a man lay down his life for his friends."

Analogously, as Christ is head of the Church, the husband is head of his wife, who should respect him as head in the marriage (Eph 5:22-24). In *Mulieris Dignitatem*, no. 24, however, "The Gospel 'innovation,'" Pope John Paul II re-interprets and applies the introduction to this husband-wife relationship differently from the way it was understood in the ancient household. In light of contemporary experience, the Pope interprets and applies this verse as the Divine Author going beyond the human author's original meaning to enjoin in this verse a *mutual* subordination in marriage. With the help of the introduction, "Be subject to one another out of reverence for Christ" (Eph 5:21), the Pope contrasts the one-sided subordination of the Church to Christ to the mutual subordination of wife and husband in the marriage union (MD, no. 24).

This biblical analogy between the husband-wife and Christ-Church relationships, like every analogy, has some elements that are the same and others that differ between the two analogs. The headship of the divine Christ over his human Church far exceeds the husband's headship in a marriage of two humans who are equal in dignity (MD, no. 24).

Even today, parental authority over teenage children can be undermined if the children can play off mother against father to get what they want. This may help explain the strange-sounding conclusion, which enjoins the husband to love but the wife to respect their spouse: "let each one of you love his wife as himself, and let the wife see that she respects her husband" (perhaps as head of the household vis-a-vis the children, despite their mutual subordination, Eph 5:33).

The translation in Ephesians 5:32 of the Greek *mysterion* as Latin *sacramentum* in the Vulgate, the western Church's official Bible throughout the Middle Ages, may have further facilitated the Catholic interpretation of God's natural creation of marriage as being made in the New Testament a sacrament. Because of Christ, God's beautiful natural marriage covenant has been elevated to a grace-giving sacrament and supernatural covenant between husband, wife, and God.[7]

Jesus on the Eschatological Meaning of Marriage after Death

The New Testament has another development of the doctrine of marriage beyond what is obvious in the Old Testament. It appears in all three Synoptic Gospels when the Sadducees, who do not believe in life after death, challenge Jesus with an example they considered a reduction to absurdity. They cited a widow who married seven brothers in an attempt to provide an heir to her dead husband (see the explanation of this custom in the section on Ruth above). "In the resurrection, therefore, whose wife will the woman be? For the seven had her as wife" (Luke 20:33 parallels Matt 22:28 and Mark 12:23).

Jesus explains that marriage and having children apply only to earthly life. In our resurrected bodies everyone will be immortal. Therefore, there will be no need to have children to carry on the next generation after the current one dies. Luke's version states this more clearly than do the parallel passages in Matthew (22:30) or Mark (12:25):

> And Jesus said to them, "The sons of this age marry and are given in marriage; but those who are accounted worthy to attain to that age and to the resurrection from the dead neither marry nor are given in marriage, for they cannot die any more, because they are equal to angels and are sons of God, being sons of the resurrection" (Luke 20:34-36).

Jesus clearly indicates that sexual intercourse and having children only pertain to our earthly life. It no longer will exist in our future lives in our resurrected, spiritualized, and immortal bodies. Although married sexual intercourse now has two main purposes, unitive for the spouses and procreative to carry on the human race, there will no longer be any reason for, or existence of, sexual intercourse in the resurrected life. This emphatically underlines the purpose for marital union given in Genesis and presumed throughout the Old Testament: "Be fruitful and multiply, and fill the earth" (Gen 1:28). Procreation is the purpose that is indispensable for true marriage, and helps explain why marriage can only be between man and woman and must be open to giving life.

St. Paul on Abstinence in Marriage in 1 Corinthians 7

Jesus' answer about the eschatological standing of marriage and married love brings out another facet of their meaning, which St. Paul will develop in his treatment of Christian celibacy in 1 Corinthians 7.

Before getting to that topic, however, Paul emphasizes that both husband and wife have equal rights and claims on each other's sexuality, while retaining the biblical and traditional belief that the husband is head of the marriage.

> The husband should give to his wife her conjugal rights, and likewise the wife to her husband. For the wife does not rule over her own body, but the husband does; likewise the husband does not rule over his own body, but the wife does. Do not refuse one another except perhaps by agreement for a season, that you may devote yourselves to prayer; but then come together again, lest Satan tempt you through lack of self-control (1 Cor 7:3-5).[8]

Pope John Paul II comments about conjugal relations and periodic abstinence:

> St. Paul clearly says that both conjugal relations and the voluntary periodic abstinence of the spouses must be a fruit of the "gift of God," which is their "own," and that the spouses themselves, by consciously cooperating with it, can keep up and strengthen their reciprocal personal bond together with the dignity that being "temple[s] of the Holy Spirit who is in [them]" (see 1 Cor 6:19) confers on their bodies (John Paul II 2006, [1986], *Man and Woman*, 85:7).[9]

A key point here is that both marital relations and voluntary abstinence come as a "gift of God," with which the spouses cooperate. In the context of Natural Family Planning (NFP), this gift would involve not only the sacramental grace of marriage but also the more particular spiritual gift of discerning when to have relations and when to abstain. This "gift of God" and this principle are critical in couples' decisions concerning, and practice of, NFP.

Paul discusses abstinence in order to "devote yourselves to prayer." Of course, he cannot envisage NFP's future use of natural fertile and infertile periods to try to achieve or temporarily avoid pregnancy. Yet, because NFP involves similar decisions to abstain from marital intercourse as those mentioned by Paul, these decisions likewise have to be mutually agreed upon by both spouses. NFP cannot work without the cooperation of both partners. Paul's concern about excessively long times of abstinence in marriage becoming temptations to sin also provides a caution regarding contemporary NFP, if or when its practice seems to require excessively long abstinence. Awareness of this concern continues to spur NFP teachers to find ever more accurate ways to determine the fertile period in attempts to shorten the periods of abstinence for couples seeking to avoid a pregnancy in their current cycle.

Celibacy & Marriage in 1 Corinthians 7

St. Paul, who, like Jesus, remained celibate, also uses Jesus' eschatological emphasis on the coming of the "End Times" to discuss celibacy as a Christian alternative to marriage. Paul would wish others to remain "as I myself am," that is, celibate. "But each has his own special gift from God, one of one kind and one of another." (1 Cor 7:7) Both Christian marriage and celibacy are gifts or vocations from God, and each must follow his or her own vocation.

Paul admits that for his advice to the unmarried, he has "no command of the Lord, but I give my opinion as one who by the Lord`s mercy is trustworthy. I think that in view of the present distress it is well for a person to remain as he is." (1 Cor 7:25-26) Reference to "the present distress" refers to Paul's belief that end of the world will occur quite soon amidst great destruction and suffering. "For the form of this world is passing away" (1 Cor 7:31). In light of this expected traumatizing end of the world, Paul's opinion is that "it is well for a person to remain as he is," without taking on new responsibilities and commitments, such as marriage and family if one is currently single.

For Paul, however, the strongest argument for remaining celibate rather than marrying is the greater opportunity that celibacy offers for completely single-minded devotion to the Lord.

> I want you to be free from anxieties. The unmarried man is anxious about the affairs of the Lord, how to please the Lord; but the married man is anxious about worldly affairs, how to please his wife, and his interests are divided. And the unmarried woman or girl is anxious about the affairs of the Lord, how to be holy in body and spirit; but the married woman is anxious about worldly affairs, how to please her husband. I say this for your own benefit, not to lay any restraint upon you, but to promote good order and to secure your undivided devotion to the Lord (1 Cor 7:32-35).

Paul's own celibacy frees him for completely "undivided devotion to the Lord" in his constant travel, frequent and mortal dangers, and considerable sufferings. This would not be as easy for him if he had to be concerned about a spouse (with children usually presupposed).

Among the important "worldly affairs, how to please his wife" (or her husband), are decisions about having and raising children.

Of course "devotion to the Lord" is the task of every Christian, and Christian love is much more inclusive than love in marriage and celibacy. Married love must be understood in the context of this greater love, as it is especially beautifully expressed in 1 John:

> Beloved, let us love one another; for love is of God, and he who loves is born of God and knows God. He who does not love does not know God; for God is love. In this the love of God was made manifest among us, that God sent his only Son into the world, so that we might live through him. In this is love, not that we loved God but that he loved us and sent his Son to be the expiation for our sins. Beloved, if God so loved us, we also ought to love one another. No man has ever seen God; if we love one another, God abides in us and his love is perfected in us (1 John 4:7-12, RSV).

"THEOLOGY OF THE BODY" AND MAGISTERIAL SUMMARIES OF BIBLICAL TEACHING

One way to organize biblical information culled from all over the canonical Bible about human cooperation with God in procreation is to use magisterial summaries of biblical teaching, including Pope John Paul II's "Theology of the Body." This is analogous to how the Church Fathers often used the Nicene Creed to organize biblical evidence scattered throughout the Bible that reveal and relate to God as Trinity of Father, Son, and Holy Spirit.

A helpful introduction, therefore, may be to quote from Vatican II's *Pastoral Constitution on the Church in the Modern World* (*Gaudium et Spes* [GS]).

> Marriage and conjugal love are by their nature ordained toward the begetting and educating of children. Children are really the supreme gift of marriage and contribute very substantially to the welfare of their parents. The God Himself Who said, "it is not good for man to be alone" (Gen. 2:18) and "Who made man from the beginning male and female" (Matt. 19:4), wishing to share with man a certain special participation in His own creative work, blessed male and female, saying: "Increase and multiply" (Gen. 1:28). Hence, while not making the other purposes of matrimony of less account, the true practice of conjugal love, and the whole meaning of the family life which results from it, have this aim: that the couple be ready

> with stout hearts to cooperate with the love of the Creator and the Savior, who through them will enlarge and enrich His own family day by day (GS, no. 50).

Marriage as by Nature Ordained toward Begetting & Educating Children

The main points that Vatican II makes, that marriage naturally tends toward the "begetting and educating of children," and that children are "the supreme gift of marriage," could hardly be more counter-cultural. Catholic tradition in this case remains quite thoroughly biblical.

In Genesis, the original intent of marriage is manifestly to "increase and multiply and fill the earth" (Gen 1:28). One of the biggest marital tragedies in Scripture is childlessness, which is regarded as a curse and disgrace, as is illustrated in several accounts of sterile wives like Sarah, Hannah and Elizabeth. Children and large families are consistently regarded as special gifts of God. In both Old and New Testaments, widows whose only children die are objects of special compassion of the prophet Elijah (1 Kings 17:17-24) and of Jesus (Luke 7:11-16). In the Old Testament, the Fourth Commandment and several wisdom passages focus on the raising and education of children and their relationships to their parents. New Testament letters similarly contain exhortation on the proper raising of children (as in Eph 6). Overall, in Scripture, marriage usually presupposes families and children and all that pertains to them.

Of course, the Bible also reports many negative examples of marriage and sexual practices that follow from the fallen conditions of human sexuality and marriage. Scripture often treats these as detrimental cases that illustrate the dire consequences of such misuse of marriage or sexuality (e.g., Sarah's taking it into her own hand to make up for her own childlessness through her maid Hagar: see Gen 16 and 21:9-21). However, the Bible often shows how God uses even these negative actions as part of his plan for nations (Hagar's exiled son thus also becomes the father of an important nation, Gen 21:13). Matthew's genealogy has the surprising insertion of four Old Testament women whose questionable sexual history or behavior God used to continue the messianic line from which came the Savior Jesus (Matt 1:1-11).

The major biblical focus regarding marriage remains on the couples' generously cooperating with God in raising and educating new human life. As Eve said when Cain was born shortly after her expulsion from Eden, "I have gotten a man with the help of the LORD" (Gen 4:1). The very atmosphere of Scripture is quite alien to widespread contemporary reluctance about having children and exaggerated attempts to limit children.

Perhaps at least partially for this reason, there is little explicit treatment in Scripture of some of the topics and foci of this conference—on how parents cooperate with God by making decisions regarding when and how many children to bring into the world. In unusual biblical situations where avoiding children is desirable, there is an example of David refusing to have children from Michal, Saul's daughter. He simply spurned intercourse with her, because she despised him when he carelessly exposed himself while wildly dancing before the Lord (2 Sam 6:16, 20-23). In context below, we will discuss a highly unusual situation in Scripture in which someone tries to avoid having children while still having intercourse (Gen 38:8-10).

BIBLICAL SUPPORT FOR COMMUNION OF PERSONS IN MARRIAGE

A major component of the biblical worldview about marriage is the importance of complete giving of self and acceptance of one's spouse as a human person in his or her own right, never as an object of one's own desires. There were some shocked objections to the argument that Pope John Paul II used to emphasize the need to treat one's spouse as a person, not an object. He quoted Jesus' statement in the Sermon on the Mount about the commandment, "You have heard that it was said, You shall not commit adultery," as contrasted with Jesus' even more radical judgment, "But I say to you that every one who looks at a woman lustfully has already committed adultery with her in his heart" (Matt 5:27-28). The Pope argued from this contrast that even in marriage, one can treat one's spouse with lust, which is sinful because it does not respect the spouse as a person. This application goes beyond the original point of Jesus' saying, but it is not incompatible with Jesus' message.

This saying of Jesus occurs in a section of the sermon that is referred to as the "antitheses" (Matt 5:21-48). In the first antithesis, Jesus refers to the commandment not to kill, which he internalizes and radicalizes to not even nursing anger at another. The second antithesis expands the commandment not to commit adultery to include not even looking at another with lust. Through these antitheses, Jesus goes beyond what the Law literally forbids, like killing and adultery, to include interior dispositions, like anger and lust.

The importance of this antithesis is that it clearly exemplifies the biblical worldview about the meaning of sexual love in marriage. It is clear that for Jesus, morality extends much deeper than external keeping of a command. Jesus demands that one's heart has the attitude required to be able to live the commandments with more honesty than mere legalistic conformity to them. The reminder that one can regard even one's spouse immorally with lust provides an attention-getting illustration of the importance of treating one's spouse with love and respect as an equal person. This instruction reinforces the biblical perspective on marriage as a communion of two persons equally worthy of respect in the dignity of each and of both together as image of God.

OPENNESS TO LIFE: JESUS, 'LET THE CHILDREN COME TO ME'

Especially because Scripture treats children as the normal result of married love and its greatest gift, married openness to conceiving life is usually presupposed. We have already repeatedly mentioned how the Bible presumes that marital sexual relations will be open to conceiving children and will do nothing to impede such conception. One secondary reason why the story of Jesus receiving children may have been preserved in the Gospels (besides its primary lesson about entering the Kingdom as children) may have been to illustrate Jesus' love of, and openness toward, children. In Mark 10:13-16 and its parallels in Matthew and Luke, Jesus rebukes his disciples for trying to keep children away from him. When the annoyed male disciples try to keep little children from bothering Jesus, he forcefully rebukes them and accepts and tenderly blesses the children (Mark 10:13-16 [parallels Matt 19:13-15 and Luke 18:15-17]). Although this incident has a different historical referent, it can also be applied to illustrate a theological argument that Jesus demonstrated a very positive attitude toward children, which can challenge the contemporary hostility toward having more than a minimum number of children.

CO-CREATING & RECEPTIVITY TO GOD'S GIFT OF LIFE IN MARRIAGE

Although the titles of several of these conference presentations use the word *co-creating*, a married Catholic student with children who is writing his Marquette dissertation on marriage strongly suggests focusing less on co-creating children with God and more on children as

God's supreme gift in marriage.[10] Focus on children as gift would help a couple be less susceptible to the temptation to try themselves to be in complete control of outcomes (like having or not having children). It would help them become more focused on remaining receptive to divine gifts regarding children as they cooperate with God's desire to give the couple the gift of children. Mary is the supreme exemplar of this kind of parental receptivity to God's gift of a child. Despite her genuine and realistic unease ("How shall this be, since I have no husband?" [Luke 1:34]), she gave God her unreserved "yes" to his offer of a child: "Behold, I am the handmaid of the Lord; let it be done to me according to your word" (Luke 1:38).

The biblical perspective on marriage certainly presupposes that spouses make decisions about having children, but that it is God who actually either gifts them with a child or leaves them childless. Natural Family Planning (NFP) provides contemporary couples more information than biblical couples had to enable them to cooperate with God more intentionally and with more comprehension, because it helps them to distinguish between the times when the woman is fertile and other times when she is not.

There is nothing in Scripture that would forbid parents to use such knowledge in efforts to cooperate with the divinely created fertility cycle of the women. At the same time, the biblical worldview does not support a "providentialist" insistence that couples should blindly use marital intercourse and leave the results entirely to providence to provide for the marriage and all children so conceived (even when this is sometimes irresponsible, as when the wife has a life-threatening illness).[11]

Nevertheless, even when using NFP, the biblical worldview presumes a situation in which couples must be open to God's will regarding whether their efforts will succeed or fail as to conception or temporary avoidance of a child. Scripture manifestly portrays God, the creator of marriage, as remaining in charge of all that issues from marriage. Couples cooperate with God's will by always acting virtuously and according to God's commandments in the ways they try to have children.

DISCERNMENT OF BRINGING NEW LIFE INTO THE WORLD

To go beyond what has already been presented requires going beyond historical exegesis to a more theological approach that takes into account not only the entire biblical canon but also how Scripture has been interpreted in Church tradition and by Catholic authors. This is the more immediate concern of other presentations in this conference. However, it is important for exegetes also to try to make at least some attempts toward a response to this topic. Since I am trained as a Jesuit, I will turn to St. Ignatius Loyola, founder of the Jesuits, for some inspiration from his very Catholic understanding and application of his genuine biblical perspective to questions of discernment.

Because my answer is more general and less directly responding to how to discern whether to try to conceive children, I will not turn to Saint Ignatius's "Rules for Discernment of Spirits." Instead, I will consult his final contemplation that summarizes the fruit of his *Spiritual Exercises*, his "Contemplation to Gain Love" (Ignatius Loyola). This contemplation for love seems particularly appropriate for couples discerning God's will with regard to having children.

St. Ignatius begins his contemplation to obtain love with two very practical presuppositions: "the first is that love ought to be put more in deeds than in words. The second, love consists in interchange between the two parties; that is to say in the lover's giving and communicating to the beloved what he has or out of what he has or can." Obviously, discernment about having children has to take place in a context of the mutual love of the spouses. This love is not primarily a matter of emotions or words, but is demonstrated in deeds of love that the couple practices toward each other. By their loving deeds, the couple strives constantly toward greater mutual love. As their love and virtue grow, they will become more able to discern God`s will about when to have children. Their love will also overflow to the children they have or will have.

Secondly, love shares what each person has with the beloved. In this case, each spouse would share with the beloved his or her insights, desires, sense of God's will for their marriage and family. They will also share in the work of maintaining a household and family. As they share generously with each other, the couple increases in the virtue of generosity, which is essential to having and raising children. Although the Bible does not tell each particular couple how many children to try for, it certainly presumes and promotes parents' generosity toward having children, and that they would not selfishly limit the number of their children merely for their personal comfort or convenience.

St. Ignatius prepares for his contemplation on love by telling the one praying "to ask for interior knowledge of so great good received, in order that being entirely grateful, I may be able in all to love and serve His Divine Majesty" (Ignatius, "Contemplation to Gain Love, Second Prelude," § 29). Before one can receive more grace from God and become more generous toward God and one's family, he or she must become ever more grateful for what God has already given. This gratitude is required to "be able in all to love and serve his Divine majesty" (Ignatius, "Contemplation to Gain Love, Second Prelude," § 29). Gratitude is one form of recognizing our dependence on God. Especially in its many accounts of frustrated sterile couples, Scripture makes eminently clear that to have children husband and wife are completely dependent on God giving them the gift of conceiving a new life.

In his "Second Point" of the contemplation, St. Ignatius instructs the one praying to "look how God dwells in creatures, in the elements, giving them being, in the plants vegetating, in the animals feeling in them, in men giving them to understand: and so in me, giving me being, animating me, giving me sensation and making me to understand." (Ignatius, "Contemplation to Obtain Love, Second Point," §29). This insight into how God lives and works in all creatures, including the married couple, provides a very important context for understanding "co-creation." Recognizing that God works in and through a couple's natural powers reminds them of their dependence on God, even when they are making love to each other and doing what they can to facilitate God's creation of a new human soul and life. It guards against the all too human temptation to think and act as if they were equal to God and in control of the results of their marital union.

CONCLUSION

Scripture does not explicitly treat the topic of this presentation—parents co-creating with God and discerning when to bring new life into the world. It does, however, provide definite (though currently countercultural) viewpoints on the meanings and purposes of marriage and having children by which to ground such discernment. The worldview of Scripture clearly demonstrates that God created marriage as very good, and that children are the supreme gift of marriage. Scripture also presupposes that married couples make decisions about trying to have children or not, but usually with the expectation of the blessing of a good number of children.

For explicit guidance on just how parents are to discern whether they should try for another child, readers of Scripture have to go beyond the Bible's historical portrayal of marriage in the ancient biblical cultures and world. A complete answer requires interdisciplinary contributions from several areas of theology, philosophy, medical, and other fields. Still, biblical specialists also ought to contribute to this effort by themselves trying to apply Scripture through theological interpretation to such contemporary questions. This presentation is one such attempt by a biblical specialist, which appears in the context of this conference alongside theological, anthropological, and other presentations making similar attempts. It is hoped that this presentation can provide some biblical grounding for the fuller answers attainable through other approaches.

END NOTES

1. On theological interpretation of Scripture, see Kurz (2007), "Developing a Theological Approach to Scripture," pp. 45-67.
2. On the "biblical worldview," see Johnson and Kurz (2002), Chapter 8 [Kurz], "Voices in the Church: Preunderstandings in Applying Scripture," pp. 182-202; see especially "Finding a Broader Context for Arguments," pp. 186-88, which treats the "biblical worldview." Compare Johnson's complementary analogy, "Imagining the World that Scripture Imagines," Chapter 5, pp. 119-142, along with Chapter 6, "Bill Kurz: Response to Luke Johnson," esp. pp. 147, 151-54.
3. Compare Holmes (2005), pp. 318-319; Curtis 1992, pp. 389-391; Goshen-Gottstein (1994), pp. 171-195.
4. See Ramsey (1988), pp. 56-86; John Paul II (2006), Audiences 29-31; see also Griffiths (2009), on post-lapsarian desire in general, pp. 27-30.
5. For the law about marrying the widow of a brother to provide the brother an heir and preserve their family property inheritance, see Deut 25:5-10. "If brothers dwell together, and one of them dies and has no son, the wife of the dead shall not be married outside the family to a stranger; her husband`s brother shall go in to her, and take her as his wife, and perform the duty of a husband`s brother to her. And the first son whom she bears shall succeed to the name of his brother who is dead, that his name may not be blotted out of Israel" (vv 5-6). If the brother refuses to do this, he faces public legal shame: "then his brother`s wife shall go up to him in the presence of the elders, and pull his sandal off his foot, and spit in his face; and she shall answer and say, 'So shall it be done to the man who does not build up his brother`s house'" (v 9). The list in 1 Chronicles 23:21-22 provides a slightly different case, but one related to this law: "The sons of

Mahli: Elea`zar and Kish. Elea`zar died having no sons, but only daughters; their kinsmen, the sons of Kish, married them").

These laws should be understood within the broader context of Old Testament laws relating to marriage and property. Thus Numbers 36:1-9 forbids marrying outside one's tribe, lest the ancestral lands of one's tribe be transferred to another tribe. See especially, "Let them marry whom they think best; only, they shall marry within the family of the tribe of their father. The inheritance of the people of Israel shall not be transferred from one tribe to another; for every one of the people of Israel shall cleave to the inheritance of the tribe of his fathers" (Num 36:6-7).

6. See Anderson (2008), pp. 31-34. Anderson points to two texts in Ruth that relate conjugal love and divine love. In Ruth 2:11-12, Boaz explains why he was helping Ruth. He had heard of all she had done for her mother-in-law Naomi. He continued, "The LORD recompense you for what you have done, and a full reward be given you by the LORD, the God of Israel, under whose wings you have come to take refuge!" (v12). In Ruth 3:9-10, when Ruth surprised Boaz at night, she both identified herself and proposed marriage: "I am Ruth, your maidservant; spread your skirt [Hebrew also means *wing*] over your maidservant, for you are next of kin" (Ruth 3:10). As Anderson explains, "God will spread his wings (*kanaf*) over Ruth through agency of Boaz's robe (*kanaf*). ... her enjoyment of divine protection will be mediated through Boaz in marriage" (p. 33).

   Anderson's conclusion is especially pertinent to our topic. "The Book of Ruth tells us that within the sacred bond of marriage there lies a symbol of the love of God for humanity. ... Human marriage is an analogical expression of the love of God for his people" (p. 33). This was already true in the Old Testament.

7. Scholarly treatments of Ephesians 5:21-33 are deeply divided, often along ideological lines, with concerns about subordination of women and the relationship of Paul's treatments of marriage and celibacy. Recent examples include Kleinig (2005) and Osiek (2002). Papal and other Catholic interpretations offer an understanding of the texts that do not distort the texts to fit one another.

8. See some helpful historical context in Peterman (1999). Another article reviews the scholarly disagreement over whether Paul is endorsing spiritual marriage, and how this thinking deeply influenced the early church (see Peters 2002).

9. John Paul II (2006), Audience 85:7, p. 456 in context of Audiences 83-85.

10. Kent Lasnoski, ABD (Marquette University, Department of Theology), made these observations in June, 2010, to my research assistant, Anne Carpenter.

11. Against "providentialism," see Curtis and Michaelann Martin (2007), pp.144-46. Compare Brugger (2010a): "The answer is 'no,' NFP is not unqualifiedly good and can be used wrongly. The reason for this is subtle and needs to be stated carefully, because there is a popular, although erroneous, belief among some Catholic couples that NFP is 'second best,' and that if a couple is seriously Catholic, they will not self-consciously plan the children they conceive, but simply 'let God send them.' I do not mean to offend anyone`s practices, but this 'come what may' attitude is found nowhere in Catholic teaching on procreation in the last 150 years. There is no decision more serious to a Catholic couple than whether or not to participate with God in bringing a new human person into existence."

Ethicist Kevin Miller makes an important distinction regarding this response in an email: "RE: ZENIT: Just Cause and Natural Family Planning," June 17, 2010. "I would say that it isn`t that NFP isn`t good when used with a wrong intention—it's that NFP is still good but the intention and therefore also the action as a whole are wrong."

In a follow-up article on ZENIT, Brugger (2010b) offers the following response: "I am happy to speak further on the question of *just causes* for spacing births. Some may believe that only extraordinary situations can constitute legitimate reasons for practicing NFP to defer pregnancy (e.g., severe illness of a spouse; extreme financial difficulties; mental breakdown, etc.). In my opinion, this extreme interpretation is incorrect and can result in avoidable harms."

"A few concrete examples of *iustae causae* for deferring pregnancy might include:

1) Physical or mental illness of one of the spouses;
2) Serious financial instability (e.g., during a period of unemployment);
3) Needs arising from caring for "high-needs" children;
4) The instability of transitional periods such as spouses in graduate school;
5) Debilitating stress that can arise from having a large family in societies where large families are no longer valued (see *Gaudium et Spes*, no. 50)."

SOURCES CONSULTED

Anderson, Gary A. 2008. "A Marriage in Full." *First Things*, 183: 31-34.

Anderson, Carl and José Granados. 2009. *Called to Love: Approaching John Paul II's Theology of the Body*. New York: Doubleday.

Benedict XVI. 2006a. *Deus Caritas Est (God Is Love)*. Papal encyclical. Boston: Pauline Books and Media.

———. 2006b. *Sunday Angelus (Oct. 8)*.

Brugger, E. Christian. 2010a. "Reasons for Postponing a Pregnancy." ZENIT. www.zenit.org/article-29757?l=english; accessed June 2010.

———. 2010b. "Response: Just Cause and Natural Family Planning." ZENIT. www.zenit.org/article-29625?l=english; accessed June 2010.

Catechism of the Catholic Church. 1997. 1993. Citta del Vaticano: Libreria Editrice Vaticana.

Congregation for the Doctrine of the Faith. February 27, 1987. *Donum Vitae* (*Instruction on Respect for Human Life*). The Holy See online. www.vatican.va/roman_curia/congregations/cfaith/documents/rc_con_cfaith_doc_19870222_respect-for-human-life_en.html.

Curtis, Edward M. 1992. "Image of God (OT)." In, *Anchor Bible Dictionary*. David Noel Freedman. Editor-in-chief. New York: Doubleday; III: 389-391.

Eberstadt, Mary. 2008. "The Vindication of *Humanae Vitae*." *First Things* 185: 35-42.

Goshen-Gottstein, Alon. 1994. "The Body as Image of God in Rabbinic Literature." *Harvard Theological Review* 87: 171-195.

Griffiths, Paul J. 2009. "The Nature of Desire." *First Things* 198: 27-30.

Hahn, Scott and Regis Flaherty. Eds. 2007. *Catholic for a Reason IV: Scripture and the Mystery of Marriage and Family Life*. Steubenville, OH: Emmaus Road Publishing.

Holmes, Stephen R. 2005. "Image of God." In, *Dictionary for Theological Interpretation of the Bible*. Vanhoozer, Kevin J. Gen. ed. Grand Rapids: Baker Academic; pp. 318-319.

Ignatius of Loyola. [no date provided] "Contemplation to Gain Love" in *The Spiritual Exercises*. Christian Classics Ethereal Library. www.ccel.org/ccel/ignatius/exercises.xvi.html; accessed June 2010.

John Paul II. 1995. *Evangelium Vitae* (*The Gospel of Life*). Papal encyclical. The Holy See online. www.vatican.va/holy_father/john_paul_ii/encyclicals/documents/hf_jp-ii_enc_25031995_evangelium-vitae_en.html; accessed May 2011.

———. 1994. *Letter to Families*. The Holy See online. www.vatican.va/holy_father/john_paul_ii/letters/documents/hf_jp-ii_let_02021994_families_en.html; accessed May 2011.

———. 2006. *Man and Woman He Created Them: A Theology of the Body*. Trans., intro., and index by Michael Waldstein. Boston: Pauline Books and Media; Rome: Libreria Editrice Vaticana; accessed May 2011.

———. 1988. *Mulieris Dignitatem (On the Dignity and Vocation of Women)*. Apostolic Letter. The Holy See online. www.vatican.va/holy_father/john_paul_ii/apost_letters/documents/hf_jp-ii_apl_15081988_mulieris-dignitatem_en.html; accessed May 2011.

Johnson, Luke Timothy and William S. Kurz, S.J. 2002. *The Future of Catholic Biblical Scholarship: A Constructive Conversation*. Grand Rapids/Cambridge, UK: Eerdmans.

Kleinig, John W. 2005. "Ordered Community: Order and Subordination in the New Testament." *Lutheran Theological Journal* 39: 196-209.

Köstenberger, Andreas J. with David W. Jones. 2010, 2004. *God, Marriage, and Family: Rebuilding the Biblical Foundation*. Second Edition. Wheaton, IL: Crossway.

Kurz, S.J., William. 2001. "Ethical Actualization of Scripture: Approaches toward a Prolife Reading." *Fides Quaerens Intellectum* 1.1: 67-94.

———. 2003. "'To Be As God': Biblical Reflections on the Sexual Revolution." *Fides Quaerens Intellectum* 3: 111-37.

———. 2004. "'To Be as God': Scriptural Links between Abortion and Natural Family Planning": 147-70. *Life and Learning XIII: Proceedings of the Thirteenth University Faculty for Life Conference at Georgetown University 2003*. Joseph W. Koterski. Ed. Washington, DC: University Faculty for Life.

———. 2007. *Reading the Bible as God's Own Story: A Catholic Approach for Bringing Scripture to Life*. Ijamsville, MD: Word Among Us.

———. 1997. "Intertextual Permutations of the Genesis Word in the Johannine Prologues": 179-90. *Early Christian Interpretation of the Scriptures of Israel: Investigation and Proposals*. Craig Evans and James A. Sanders. Eds. *Journal for the Study of the New Testament Supplement Series 148; Studies in Scripture in Early Judaism and Christianity* 5. Sheffield, UK: Sheffield Academic Press.

Louth, Andrew. 2007. *The Origins of the Christian Mystical Tradition: From Plato to Denys*. New York: Oxford University Press.

Martin, Curtis and Michaelann Martin. 2007. "Super-Natural Family Planning": 137-150. In Hahn, Scott and Regis J. Flaherty, Eds. *Catholic for a Reason IV: Scripture and the Mystery of Marriage and Family Life*. Steubenville, OH: Emmaus Road.

Martin, Francis. 1994. *The Feminist Question: Feminist Theology in the Light of Christian Tradition*. Grand Rapids: Eerdmans.

McDermott, S.J., John M. & John Gavin, S.J. 2007. Eds. *Pope John Paul II on the Body: Human, Eucharistic, Ecclesial: Festschrift Avery Cardinal Dulles, S.J.* Philadelphia: Saint Joseph's University Press.

Miller, Kevin. 2010. Email response: "RE: ZENIT: Just Cause and Natural Family Planning," June 17, 2010.

Osiek, Carolyn. 2002. "The Bride of Christ (Ephesians 5:22-33): A Problematic Wedding." *Biblical Theology Bulletin* 32: 29-39.

Peterman, G. W. 1999. "Marriage and Sexual Fidelity in the Papyri, Plutarch, and Paul." *Tyndale Bulletin* 50: 163-172.

Peters, Greg. 2002. "Spiritual Marriage in Early Christianity: 1 Cor 7:25-38 in Modern Exegesis and the Earliest Church." *Trinity Journal* 23: 211-224.

Paul VI. 1968. *Humanae Vitae* (*Of Human Life*). Papal encyclical. The Holy See online www.vatican.va/holy_father/paul_vi/encyclicals/documents/hf_p-vi_enc_25071968_humanae-vitae_en.html; accessed May 2011.

Pius XII. 1943. *Divino Afflante Spiritu*. Encyclical Letter. The Holy See online www.vatican.va/holy_father/pius_xii/encyclicals/documents/hf_p-xii_enc_30091943_divino-afflante-spiritu_en.html; accessed May 2011.

Ramsey, Paul. 1988. "Human Sexuality in the History of Redemption." *Journal of Religious Ethics* 16: 56-86.

Scola, Angelo Cardinal. 2005. *The Nuptial Mystery*. Grand Rapids: Eerdmans.

Second Vatican Council. 1964. *Lumen Gentium* (*Dogmatic Constitution on the Church*). The Holy See online. www.vatican.va/archive/hist_councils/ii_vatican_council/documents/vat-ii_const_19641121_lumen-gentium_en.html; accessed May 2011.

———. 1965a. *Gaudium et Spes* (*Pastoral Constitution on the Church in the Modern World*). The Holy See online. www.vatican.va/archive/hist_councils/ii_vatican_council/documents/vat-ii_cons_19651207_gaudium-et-spes_en.html; accessed May 2011.

———. 1965b. *Dei Verbum* (*Dogmatic Constitution on Divine Revelation*). The Holy See online. www.vatican.va/archive/hist_councils/ii_vatican_council/documents/vat-ii_const_19651118_dei-verbum_en.html; accessed May 2011.

Smith, Janet E. Ed. *Why* Humanae Vitae *Was Right: A Reader*. 1993. San Francisco: Ignatius Press.

Von Balthasar, Hans Urs. 1993. "A Word on *Humanae Vitae*." *Communio* 20: 437-450.

West, Christopher. 2003. *Theology of the Body Explained: A Commentary on John Paul II's "Gospel of the Body."* Boston: Pauline Books and Media.

Whitehead, Kenneth D. Ed. 2007. *The Church, Marriage, and the Family. Proceedings from the 27th Annual Convention of the Fellowship of Catholic Scholars, September 24-26, 2004.* South Bend, IN: St. Augustine's Press.

Williams, A. N. 2007. *The Divine Sense: The Intellect in Patristic Theology.* Cambridge, UK: Cambridge University Press.

15

Co-Creating with the Creator

A Virtue-Based Approach

MELANIE SUSAN BARRETT, PHD

Assistant Professor, Department of Christian Life, Mundelein Seminary, University of St. Mary of the Lake, Archdiocese of Chicago

ABSTRACT

The Roman Catholic Church counsels married couples concerning the *means* for planning one's family (Natural Family Planning rather than contraception), but says relatively little concerning *when* to have children and *how many* to have. What resources can be found in the Catholic (and broader Christian) tradition to further assist couples undergoing this process of discernment? This essay contends that the virtues—including but not limited to those mentioned within the Church's documents on marriage—help constitute an ethical framework for a couple's discernment in seeking to cooperate with the Creator. The argument proceeds in two parts. Part One explains the Church's teaching concerning Natural Family Planning, in order to clarify its underlying rationale. The goal there is twofold: first, to correct misunderstandings of this teaching, emerging both from the theological "left" (in its concern to maximize freedom and empower women) and from the theological "right" (in its concern to uphold traditional family values and ways of life); and second, to illuminate the centrality of the virtues of prudence, chastity, and charity to the practice of periodic abstinence. Part Two investigates the undertheorized questions of when to have children and how many to have: first, by mining Church teaching for useful reflections; second, by surveying the various circumstances (physical, psychological, economic, and social) that pose genuine constraints on family size; and third, by specifying some of the additional virtues that spouses need to cultivate in order to maximize their ability to make prudent moral choices regarding family size.

INTRODUCTION

For married Catholic couples today, negotiating their fertility—when to have children, how many to have, and what means to use for spacing them—can become a harrowing process. Even those who look to the Roman Catholic Church for guidance in this area often find themselves bereft of support. Moral principles articulated by the Magisterium are relatively limited in scope, focusing almost exclusively on the means for planning one's family (Natural Family Planning versus contraception or *in vitro* fertilization) with little attention given to other considerations.

Additionally, certain features of the contemporary cultural milieu converge to make child-rearing appear a risky enterprise at best, a harmful one at worst. In a time marked by economic uncertainty, a high divorce rate, an exaggerated emphasis on the need for personal freedom, and all-too-painful examples of unruly, undisciplined, and spoiled children, parenting's promise to bring deeper meaning and fulfillment to those couples who boldly embark upon it often seems to ring hollow. In light of this, the following question becomes poignant: What resources can be found in the Catholic (and broader Christian) tradition to further assist couples undergoing this process of discernment?

It is my contention that the virtues—including but not limited to those mentioned in the Church's documents on marriage—help constitute an ethical framework for a couple's discernment in seeking to cooperate with the Creator. In Part One, I will explain what the Church advises concerning the means for planning one's family—periodic abstinence rather than contraception—in order to clarify its underlying rationale. My goal there is twofold: first, to correct misunderstandings of this teaching, emerging both from the theological "left" (in its concern to maximize freedom and empower women) and from the theological "right" (in its concern to uphold traditional family values and ways of life); and second, to illuminate the centrality of the virtues of prudence, chastity, and charity for the practice of periodic abstinence. In Part Two, I will investigate the under-theorized questions of "when" and "how many": first, by mining Magisterial teaching for useful reflections; second, by surveying the various circumstances (physical, psychological, economic, and social) that pose genuine constraints on family size; and third, by specifying some of the additional virtues that spouses need to cultivate to maximize their ability to make good moral choices.

PART ONE: USING MORAL MEANS

In Part One, I will explain three things: (1) why, in the Church's view, Natural Family Planning (NFP) is morally good and contraception is morally evil, even in cases where both are accompanied by a justifiable reason to not conceive; (2) what virtues are associated with the practice of NFP; and (3) why NFP is *not* an anti-life practice that impedes God's will, as some claim, by privileging rational discernment and personal choice over heroic trust in God.

Contraception versus Natural Family Planning

Critics on the theological left, attentive to the ethical imperative to respect women's dignity, seek to empower women by expanding their arena of freedom over their internal selves (both body and soul) and over the external circumstances that shape their lives. Such a concern is completely reasonable. Human beings are fulfilled when they attain happiness—that life of well-being and well-doing that the ancient Greek philosophers (such as Socrates, Plato, Aristotle, and the Stoics) describe as *eudaimonia*. The medieval theologian St. Thomas Aquinas, building on Aristotle, further develops this idea. While perfect happiness can be found in God alone (in the beatific vision, seeing God face-to-face in heaven), explains Aquinas, the imperfect happiness of this life requires both virtue (including the soul's ability to transcend the bodily organs) and external goods (like food, drink, money, and political power) which support the body and help one to live virtuously, either through action or contemplation or both (Aquinas 1981, *S.T.* I-II 5-7). Happiness in this life also requires good friends, for we delight in helping our friends and seeing them thrive, and we often rely upon their help as well (Aquinas 1981, *S.T.* I-II 8).

All of these pre-requisites for happiness entail a certain measure of freedom. An uneducated woman in a traditional culture whose husband marries her solely for the purpose of siring his children and carrying on the family line, and who keeps her strictly isolated at home bound to domestic duties, is thereby limited in her ability to flourish. Attaining happiness is considerably more difficult, in that she lacks the comfort and support of close friends, leisure time to contemplate God, opportunities to develop her intellect through education, and the ability to choose a spouse who genuinely loves her and treats her with equal regard.

Freedom is thus a necessary component of happiness. As Pope John Paul II asserts, "Human nature ... is made for freedom. ... Where society is so organized as to reduce arbitrarily or even suppress the sphere in which freedom is legitimately exercised, the result is that the life of society becomes progressively disorganized and goes into decline" (*Centesimus Annus*, no. 25). Seen in this light, the desire to better the lives of women by expanding their freedom is entirely legitimate.

But certain caveats are also in order. For while freedom is a genuine good, like most goods, it has its limits. As we know from experience, chocolate is altogether pleasant and enjoyable, yet too much of it can cause obesity and heart disease; leisure time is necessary but an excessive amount of it can sap one's motivation and make one lazy; physical exercise is generally conducive to health but overdoing it can damage one's health or cause injuries. So too with freedom, although it becomes harmful not when we have too much of it, but when it is exercised in ways that are destructive. Children who are free to pursue all their desires without being reined in by their parents become self-centered rather than generous. Businesses freed from any legal requirements to respect the rights of workers or the integrity of the natural environment tend to exploit both when it is profitable to do so. "Although each individual has a right to be respected in his own journey in search of the truth," notes John Paul II in *Veritatis Splendor*, "there exists a prior moral obligation, and a grave one at that, to seek the truth and to adhere to it once it is known" (no. 34; cf. Vatican II, *Dignitatis Humanae*, no. 2). Freedom is genuinely good for human beings, but only insofar as it retains its "essential and constitutive relationship to truth" (*Veritatis Splendor* [VS], no. 4).

With this framework in mind, how should we think about contraception? Does the use of contraception constitute an appropriate use of freedom, by enabling married couples to act virtuously in relation to their fertility? Or is it an expression of freedom severed from truth, resulting in actions that are harmful rather than helpful? It is the latter, according to Magisterial teaching. Why? To solve this mystery, we must look to Pope Paul VI's 1968 encyclical *Humanae Vitae* (hereafter HV) for instruction.

Echoing the personalist orientation found in numerous theological writings in the latter half of the twentieth century, Paul VI provides an ethical analysis of human fertility based not on a physicalist understanding of natural law—which judges moral actions primarily on their ability to adhere to biological imperatives—but on a personalist approach that situates sexuality squarely within the context of the vocation of marriage and its relation to human fulfillment. To grasp the moral significance of the sexual act, he focuses our attention not on the biological reality—the natural physical destination of human sperm in their singular quest to fertilize human ova—but on the overall human reality, which includes the biological reality but is not solely defined by it. In particular, he underscores the spiritual significance of human love in the divine plan.

According to Paul VI, conjugal love—the love characteristic of spouses—has four attributes. First, it is *human*, "a product not only of natural instinct and inclinations [but] also and primarily ... an act of free will" in which spouses resolve not simply to "persevere through daily joys and sorrows" but also to increase their love to the point of becoming "one in heart and soul, [obtaining] together their human perfection" (HV, no. 9). Second, conjugal love is *total*, "a very special form of personal friendship whereby the spouses generously share everything with each other without undue reservations and without concern for their selfish convenience." To love truly is to love the other for their sake—not for what we receive from them—and to do so "joyfully," enriching the beloved with one's own gift of self (HV, no. 9).

Third, spousal love is *faithful and exclusive*. Although lifelong fidelity can be a challenge at times, Paul VI acknowledges, nevertheless, it is the pre-requisite for "intimate and lasting happiness," which flows out of fidelity "as from a fountain" (HV, no. 9). Fourth, spousal love is *fruitful*: it "looks beyond itself and seeks to raise up new lives," through being ordained to the procreation and education of children. Children are not incidental to marriage; they are its "supreme gift, a gift that contributes immensely to the good of the parents themselves" (HV, no. 9; *Gaudium et Spes* [GS], no. 50).

Conjugal love is the proper context for the sexual act; thus, any moral evaluation of the sexual act must necessarily begin with conjugal love as its primary reference point. Proceeding accordingly, sexual acts that fail to express the true character of spousal love, in at least one respect, are thereby morally deficient. With respect to the first three dimensions of conjugal love, the following acts naturally come to mind as inherently sinful: fornication (because it is not spousal); rape (because it is not loving); adultery (because it is neither faithful nor exclusive); pornographic sex (because objectifying one's spouse or entirely rejecting one's spouse in favor of self-gratification falls short of the total love expressed by mutual self-gift); and, all forms of unchaste sex (because it is not fully human to seek sexual release like an animal who is driven solely by biological need and lacks the virtuous capacity to restrain that desire where necessary to deepen friendship).

But what about the fourth criteria, that of fruitfulness? What kinds of conjugal acts are immoral because they violate love's *fruitful* dimension? For Paul VI, the answer is contraceptive acts: acts that make an otherwise fertile act infertile, in order to prevent conception. Condoms, diaphragms, sponges, and birth control pills all generally fall into this category of being morally impermissible for spouses to use because they are contraceptive. They become morally permissible only if it can be objectively demonstrated that such means are being used with a therapeutic intention. In that case, such means would not truly be "contraceptive" (against conception), because the proximate end of one's act would not be "to prevent conception" but rather "to cure a disease." As Paul VI asserts, "such treatment is permissible even if the reduction of fertility is foreseen, as long as the infertility is not directly intended for any reason whatsoever" (HV, no. 15).

At first glance, this overall teaching appears to unfairly restrict human freedom. Without recourse to contraception, married couples who wish to engage in the conjugal act to express love and deepen friendship would necessarily be forced to accept large families even in cases where they are physically, financially, or psychologically unable to care for them. However, this is not the intention either of Paul VI or of his successors. Immediately following his explication of the four dimensions of spousal love, Paul VI launches into a discussion of "responsible parenthood." Echoing his previous assertion that the human aspect of spousal love mandates that sex must be "a product not only of natural instinct and inclinations [but] also and primarily ... an act of free will," he states explicitly that if parents are to act responsibly, "reason and will [must] exercise mastery over [the innate] impulses and inclinations of the soul" (HV, nos. 9-10; cf. no. 21).

Mastery over the soul's inclinations is another way of talking about virtue, in this case the virtues of prudence and chastity. Chastity is a species of temperance, the virtue of moderation (Aquinas 1981, *S.T.*, II-II 41). When we act temperately, we order our sense appetites in accord with what is reasonable. For example, a person who is on a diet might abstain from dessert altogether, or restrict himself to just one serving per week, in order to lose weight. A single woman at a bar might limit herself to only one or two alcoholic beverages, to prevent lapses of judgment resulting in sexual impropriety. A couple who is dating might abstain altogether from sex until their wedding day, in order to protect each other's hearts and establish a stable environment for any future children. All of these are examples of temperate behavior because one "tempers" or moderates one's natural desire for food, alcohol, or sex in accord with what reason prescribes.

How do we discern what is reasonable? By intending a good end (such as being healthy or guarding one's heart), deliberating about the best means to this end (taking counsel from experts or other pertinent authorities), applying any relevant moral principles to the situation at hand, and finally making a judgment about what we think is right and committing ourselves to act on it. To do this well, is to exercise the intellectual virtue of prudence (Aquinas 1981, *S.T.* II-II 47.8).

So the thrust of Paul VI's argument is that married couples who wish to act responsibly in regard to their fertility need at least two virtues: chastity (the ability to moderate sexual desires) and prudence (the capacity to make good judgments about *when* and *how* to moderate them). He then offers counsel, based on the teaching authority given by Christ to the original apostles and their successors (the bishops). The Pope's counsel is intended not as a cultish exercise in brainwashing, but as a logical argument that is accessible by reason and that accords with divine revelation. He counsels that spouses who have serious reasons "not to have another child either for a definite or an indefinite amount of time" can abstain from sexual intercourse during fertile times (HV, no. 10). Practicing temporary abstinence in order to prevent conception is morally acceptable, he argues, because it respects the act's intrinsic relationship to procreation, by not suppressing it (HV, no. 11).

According to Paul VI, the fundamental nature of the conjugal act, its overall significance, is comprised of two essential aspects: one unitive and one procreative (HV, no. 12). The "unitive" significance (or meaning) of the conjugal act refers to the act's ability to unite the spouses by strengthening their friendship and deepening their love for one another. The "procreative" significance (or meaning) refers to its generative capacity during fertile times to co-create a unique human being in cooperation with God, the ultimate author of all life. The unitive meaning is violated when sex occurs in a way that is contrary to friendship, for example, by treating one's spouse as an object rather than a unique person with intrinsic dignity, or by raping him or her. The procreative meaning is violated when sex occurs in a way that directly impedes procreation, for example, by contracepting either before, during, or immediately after the conjugal act.

Notably, these two constitutive aspects of the conjugal act are grasped not by analyzing the physical material of sex (human sperm and ova) in isolation from other concerns, but by considering the act in the broader context of human fulfillment. For as John Paul II explains in *Vertiatis Splendor*, the good of the body is subordinate to the good of the soul, so we can discern the body's moral significance only in "the light of reason, [supported by] virtue, [expressive of] the gift of self, in conformity with the wise plan of the Creator" (VS, 1993, no. 48).

John Paul II's personalist approach to natural law, in contrast to a simple physicalist approach, is precisely the methodology that Paul VI himself utilizes. Paul VI maintains that the two inherent meanings of the marital sexual act, unity and procreation, must be respected at all times because they are constitutive of human fulfillment. To begin with, by aiming at spousal unity, "the conjugal act fully maintains its capacity for fostering true mutual love" (HV, no. 12). Fostering love is the main purpose of both marriage and the human vocation broadly construed. Love is both a commandment ("love thy neighbor as thyself ... love is the fulfillment of the law" [Rom 13:9-10]), and the sole means to true self-realization and growth in holiness. Made in the image and likeness of a God who is love (Gen 1:27; 1 Jn 4:8), the human person "cannot fully find himself except through a sincere gift of himself," as the Second Vatican Council professes (GS, no. 24).

Additionally, human beings, at least those in the married state, are called by God to "be fruitful and multiply" (Gen 1:22, 9:7), or in Paul VI's words, to undertake the "mission" of parenthood (HV, no.

13). And mission, as Swiss theologian Hans Urs von Balthasar affirms, is the fundamental path of Christian discipleship. Jesus is God as mission—the literal embodiment of the Father's act of sending himself forth. As his disciples, we too are sent forth (von Balthasar 1992, pp.150ff). Carrying out God's mission inevitably involves some form of suffering, as was the case with the prophets of old (e.g., Job, Jeremiah, Elijah) and with Jesus himself, but such suffering is always in the service of love (von Balthasar 1983, pp. 407-408). As to the family's mission, it too is love, specifically "to guard, reveal, and communicate love" so as to reflect and share in God's love for humanity and Christ's love for his Church (*Familiaris Consortio* [FC], no. 17). Not only the unitive but also the procreative meaning of the conjugal act, therefore, has love as its defining context.

What does this imply about controlling human fertility? Does respecting the procreative meaning of the conjugal act mean that couples must subjectively desire to conceive a child each and every time they engage in intercourse? No, because not all acts are naturally fertile to begin with. In fact, the majority of conjugal acts are naturally infertile—those during menopause, pregnancy, menstruation, and on most days in a healthy female menstrual cycle prior to menopause.

Consequently, a couple who has made a prudent judgment not to have a child at a particular time, on the basis of justifiable reasons, is free to engage in the conjugal act during infertile times. Moreover, their subjective choice to engage *only* in those conjugal acts that are naturally infertile (non-procreative) can in no way be considered "anti-procreative." Only by willfully choosing to make an otherwise fertile act infertile would the procreative meaning of the conjugal act be violated. Whereas periodic abstinence (NFP) *respects* the procreative meaning of the conjugal act by abstaining during fertile times, contraception *contravenes* it.

Let us now return to our earlier concern regarding freedom as a means for advancing human flourishing. Assuming prudent reasons not to conceive, are spouses who engage in contracepted sex more free than those who practice periodic abstinence? At first glance, the answer appears to be "yes." After all, couples who contracept can be more spontaneous with regard to their sexual activity. They can enjoy the unitive benefits of spousal intercourse even during fertile times of the month. Women in particular are blissfully free from the irritating tasks of observing vaginal mucus for signs of fertility, charting out daily changes in body temperature, and/or urinating on a stick ten days a month while using a fertility monitor. Additionally, the use of barrier methods (like condoms) enables a woman to have sex precisely when she is most interested—when her hormone levels peak at ovulation—without having to restrain her desire in the least. Assuming her husband is a willing participant, her increased level of interest is experienced as a boon for him as well.

But is the wife in this scenario truly more free than one who practices NFP? On closer investigation, the answer seems to be "no." Barrier forms of contraception can inhibit a couple's sense of intimacy and closeness precisely by placing an artificial "barrier" between them. Reliance on hormonal methods requires women to take a pill daily or receive hormone shots regularly, and also subjects them to unpleasant side effects: some of them potentially life-threatening, such as the increased risk of breast cancer or stroke. Moreover, being on the pill frees a woman *in theory* to have sex with her husband during fertile times, but *in practice* the benefit no longer exists because her self-imposed infertility means no ovulation and therefore no increased sexual desire. In addition, oral contraceptives can further reduce the sex drive by elevating a protein (SHBG) that binds itself to testosterone, a side effect that can persist even after contraceptives have been discontinued.[1] Finally, in cases of breakthrough ovulation resulting in an unplanned pregnancy, the pill can unwittingly function as an abortifacient.

Perhaps most notably, for a woman whose husband seeks to engage in sex with her on a frequent (almost daily) basis, by choosing to use contraception instead of NFP, she forgoes an indispensable tool to help him develop the virtue of chastity. Consequently, she is more likely to be objectified by her husband, treated reductively as a sexual outlet for his insatiable need rather than as an equal partner with whom he endeavors to deepen friendship.[2] For as John Paul II contends, self-gift presupposes self-possession. One who lacks the virtue of chastity is not truly free to give himself to others. Though culturally masked as authentic freedom, in reality sexual licentiousness is a form of enslavement, incapable of producing genuine communion and the profound sense of joy that is concomitant with it.

NFP promotes authentic human freedom in a second respect as well, by increasing the likelihood that couples will have children (and more of them) and thereby attain a deeper level of personal fulfillment. Contraception, by contrast, provides no such benefit. How does this work? Once spouses have made a prudent decision to postpone childbearing at a particular time, what happens next? At what point will they revisit the issue? A great deal depends on the practice they choose. If they habitually use contraception, the question might not arise at all. For childless couples who live busy lives filled with the activities of advancing in careers, socializing with friends, spending time with extended family members, attending cultural events, going on vacations, and remodeling their homes, an existential "space" for children might not naturally present itself. Their original circumstances might change, clearing the roadblocks to starting a family, yet they might be too busy even to notice. For spouses who already have at least one child to care for, the busyness factor is even more overwhelming.

By contrast, if the spouses practice NFP, then the question of parental readiness arises much more frequently. Every month that they desire sexual union during their week of shared fertility is experienced as a struggle. This naturally gives rise to the question, "Why are we abstaining? Is it still necessary?" If their original circumstances have changed, then they will recognize this more quickly. If the initial impediments remain but are within their power to change, their motivation for doing so will be greater. For example, a couple who needs to pay off substantial credit card debt will be more frequently reminded to forgo unnecessary luxuries in order to attain financial stability and start a family.

Theoretically, contracepting couples are quite capable of evaluating parental readiness on a regular basis. But as was the case with cultivating chastity, without a practice of periodic abstinence to prod them, they are much less likely to do so. Consequently, healthy spouses who practice NFP during their childbearing years are more likely to become parents and also to have more children. Though being a parent certainly limits one's freedom in certain respects, particularly where infants are concerned, overall the practice of parenting is more conducive to authentic freedom because it tempers selfishness and increases one's freedom to love.

An illustrative example: although attending the symphony in the park in the summer with their dog gives childless spouses the opportunity to express love—both to one another and to their beloved pet—such an outing pales in comparison to the degree of love that arises from bringing one's children to the same event. While communing with a well-behaved dog who requires little supervision might subjectively be experienced as more romantic, in the objective order it involves a less profound act of love, because less of the soul is engaged. As with a dog, caring for children involves feeding them, monitoring their health, training them to be quiet and still, and giving them physical affection. Parenting however, also involves much more. Children must be taught to be self-sufficient; to reason well and make prudent choices; to be temperate, chaste, and brave; to treat strangers with profound respect for their dignity as persons made in God's image; to be patient and forgiving, even with their siblings; to be generous of spirit and care for the poor; and to have faith in a God who loves them radically and calls them to radical love of others in response. Every moment of parenting, whether at the symphony, the grocery store, a family reunion, or a simple dinner, requires this high degree of loving attentiveness, and all the forethought, planning, creativity, and humility that make it efficacious.

Family life is not merely one consumer choice among other equally good lifestyle choices; it is a "communion of persons" whose inner principle … permanent power and … final goal is love" (FC, no. 18). Marriage is a vocation created by God to bring about growth in holiness through self-giving. Practically speaking, a spouse who is also a parent has greater opportunities for self-gift, and thus for becoming holy, especially if he or she parents more than one child. This is not to imply that other social arenas, such as the workplace, do not also provide opportunities for married people to act in loving ways and grow in virtue. It is simply to acknowledge that the deeply personal and profoundly intimate character of caring for another human being as his or her parent enables love to flourish. For this reason, it is greatly conducive to personal fulfillment. By increasing the likelihood that spouses will choose to become parents and attain this greater happiness, the practice of NFP can be regarded as reinforcing authentic freedom rather than hindering it.

Virtues Associated with Natural Family Planning

In addition to prudence and chastity, spouses who practice NFP cultivate and deepen other important virtues as well, most notably charity, by being united to God in friendship and loving others in God. Aristotle famously categorized three different types of friendships: (1) those for the purpose of obtaining some useful good; (2) those for the purpose of obtaining pleasure; and (3) those between good people based on mutual regard for one another as persons. The first two forms of friendship occur frequently but are fleeting. Once there is no longer something useful or pleasurable to be gained, there is no reason to continue the friendship. The third type of friendship is perfect but rare, because good people are hard to find and because they require "time and familiarity" to cultivate. This love of true friendship is not a feeling. It is a choice springing from character wherein we "wish well to those whom [we] love, for their sake," and they make "an equal return in goodwill and in pleasantness to us" (Aristotle 1962, 8.3-5).

Extending Aristotle's definition to the theological realm, Aquinas characterized our love for God as one of friendship (*caritas*) because God wishes us well and actively communicates his happiness to us. *Caritas*, the virtue of charity, not only unites us to God; it is the very life of the soul, just as the soul is the life of the body. Consequently, our love for others is always a participation in divine charity (Aquinas 1981, *S.T.*, II-II 23.1-2). To love another person for his or her sake is not simply to wish that person well, but to wish that he or she may be in God—the only authentic path to complete and everlasting happiness—and to be affectively united with that person (Aquinas 1981, *S.T.*, II-II 25.1, 27.2).

Apart from this explicit reference to God, our predominant contemporary understanding of marital friendship is not altogether different from that of Aristotle and Aquinas. A national survey on love and marriage asked men and women which model of love best correlates with good marriages and families. Respondents chose among three classical models found in the Western theological and philosophical tradition: "marital love as *mutuality or equal regard* ('giving your spouse and children the same respect, affection, and help as you expect from them') ... marital love as *self-sacrifice* ('putting the needs and goals of your spouse and children ahead of your own') ... [and marital love] as serving *self-fulfillment* ('fulfilling your personal needs and life goals')" (Browning et al. 2000, p.18). Among the 1,019 respondents polled, 55% chose mutuality, 38% chose self-sacrifice, and only 5% chose self-fulfillment (Browning et al. p.19). Thus, despite the general current of selfishness pervading our culture, most people readily acknowledge that a good marriage involves mutual regard for one another as persons, and an active readiness to help one another, even at some cost to oneself.

An argument can be made that the practice of NFP deepens marital friendship—and thus the virtue of charity—in a way that contraception does not, precisely by cultivating these two dispositions (mutual regard and self-sacrifice). After all, contraception is almost always the woman's responsibility alone. According to recent statistics, only 17% of contraception is used by men (either condoms or a vasectomy), whereas 67.7% is used by women (the pill, tubal sterilization, IUD, injectables, vaginal ring, implant, patch, female condom, foam, cervical cap, sponge, emergency contraception, or other methods).[3] Because the woman is primarily responsible for contraception, she alone must endure its burdens and health risks. It is a sacrifice she makes for the sake of her marriage, but it is one-sided.

By contrast, practicing NFP requires mutual self-sacrifice. Both husband and wife are required to abstain from sexual intercourse approximately one week each menstrual cycle. This can be subjectively experienced as difficult, especially for the wife whose sexual desire is particularly intense that week due to hormonal changes. If the couple is used to having intercourse on a regular basis, however, taking a time out can be fruitful by encouraging them to become more romantic in their affections, to express their love in alternate, non-genital ways. This can result in better quality foreplay when they subsequently return to intercourse. Most notably, as discussed earlier, practice at sexual restraint helps spouses cultivate the virtue of chastity, so their future sexual encounters are more likely to be intentional and deeply personal expressions of love rather than simple opportunities for sexual release. This is not to imply that contracepting couples are doomed to impersonal sex; it is simply to acknowledge that chaste individuals have a greater capacity to express love through sex. The practice of periodic abstinence helps non-chaste spouses cultivate the virtue of chastity, whereas contraception provides no such benefit.

NFP's contribution to mutuality—and thus to the virtue of charity—can also be seen in the meaning it expresses as a symbolic language between the spouses. As John Paul II maintains in his *Theology of the Body*, sexual intercourse, by its very nature as a profoundly intimate exchange with the potential to be life-giving, objectively bespeaks a total gift of self: "I give you my whole self, and I accept your gift of self in return, now and always." Engaging in intercourse, while holding something back, is thus an inherent contradiction. Such is the case with fornication ("I give you my whole self ... but just for tonight");

adultery ("I give part of myself to you … but the other part to my mistress"); fantasy sex ("I accept your gift of self but only if we role-play and pretend you're really somebody else"); and pornographic sex ("I'm not really interested in you as a person right now, just your body parts"). A similar contradiction occurs when married couples use contraception: "I give you my whole self … except my fertility" or "I accept your whole gift of self in return … except your fertility." NFP, by contrast, preserves the objective language of self-gift because spouses do not actively withhold their fertility from one another during their acts of intercourse.

In sum, there is a discernible moral difference between practicing contraception and practicing periodic abstinence in order to prevent conception. Whereas contraception violates the procreative meaning of the conjugal act—by explicitly acting to make an otherwise fertile act of intercourse infertile—periodic abstinence respects the procreative meaning because spouses altogether abstain from intercourse during fertile times. Moreover, despite the fact that it limits sexual spontaneity, NFP is more conducive to authentic freedom—which promotes human fulfillment—in several respects: it encourages spouses to evaluate their parental readiness more frequently, increasing the likelihood they will become parents and grow in holiness through parenting; its sacrificial dimension promotes the virtue of chastity, helping to ensure the personal quality of the sexual act; and it deepens the virtue of charity, which sustains marital friendship by enhancing mutuality and helping to preserve sex's objective meaning as total self-gift.

Critics of Natural Family Planning

Having responded to theological critics on the left (who contend that contraception should be acknowledged as morally valid), I will now respond to theological critics on the right (who contend that *both* contraception *and* Natural Family Planning should be acknowledged as morally deficient). Critics on the theological right, in a laudable but mistaken effort to be "true to Church teaching," often deem NFP to be morally problematic for two reasons: (1) it is relatively "new" in the history of Catholic moral theology, and thus an object of suspicion; and (2) it resembles contraception (which the Church wholeheartedly condemned in *Humanae Vitae*) because both are chosen on the basis of the same judgment: to prevent conception with rational planning, and this is seen as impeding rather than discerning God's will for them as a couple. To correct this error, I will explain why a couple can choose to engage in the conjugal act only during infertile times, on the basis of justifiable reasons to not conceive, without thereby committing a sin; and why the contemporary Church teaches that rational planning about *when* to have children and *how many* to have is consistent with responsible parenthood.

The Church's teaching regarding periodic abstinence is relatively new in the history of Catholic moral theology. Conservative critics of the practice regard this as grounds for suspicion. They worry that the Church is gradually conforming herself to a culture that overemphasizes freedom, individual autonomy, and personal fulfillment at the expense of traditional family values and duties. In addition, cognizant of the culturally dominant "contraceptive mentality"—the view that sex is primarily not about children but about something else, like pleasure—which has resulted in millions of unplanned and unwanted pregnancies and frequent recourse to abortion, they regard Catholic couples who consciously endeavor to limit their family size through periodic abstinence as infected with a mild version of this same self-centered, anti-life worldview, even when couples practicing NFP possess demonstrably serious reasons to not conceive at a particular time.

From their perspective, to be fully open to life and to doing God's will, spouses must subjectively *desire* to procreate each and every time they engage in the conjugal act, at least to some degree. Circumstances that seem inopportune for conceiving another child (such as financial constraints, grave health impediments, or serious marital difficulties) call for heroic trust in God, whose providence ensures that divine care will supplement whatever the parents themselves might be lacking. To consciously choose—and subsequently plan—*not* to conceive under such circumstances is seen as potentially defying God's will for them as a couple. After all, God might *want* them to conceive a child at this time, despite the difficulties, and the only way to be sure is to maximize the space in which God can act: by neither contracepting nor periodically abstaining. If conception does occur, this can be taken as proof that God specifically willed it to take place *at that time*; determining whether it is a good time to conceive (or not) is always God's responsibility *alone*. In their view, spouses themselves never participate in the decision (unless they are acting immorally). Consequently, despite the fact that the Church now officially endorses periodic abstinence for those who have justifiable reasons not to conceive, faithful Catholics who desire to perfectly obey God's will should *never* practice it.

In my estimation, this misunderstanding stems in part from a misreading of *Humanae Vitae*. Paragraph 11 of the current standard English translation states that "each and every marital act must of necessity *retain its intrinsic relationship* to the procreation of human life." An alternate but equally useful translation is found in Janet Smith's translation: "it is necessary that each conjugal act remain *ordained in itself [per se destinatus]* to the procreating of human life." What does it mean for an act to be "intrinsically related" or "ordained in itself" to procreation? The answer is found is paragraph 16, which clarifies the difference between periodic abstinence and contraception. In practicing periodic abstinence, "the spouses rightly use a faculty provided them by nature," whereas in contracepting they "obstruct the natural development of the generative process." The central issue at stake is not whether the spouses *desire* to conceive (or not), but whether, based on that desire, they *impede* the act from attaining its natural end.

Earlier English translations of the document were less clear, however, because they based themselves on the Italian version of the encyclical rather than the Latin text. As Smith has pointed out, paragraph 11 of the Latin text utilizes the phrase *per se destinatus*, whereas the Italian text uses the simple verb *aperto*, which is less philosophically precise yet was subsequently translated into English, as "open" (Smith 1991, pp. 78-79, 269-270). Herein lies the confusion, for what does it mean to say that each and every conjugal act must remain "open" to procreation? How can an act that is naturally infertile be open to procreation? For many English readers of the document the answer was simple: spouses are required to be continually *open* to the *idea* of having children, at least to some degree. In the minds of such readers, this attitude is also more pro-life because it ensures that couples faced with an unplanned pregnancy will never be tempted to have an abortion.

With this false interpretation of paragraph 11 in mind, the encyclical's later permission to practice NFP appears either as an outright contradiction by a wishy-washy Church, striving on the one hand to resist modernity, and on the other to concede to it; or as a singular exception to an otherwise exceptionless general moral principle, intended pastorally to assist those couples whose faith is too weak or whose commitment to Christ is too tenuous to endure the rigors of conforming to the principle with total devotion. To proponents of this latter view, the practice of periodic abstinence amounts to a "Catholic-lite" alternative for those who rightly reject contraception as morally bankrupt yet ultimately fall short of the heroic trust in God—and the concomitant willingness to suffer for God's sake—that constitutes true discipleship.

Another basis for the conservative critique of NFP lies in the inability of many traditional Catholics to fathom why the contemporary Church suddenly placed the procreative and unitive meanings of the conjugal act on equal footing, after centuries of Church teaching that upheld the procreative purpose as primary. To resolve this confusion, a brief historical excursus is in order.

In the early Church, many impassioned exhortations in the area of Christian apologetics, subsequently codified as official theological doctrine, sought to uphold the reality of both the Incarnation and the Resurrection—and the intrinsic goodness of the human body by implication—against those who held that evil matter could never serve as the bearer of divinity. St. Augustine of Hippo was one of the heralds of this teaching, defending, among other things, the inherent goodness of procreation in marriage. Despite this laudable trajectory, however, Augustine's personal struggle with sexual lust, coupled with a profound appreciation of the persistent capacity for human sinfulness, converged in a deep pessimism toward sexual intercourse in general.

In his treatise, *On Marriage and Concupiscence*, Augustine upheld the goodness of procreation and defended marriage as an honorable institution, yet deemed the conjugal act inherently shameful on account of the sexual pleasure involved (Augustine 1887b, Ch. 27). In stark contrast to contemporary Church teaching, which underscores the act's unitive dimension—its capacity to express love and thereby deepen marital friendship—Augustine held that all sexual pleasure is indelibly rooted in lust. Consequently, all conjugal acts are sinful, unless done for the explicit purpose of procreation (Augustine 1887b, Ch. 17). Even then, they remain shameful. Although the intense ardor required to complete the sexual act "is no longer accounted sin in the regenerate," it nevertheless remains "the daughter of sin"—a direct consequence of the Fall—and the precise vehicle through which Original Sin is transmitted from parent to child (Augustine 1887b, Ch. 27). Thus, whereas Catholics today profess that Jesus was born without Original Sin because Mary herself was immaculately conceived, Augustine attributes Jesus' purity to the fact that Mary experienced no sexual pleasure by conceiving him as a virgin (Augustine 1887b, Ch. 27).

Had Augustine been privy to our modern scientific understanding of fertility, he would have had to deem most conjugal acts in most marriages as not merely shameful but sinful (at least venially). For as we recognize today, nature is designed in such a way that procreation is possible only for a few days each month and only in the years prior to menopause. Viewed across the entire lifespan of a lasting marriage, this adds up to very few days indeed. Spouses seeking to follow Augustine's teaching to the letter would have to restrain themselves far beyond what is required for the virtue of chastity. Moreover, for faithful spouses who marry later in life (post-menopause), consummation on their wedding night (or at any point thereafter) would necessarily have to be followed by a trip to the confessional: repenting of their venial sin (engaging in sex when procreation was impossible) and re-committing themselves never to have sex again. Such excessive restraint can be morally justified only if Augustine is correct in his belief that *all* sex is necessarily an expression of lust. But to agree with Augustine would be to reject St. Paul's assertions—which Augustine himself seems to have missed—that our old selves were crucified with Christ (Rom 6:6-8), and that in Christ we become a new creation (2 Cor 5:17), prompted by the Spirit to crucify all our self-indulgent passions and desires (Gal 5:24-25), and re-created in the goodness and holiness of the truth (Eph 4:22-24).

Moving forward in history, Aquinas implicitly grasps the redemptive possibility of sex without lust, though he does not yet fully develop it. Contra Augustine, he maintains that sexual desire is not problematic in and of itself; like all desires, it becomes virtuous once it is ordered by reason. "Just as the use of food can be without sin, if it be taken in due manner and order, as required for the welfare of the body," Aquinas explains, "so also the use of venereal acts can be without sin, provided they be performed in due manner and order, in keeping with the end of human procreation" (Aquinas 1981, *S. T.*, II-II 153.2). The virtue of chastity is a mean between the vicious extremes of lust (excessive sexual desire unrestrained by reason) and insensibility (insufficient sexual desire rendering one unable to pay the marriage debt) (Aquinas, *S. T.*, II-II 153.3). Conjugal intercourse can be practiced chastely—virtuously—because it does not intrinsically corrupt the faculty of reason; it merely causes spouses to shift their focus from the good of contemplation to a good action (Aquinas 1981, *S. T.*, III *Suppl.* 49.4.1; cf. *S.T.*, I-II 34.1.1). The intensity of passion experienced in the conjugal act does not exceed the bounds of reason because it is a reasonable thing for a married couple to do (Aquinas 1981, *S.T.*, III *Suppl.* 49.4.3). Sexual pleasure, like all natural pleasures, is morally good as long as the act that produces it is morally good (Aquinas 1981, *S.T.*, I-II 34.1; cf. Grabowski 2003, p. 79).

Aquinas' recognition of chaste conjugal sex as a genuine possibility in a world redeemed by Christ significantly departs from Augustine's view that all sex is tainted by lust, but both theologians affirm procreation as the purpose of the conjugal act. Neither explicitly proposes a unitive purpose of sex to supplement its procreative purpose. Aquinas sets the stage for later theologians to do so, however, by removing shame from the conjugal act and by asserting that the one-flesh union leads a husband to love his wife more intensely than he loves his parents (Aquinas 1981, *S.T.*, II-II 26.11).

The practice of periodic abstinence came into fashion in the mid-nineteenth century, when science began to clarify the patterns of fertility surrounding a woman's menstrual cycle.[4] The Church lent its official approbation to the practice relatively quickly. In 1853 and 1880, under popes Pius IX and Leo XIII, the Apostolic Penitentiary—the tribunal in the Roman Curia that handles internal forum matters such as the forgiveness of sins—instructed confessors as follows: to not "disturb" couples who are practicing periodic abstinence, and to cautiously recommend the practice as an alternative to those who are practicing Onanism (early withdrawal, possibly coupled with masturbation; see Noonan, 1986, p. 439 and p. 441).

The beginnings of an official theological justification for NFP can be found in the *1917 Code of Canon Law*, which states that along with the procreation and education of children, marriage has a secondary end: "mutual help and the allaying of concupiscence" (*1917 Code of Canon Law*, c. 1013, §1). Although Augustine (and later medieval canonists) had counted marriage's ability to remedy concupiscence among its intrinsic goods—since sex with one's spouse ensures fidelity by helping one avoid the greater evils of adultery and divorce—the concept of "mutual help" in marriage was substantially more positive.

But can the conjugal act *itself* promote marriage's goal of mutual help between the spouses? Yes and more, according to Pope Pius XI in *Casti Connubii*, his 1930 encyclical on Christian marriage. Pius XI defends the practice of periodic abstinence by asserting that those who do not procreate "on account of natural reasons ... of time" are not acting against nature because a non-procreative conjugal act can still further secondary ends "such as mutual aid, the cultivating of mutual love, and the quieting of concupiscence" (CC, no. 59).[5] Among these ends, recognition of the second—*the cultivating of mutual love*—constitutes a significant development in magisterial teaching, one that helped to codify the emerging personalist approach to sexual ethics. In the 1920s and 1930s, theologians like Dietrich von Hildebrand and Herbert Doms contended that sex can be a privileged form of self-giving between spouses that both expresses and fosters their communion of love (Grabowski 2003, pp.85-86).

More recent Church documents reflect this change: by characterizing the good of the spouses—which includes, above all, their growing in love through a mutual gift of self—as an end of marriage on par with the procreation and education of children; and by placing the unitive meaning of the conjugal act on par with its procreative meaning. The Second Vatican Council, in its pastoral constitution *Gaudium et Spes*, highlights the importance of parenthood "while not making the other purposes of matrimony of less account," because "marriage ... is not instituted solely for procreation" and even the welfare of the children themselves demands "that the mutual love of the spouses be embodied in a rightly ordered manner, that it grow and ripen" (GS, no. 50). The couple's union is "a mutual gift" of both their persons and their actions, enabling them to "experience the meaning of their oneness and attain to it with growing perfection day by day" (GS, no. 48).

In *Humanae Vitae*, written two and a half years later, Paul VI further develops this framework by proposing four defining characteristics of conjugal love, by regarding the conjugal act as the most apt expression of conjugal love, and by explicitly describing the conjugal act as constituted by two inseparable aspects or meanings—one unitive and one procreative. Fifteen years after *Humanae Vitae*, the *1983 Code of Canon Law* characterizes marriage as naturally ordered "to the good of the spouses and the procreation and education of offspring" (*1983 Code of Canon Law*, c. 1055, § 1). This contrasts with the *1917 Code of Canon Law* that described procreation as primary and other goods of marriage as secondary. The 1994 *Catechism of the Catholic Church*, discussing the love of husband and wife, proclaims sexuality to be "a source of joy and pleasure" established by the Creator, affirms conjugal acts that intimately and chastely unite the spouses to be "noble and honorable," and declares that "the truly human performance of these acts fosters the self-giving they signify and enriches the spouses in joy and gratitude" (CCC, no. 2362). It then explicitly asserts that "the spouses' union achieves the twofold end of marriage: the good of the spouses themselves and the transmission of life" which "cannot be separated without altering the couple's spiritual life and compromising the goods of marriage and the future of the family" (CCC, no. 2363).

The gradual shift from understanding procreation as the *sole purpose* of the conjugal act to *one aspect* of the conjugal act, along with its unitive aspect, should not be interpreted as a devaluing of the vocation of parenting. Children remain marriage's "supreme gift" (GS, 1966, no. 50). Rather, what has taken place is a broadening of the Church's understanding of both sex and marriage to include *all* the ways in which spouses are called to express love. Marriage's sacramental dimension reminds us that we stand before God both as sinners and as disciples who have been internally transformed by grace and commissioned by Christ to heal a broken world. Spouses enact this mission both by raising children and through other acts of love (including sexual intercourse) that constitute a gift of self. The entire spousal relationship, as constituted by such self-giving acts, mirrors Christ's love for his Church, just as the love of family members for one another reflects the communion of life and love among the persons of the Trinity. Seen from the vantage point of love and discipleship, conjugal acts that endeavor to express love and deepen friendship are morally praiseworthy, even when enacted during infertile times.

PART TWO: DISCERNING "WHEN" AND "HOW MANY"

Having explained the Church's rationale for recommending the practice of periodic abstinence as a means for planning one's family, let us now set forth the conditions under which that practice is legitimate. When is it prudent to avoid procreating, and when is it prudent to actively strive for it? How do spouses discern the "right time," either to start having children or to expand the size of their family? What kinds of considerations ought to be taken into account? Such questions are pressing both for fertile couples—particularly those whose regular practice of NFP makes it a monthly topic of discussion—and for those who are permanently infertile (on account of illness, dysfunction, or menopausal stage of life) yet desire children and wonder whether God is calling them to be adoptive or foster parents.

I will address the question of "when" and "how many" in three phases: (1) by surveying Magisterial teaching on these matters; (2) by categorizing common constraints on parenting and their prospects for resolution; and (3) by describing some of the moral virtues needed for discernment to be both rational and spiritually fruitful.

Magisterial Teaching: Pius XII, Vatican II, Paul VI, John Paul II, & Canon Law

Church teaching provides couples with relatively little practical guidance concerning when to have children and how many to have. It does offer some general guidelines, however. First, individuals who intend *never* to give their spouse the right to perform acts that lead to procreation *regardless of circumstance* cannot validly enter into marriage to begin with. The current *Code of Canon Law* (1983) stipulates that "in order for matrimonial consent to exist, the contracting parties must be at least not ignorant that marriage is a permanent partnership between a man and a woman ordered to the procreation of offspring by means of some sexual cooperation" (CCL, 1983, c.1096 §1), and a person who, "by a positive act of the will [excludes] ... some essential element ... or property of marriage, contracts invalidly" (CCL, c.1101 §2). The law's emphasis on *willful* exclusion means that sterile individuals are not thereby prohibited from marrying (CCL, c.1084 §3). The same permission does not apply, however, to those suffering from "antecedent and perpetual impotence," which "nullifies marriage by its very nature" because it prevents both consummation (CCL, c.1084 §1; cf. cc.1141-1142) and the fulfillment of spousal rights "to those things which belong to the partnership of conjugal life" (CCL, c. 1135).

Second, assuming neither sterility, nor permanent impotence, nor a will permanently set against having children, spouses act "responsibly" in one of two ways, according to Paul VI: either by electing "to accept many children ... guided by prudent consideration and generosity," or by deciding "not to have another child for either a definite or an indefinite amount of time" on account of "serious reasons" [*seriis causis*] or "well-grounded reasons" [*iustae causae*]" (HV, nos. 10, 16). The phrases "prudent consideration" and "well-grounded reasons" imply that in either case, whether choosing to have children or to postpone childbearing, spouses must arrive at their decision on the basis of reason: thoughtfully determining what is rationally appropriate in light of their current circumstances. God's will for them as a couple is ascertained *not* by mere instinct, impulse, whim, or desire—whether biological or emotional or both—but rather on the basis of careful and rigorous intellectual discernment guided by a spirit of generosity rather than selfishness.

Paul VI's emphasis on prudence reflects a Thomist approach to moral discernment rather than an intuitionist or physicalist approach. As Aquinas contended, human beings participate in God's eternal law—God's overarching plan for the universe—through the natural law: the exercise of human reason within the context of the person's fundamental orientation to do good and avoid evil. From a natural law perspective, determining what is right to do in terms of family size requires the same kind of analysis as other moral quandaries. Applying the stages of prudence discussed earlier, spouses must first intend a good end (i.e., to faithfully live out the vocation of marriage); deliberate about the best means to this end (i.e., by taking counsel from Paul VI that parenting is an "extremely important mission" with which "God has entrusted spouses," (HV, no. 1); consider any relevant moral principles (i.e., that spouses should be generous rather than selfish about accepting children, that they ought to act responsibly, and that NFP is a morally legitimate practice for avoiding conception); and then apply those principles to the situation at hand (their current circumstances).

This latter stage—evaluating their current circumstances—is an essential component of prudent decision-making that cannot be sidestepped. A strong desire to have another child, or to have sex during a fertile period, is not in itself a reliable indicator of God's will. After all, humans are not fundamentally desiring beings but rational beings, for only when our desires are guided by reason do they reliably orient us to fulfillment. For example, a particularly strong desire for sexual union could indicate a lack of chastity rather than a divine mandate to have another child; accordingly, that desire should not simply be acted upon without further critical reflection. To do so would be patently imprudent.

Assuming one strives to reason prudently, what kinds of circumstances qualify as "serious" or "well-grounded" reasons for deciding "not to have another child for either a definite or an indefinite amount of time" (HV, no. 10)? Writing in 1951 to Italian Catholic midwives, Pope Pius XII cites four types of circumstances—medical, eugenic, economic, and social—though his list is not meant to be exhaustive and he provides little further specification, aside from noting that such reasons could pertain "for a long period or even for the entire period of matrimonial life." Seven years later, in an address given to the Seventh International Congress of Hematology in Rome, Pius XII further elaborates on the question of eugenic considerations when he cites as a valid reason for using NFP the desire to not pass on a hereditary defect (such as hematological Mediterranean sickness) to one's children.

The Second Vatican Council, for its part, suggests that spouses must "take into account both their own welfare and that of their children, those already born and those which the future may bring, [reckoning] with both the material and the spiritual conditions of the times as well as of their state in life, [and consulting] the interests of the family ... society ... and the Church herself" (GS, no. 50). Moreover, according to the Council, it is "the parents themselves and no one else [who] should ultimately make this judgment in the sight of God," albeit while "trusting in divine Providence, refining the spirit of sacrifice," and reasoning on the basis of a conscience that conforms to the divine law and takes counsel from the Church's teaching office, "which authentically interprets that law in the light of the Gospel" (GS, no. 50).

In *Humanae Vitae*, Paul VI restates this same basic argument regarding reasons not to conceive, but in a more compressed form. After exhorting spouses to "maintain a correct set of priorities" by recognizing "their duties toward God, toward themselves, toward the family, and toward human society," he cites four reasons not to conceive: two internal to the marriage—the physical and psychological condition of the spouses—and two external: their social and economic circumstances (HV, nos. 10, 16).

John Paul II, in his *Theology of the Body*, places particular emphasis on the social dimension, exhorting spouses not to forget the needs of the various communities in which they are situated. To discern "the morally just level of births in [one's] family," he explains, one must take "into account not only the good of one's family ... the state of one's health ... [and the family's economic] means, but also the good of the society to which they belong, the good of the Church, and even of humanity as a whole" (John Paul II 2006, *Man and Woman*, p. 637). In his apostolic exhortation *Familiaris Consortio*, John Paul II contrasts such prudential reasoning with an "anti-life mentality" characterized by *future anxiety and despair* (wondering whether "it is a good thing to be alive or if it would be better never to have been born" and casting doubt on the value of bringing others "into life [who might] curse their existence in a cruel world with unforeseeable terrors"); or *panic* (stemming from population growth studies that "sometimes exaggerate the danger of demographic increase to the quality of life"); or a *consumer mentality* ("whose sole concern is to bring about a continual growth of material goods" and thereby "refusing the spiritual riches of a new human life"). The ultimate cause of such anti-life attitudes, he contends, "is the absence in people's hearts of God, whose love alone is stronger than all the world's fears and can conquer them" (FC, no. 30).

Bearing these cautions in mind, what more can be said about the objective difficulties and impediments that married couples face in choosing to be parents? To develop a practical framework that makes the Church's principles more concrete, I will proceed in two phases. First, building on Paul VI's four-fold schema, I will survey the various constraints on family size in the contemporary milieu. Second, taking seriously Vatican II's assertion that only spouses themselves can plan the size of their family, I will indicate some of the additional virtues that spouses need in order to reason prudently.

Constraints on Family Size: Physical, Psychological, Economic, & Social

As discussed earlier, Paul VI stipulates four types of good reasons for not conceiving: physical, psychological, social, and economic. In terms of the first two criteria, I propose as possible constraints: the physical health of the spouses, their psychological well-being, the overall strength of their marriage, their knowledge concerning how to be good parents, and the well-being of their current children. Each of these impediments could be either temporary or permanent, and couples are enjoined to make every possible effort to resolve them.

For example, a woman who cannot carry a pregnancy to term without grave risk to herself or her baby should make the prudent judgment not to conceive. If the cause of her illness is within her power to remedy, however, she should make every effort to do so, perhaps by quitting smoking and junk food, dieting under a doctor's supervision, exercising, or reducing stress in her life. Similarly, a husband who suffers from extreme depression, which causes him to turn inward to the point of being physically and emotionally unavailable to his wife and children, should prudently discern not to conceive another child for the time being. He too, however, is enjoined to do what is necessary to resolve his depression, perhaps by undergoing counseling, receiving medication for his illness, improving his mood through aerobic exercise, going on a spiritual retreat, engaging in community service-oriented activities that give him a renewed sense of purpose, or switching to a more fulfilling job.

Couples whose marriages are in crisis, perhaps because of abuse (either physical or emotional), adultery, addiction, or high-level conflict, or who are actively contemplating divorce, should make the prudent judgment not to conceive in their current circumstances. They must *also* strive to change their current circumstances, however, by seeking help from outside specialists, such as marriage and family therapists or addiction treatment programs; or by receiving training in either relationship skills or parenting skills or both.

In terms of economic criteria, I propose as possible constraints: the family's overall financial stability, as measured by steady employment for a living wage; access to good child care (if needed); the affordability of housing, education and medical care; the cost of caring for one's own aging parents (if applicable); current savings (or lack thereof); the family's overall level of indebtedness; and the character of work outside the home.

Financial stability is a difficult measure to gauge, for at least two reasons. First, spouses must assess not only their present situation, but also their future earnings and expenses—for roughly the next two decades as a prospective child grows into adulthood—which can be very difficult to predict. Second, in making such assessments, couples must clearly distinguish between necessities and luxuries, a challenging task within a culture of personal entitlement in which nearly all things available for purchase are marketed to consumers as goods that they deserve to have.

The Church, for its part, provides neither a looking glass into the future economy, nor a practical tool for distinguishing necessities from luxuries. I believe however, that couples can be assisted in their assessments if they bear in mind the following guidelines. To begin with, the quest for perfect financial stability is an illusory enterprise. If spouses worldwide were to postpone child-bearing until they were permanently situated in a large house in a good neighborhood, with no debt and significant savings in the bank, and employed in exciting careers that also happen to pay a living wage, with substantial money set aside for retirement, already robust college trust funds, and the wherewithal to financially support their own aging parents, then the human race might soon find itself in danger of extinction. At the very least, childbearing would become an exclusive practice for those who attain substantial wealth before the age of forty. In reality, however, most parents lack many of these things, yet somehow find a way for their children to grow up well-nourished, healthy, and well-educated. Spouses should thus be wary of holding the bar too high when assessing whether or not they can afford another child.

As to the difficult task of distinguishing between necessities and luxuries, no simple formula or technique exists. At the very least, however, families should avoid two extremes: either striving to live the equivalent of a religious vow of poverty but in the married state—disdaining all worldly goods as irrelevant to fulfillment—or pursuing an excessively materialistic lifestyle.

The first is unreasonable because human beings have a natural right to private property: not an unlimited right (for it would be unjust to retain excess goods while other people lack basic necessities) but a genuine right nevertheless. This right exists because certain basic goods are necessary for human fulfillment: such as nutritious food; adequate water; shelter from adverse weather conditions; clothing and shoes; hygienic items for basic cleanliness; medical care (both preventive and curative); adequate opportunities for recreation and contemplation; and the means to be both safe from harm and well-educated. Lacking the support of a religious community, parents themselves must financially provide such things for their children; hence, intentional extreme poverty would be irrational. As the *Code of Canon Law* stipulates, parents possess not only "the primary right" but also "the most grave duty ... to take care as best they can for the physical, social, cultural, moral, and religious education of their offspring" (CCL, 1983, c. 1136).

At the same time, spouses must also avoid the other extreme of habitually purchasing everything desirable that they can afford without first reflecting on whether they truly need it or not. Spouses who become addicted to luxury items might find it difficult to forgo a fancy car or expensive resort vacation in order to welcome another child into their family. Such materialism should be avoided not only because it limits spouses' generosity with regard to children—thereby impeding their own true happiness—but also because it inhibits their spiritual freedom by enslaving them to mere things. As Jesus exhorted his disciples, "it will be hard for one who is rich to enter the kingdom of heaven" (Mt 19:23).

In addition to the family's overall financial stability, the character of work outside the home can also pose a genuine obstacle to having more children. In the United States, gone are the days when most families can afford a home large enough to house a big family, and located in a good neighborhood with good schools, on only one salary. The current cost of housing relative to income is substantially higher than in previous generations. Consequently, with both parents working full-time, the added expense of child care for infants and toddlers can make an additional child seem truly cost-prohibitive. Moreover, the high costs of legal and agency fees for those wishing to adopt a baby are similarly discouraging. This is one of those areas where pro-life issues cannot be separated from social justice concerns. Aside from parents doing their part to forgo unnecessary luxuries, society needs to do its part to better support growing families.

To begin with, the American 80-hour work week, split 40/40 between husband and wife, needs to change. Not only does it artificially constrain family size; it also diminishes family closeness because "parents spend less time with children ('the parenting deficit'), and [spouses] spend less time with each other" (Browning et al. 2000, p. 316). In their book *From Culture Wars to Common Ground*, Don Browning and other theologians propose an alternative model: a maximum 60-hour work week for both husband and wife combined "that could be divided between the partners as 30/30 or 40/20" (Browning et al. 2000, p. 317). This solution is based on evidence showing that

> [T]he happiest families are those in which both husband and wife have some paid employment, share household chores and childcare, and work less than two full-time positions. There is arresting new evidence that fathers are happier and healthier if involved in childcare, just as mothers are happier and healthier if they participate in paid work (Browning et al. 2000, p. 317).

Pro-family employers can support this shift by offering more flexible schedules for parents of young children; by offering medical benefits to 30-hour employees, perhaps in exchange for a slight salary reduction if necessary; and by agreeing to hire two 20-hour employees in lieu of one 40-hour position in cases where such demand exists.

Related to this, in situations where workers are paid less than a living wage, governments, employers, and other non-state institutions—such as unions—should work together to rectify the situation. After all, no parent should be forced to work an unreasonable amount of hours simply in order to feed his or her children and supply them with the basic necessities of life.

Finally, in discerning how many children to have, spouses must take their social context into account, by examining the various communities in which they are situated. For example: within the family, might having a new brother or sister make one's current children more generous and less self-centered? Outside the family, would having another child make spouses more involved in their neighborhood, given that play dates and team sports are natural places for parents to meet one another and discuss topics of common concern? Even more broadly, could the addition of another unique human being who grows up in a loving family positively contribute to humanity as a whole? Such considerations ought to be part of a couple's discernment process as well.

Virtues Necessary for Ongoing Discernment

In evaluating the four types of constraints discussed above (physical, psychological, economic, and social), spouses need certain virtues to maximize their capacity for good discernment—the virtues of prudence and chastity, as well as other forms of temperance, liberality, patience, humility, faith, hope, and love. I will discuss each of these in turn.

First, when analyzing one's financial situation, the art of distinguishing between necessities and luxuries requires more than just intellectual skill. It also requires a certain level of spiritual detachment from material possessions and the pleasures associated with them. The pleasures of the senses are particularly addictive. Just as the ability to abstain from sex requires the virtue of chastity, so too the ability to refrain from other sensory pleasures requires other forms of the virtue of temperance (Aquinas 1981, *S.T.*, II-II 141.4). A person who is thoroughly addicted to eating gourmet food at expensive restaurants will undoubtedly have a difficult time viewing that practice as a luxury. A husband who is ecstatic about drinking fine wines might regard his hobby as something he simply cannot live without. A wife who is overly enthusiastic about receiving massages at her local spa might falsely regard her indulgence as an absolute necessity. Each of these things—gourmet food, fine wine, and spa massages—are genuine goods, but if we become too attached to them, then we will not be able to reason prudently in regard to them. Consequently, the virtue of temperance in all its forms is needed.

Related to this is the virtue of liberality: the ability to make good use of money, by *spending* it on things that are suitable and fitting (Aquinas 1981, *S.T.* II-II 117.3.2). While *saving* money is also important—to plan ahead for mortgages, college funds, family emergencies, or retirement—Aquinas cautions us against saving too much rather than putting our money to good use. He warns that a person who loves money immoderately tends to hoard it for themselves rather than giving it to others who need it (Aquinas 1981, *S.T.* II-II 117.3.3). Not only is this an act of injustice—a failure to give others their due—hoarding also impedes our ability to reason effectively. After all, to a person who lacks the virtue of liberality, the prospect of expanding their family looks a lot like an unwelcome drain on their bank account.

Another virtue needed for prudent discernment is patience. Being a mother or father inevitably involves numerous disappointments, even in cases where spouses have received substantial training in effective parenting. Not only must parents forgo certain luxuries in order to better support their children financially, at times they must also sacrifice other hopes and dreams. For example, more time parenting means less time available for other enjoyable or valuable pursuits, such as going back to school for a second degree, or spending leisurely mornings reading the paper. The loss of such activities in one's life can be truly disheartening. In addition, the reality of human sinfulness means that children will inevitably disappoint their parents at some time or another, by acting hurtfully or immorally.

To endure such disappointments without becoming overly distraught requires the virtue of patience. Because "sorrow and pain are ... displeasing to the soul," Aquinas observes, we "would never choose to suffer them for their own sake" but only for the sake of some good" (Aquinas 1981, *S.T.*, II-II 136.3). Raising children truly is one of those goods worth suffering for, but without the virtue of patience to bolster us, the difficulties of parenting quickly become too arduous to bear. Patience is required for prudent decision-making because an inability to endure disappointment with one child inevitably decreases one's motivation to welcome additional children into one's family.

Whereas the virtues of temperance, liberality, and patience generally help spouses become more receptive to bigger families, by moderating various forms of selfishness and depression, at the other end of the spectrum, the virtue of humility helps spouses by preventing them from undertaking far more than they can handle. Although it is praiseworthy to aim at great things, one must always do so in a way that accords with reason, being careful not to over-estimate one's own abilities (Aquinas 1981, *S.T.*, II-II 161.1.3; and 2.3). Raising a large family is a noble enterprise, one that requires great generosity of heart and personal sacrifice. As such, it is an inspiring goal. But spouses who face genuine problems should not simply dismiss them. It is one thing to trust in God's help to overcome obstacles; it is another thing to patently disregard the limits of our creatureliness: limits not just of financial resources but also of time, energy, and attention, all of which are needed in ample supply in order to be an effective parent. The virtue of humility restores our proper subjection to God by suppressing excessive self-confidence: restraining us from aiming at great things in cases where it would be presumptuous for us to do so (Aquinas 1981, *S.T.*, II-II 161.2.3).

Finally, the theological virtues of faith, hope, and love are indispensable to prudent decision-making regarding family size. Without faith (belief in God and in the truth of revelation) and hope (trust in God), raising children in a world marked by scarcity, selfishness, and, above all, death would seem an altogether fruitless enterprise. Moreover, without the virtue of charity (loving God and loving one's neighbor for God's sake), one's motivation for raising children would become primarily self-serving. For example, one might desire children in order to extend one's ego further in the world, so that one's own eventual death seems less daunting; or one might seek to be admired by others for contributing a new individual who is attractive, interesting, or socially useful; or one might simply want personal benefits like cheap labor to help run the family business or added tax benefits. By contrast, when one's desire to raise children is rooted in the virtue of charity, children are valued for their own sake—as unique individuals with their own needs and goals—rather than as mere extensions of their parents.

CONCLUSION

As we have seen, a myriad of virtues are necessary for prudent discernment regarding family size: not only the virtues of prudence and chastity, but also the virtues of faith, hope, love (*caritas*), humility, patience, liberality, and temperance in all its forms. Spouses who are supported by all these virtues are more apt to regard parenting as a worthy enterprise to begin with, to desire children for the right reasons, to refrain from over-extending themselves when faced with objective impediments, to endure the inevitable disappointments of parenting without disparaging the practice as a whole, to curtail the urge to be overly conservative about saving for the future, and to properly distinguish between necessities and luxuries when evaluating their financial readiness.

Also needed is greater support of families on the part of society at large. Governments, employers, and other non-state institutions must work together to ensure that all employees are paid a living wage, that health care is affordable and accessible, and that more flexible work schedules are available to parents who work outside the home. A sizable reduction in the current cost of housing is vitally important as well.

Armed with such social supports, as well as with the full range of virtues needed to exercise prudence, spouses can make good decisions regarding not only the best *practice* for spacing out their children (NFP rather than contraception), but also concerning *when* to have children and *how many* to have. In this way, procreation becomes not merely a natural activity—one in which both human beings and animals participate—but also a spiritual practice: one in which human beings freely and actively cooperate with their Creator.

END NOTES:

1. C. Panzer, et al. (2006), "Impact of Oral Contraceptives on Sex Hormone-Binding Globulin and Androgen Levels: A Retrospective Study in Women with Sexual Dysfunction," *Journal of Sexual Medicine* 3(1): 104-113. See also Julia K. Warnock, et al., "Comparison of androgens in women with hypoactive sexual desire disorder: those on combined oral contraceptives (COCs) vs. those not on COCs," (2006), *Journal of Sexual Medicine* 3(5): 878–882.

2. The reverse situation is also possible; a wife could be unchaste and treat her husband reductively as a sexual object, rather than relating to him as a whole person in the context of self-gift.

3. W. D. Mosher and J. Jones, (2010), "Use of contraception in the United States: 1982–2008," National Center for Health Statistics, *Vital and Health Statistics* 23(29).

4. Étienne Van de Walle and Elisha P. Renne, (2001), *Menstruation: Beliefs, Practices, Interpretations,* (University of Chicago Press), see pp. 41-43 and 45-46.

5. Initially, some interpreters argued that Pius XI did not specifically intend to defend the practice of periodic abstinence when he used the phrase "natural reasons of time." This controversy was eventually put to rest by his successor, Pius XII, in his 1958 address to hematologists, when he stated, "We have spoken on this subject in Our address of October 29, 1951, not to expound on the biological or medical point of view, but to allay the qualms of conscience of many Christians who used this method in their conjugal life. Moreover, in his encyclical of December 31, 1930, Pius XI had already formulated the position of principle: "*Neque contra naturae ordinem agere ii dicendi sunt coniuges, qui lure suo recte et naturali ratione utuntur, etsi ob naturales sive temporis sive quorundam defectaum causas nova inde vita oriri non possit*" (Pius XII, 1958).

SOURCES CONSULTED

1917 Pio-Benedictine Code of Canon Law in English Translation with Extensive Scholarly *Apparatus*. See also "Codex Iuris Canonici." In *Acta Apostolicae Sedis* 9/II (1917): 3-521. Translated by Edward Peters. San Francisco: Ignatius Press: 2001.

1983 Code of Canon Law. See also "Codex Iuris Canonici." In *Acta Apostolicae Sedis* 75/II (1983): 1-320. Translated by the Canon Law Society of America. Vatican City: Libreria Editrice Vaticana.

Aquinas, Thomas. 1981, c1948. *Summa Theologica*. Volumes 1-5. Translated by Fathers of the English Dominican Province. Westminster, MD: Christian Classics.

Aristotle. 1962. *Nicomachean Ethics*. Translated by Martin Ostwald. London: Collier Macmillan.

Augustine. 1887a. "Of the Good of Marriage." Translated by C. L. Cornish. In *Nicene and Post-Nicene Fathers*, first series. Volume 3. Philip Schaff. Ed. Buffalo, NY: Christian Literature Publishing Co.

———. 1887b. "On Marriage and Concupiscence." Translated by Peter Holmes and Robert Ernest Wallis. Revised by Benjamin B. Warfield. In

Nicene and Post-Nicene Fathers, first series. Volume 5. Philip Schaff, Ed. Buffalo, NY: Christian Literature Publishing Company.

Balthasar, Hans Urs Von. 1983. *The Christian State of Life*. Translated by Sr. Mary Frances McCarthy. San Francisco: Ignatius Press.

———. 2003. *The Laity and the Life of the Counsels: The Church's Mission in the World*. Translated by Brian McNeil, C.R.V. with D. C. Schindler. San Francisco: Ignatius Press.

———. 1992. *Theo-Drama: Theological Dramatic Theory. Volume III. Dramatis Personae: Persons in Christ*. Translated by Graham Harrison. San Francisco: Ignatius Press.

Browning, Don S., Bonnie J. Miller-McLemore, Pamela D. Couture, K. Brynolf Lyon and Robert M. Franklin. 2000. *From Culture Wars to Common Ground*. Second edition. Louisville: Westminster John Knox Press. First published 1997.

Catechism of the Catholic Church, 1994. Translated by the United States Catholic Conference. New York: Doubleday.

Denzinger-Schönmetzer. 1996. "L'observance des périodes inféconds." In *Enchiridion Symbolorum et Definitionum*, edition 37, par. 3148. See also *Nouvelle Revue Theologique* 13 (1881): pp. 459-460; and *Analecta Iuris Pontificii* 22 (1883): p. 249.

Grabowski, John S. 2003. *Sex and Virtue: An Introduction to Sexual Ethics*. Washington, DC: The Catholic University of America Press.

John Paul II. 1991. *Centesimus Annus (On the Hundredth Anniversary of Rerum Novarum)*. Washington, DC: United States Catholic Conference.

———. 1981. *Familiaris Consortio (The Role of the Christian Family in the Modern World)*. Translated by Vatican Polyglot Press. Boston: Pauline Books and Media.

———. 2006. *Man and Woman He Created Them: A Theology of the Body*. Translated and introduced by Michael Waldstein. Boston: Pauline Books and Media.

———. 1993. *Veritatis Splendor (The Splendor of Truth)*. Boston: St. Paul Books and Media.

Kochuthara C. M. I., Shaji George. 2007. *The Concept of Sexual Pleasure in the Catholic Moral Tradition*. Rome: Editrice Pontificia Università Gregoriana.

Makowski, Elizabeth M. 1977. "The Conjugal Debt and Medieval Canon Law." *Journal of Medieval History* 3: 99-114.

Paul VI. 1968. *Humanae Vitae (Of Human Life)*. Translated by Janet Smith. In *Humanae Vitae: A Challenge to Love*. New Hope, KY: New Hope Publications. See also *Acta Apostolicae Sedis* 60: 481-503.

Pius XI. 1930. *Casti Connubii (On Christian Marriage)*. Translated by Gerald C. Treacy. New York: Paulist Press. See also *Acta Apostolicae Sedis* 22: 545-546.

Pius XII. 1951. "Address to the Italian Association of Catholic Midwives." In *Acta Apostolicae Sedis* 43: 835-854.

———. 1958. "Address to the Seventh Congress of International Society of Hematology." In *Acta Apostolicae Sedis* 50: 734-736.

Smith, Janet. 1991. *Humanae Vitae: A Generation Later*. Washington, DC: The Catholic University of America Press.

Vatican II. 1965. *Dignitatis Humanae (Declaration on Religious Freedom)*. Boston: St. Paul Books and Media.

———. 1966. *Gaudium et Spes (Pastoral Constitution on the Church in the Modern World)*. Boston: St. Paul Books and Media.

PANEL II

LIFE-GIVING LOVE IN AN AGE OF TECHNOLOGY

16

With All Due Respect

REV. J. DANIEL MINDLING, OFM CAP, STD

Academic Dean, Professor of Moral Theology, Mount St. Mary's Seminary, Archdiocese of Baltimore

ABSTRACT

The frustrated desire for children experienced by an infertile couple challenges them emotionally and spiritually. Pastoral care for such couples includes the formation of conscience to equip them to face decisions concerning methods of enhancing fertility that may impinge on the dignity of their marriage and the life of their offspring. One approach to this formation is an evangelization of the heart that clarifies what constitutes an upright desire for children and what sorts of actions can embody this desire. Couples can come to see how legitimate desire for children is enmeshed in seeing the child as a gift which fulfills their marriage, in celebrating the vocation to parenthood inscribed in their conjugal love, and in upholding the sanctity of life of their offspring. Only conjugal acts can embody the legitimate desire for children, and so treatments or technologies which substitute for the conjugal act are illicit, and their underlying attitude even arrogant. Under the stress of a diagnosis of infertility, couples may be tempted to seek immoral acts because these acts promise the child they so very much desire. Such immoral actions, however, embody illicit desires because they separate the desire for children from the very values from which procreation must spring. *Life-Giving Love in an Age of Technology* (United States Conference of Catholic Bishops 2009) is a pastoral tool to facilitate the formation of conscience of all those seeking help to conceive a child.

INTRODUCTION

The Catholic teaching on reproductive technologies is addressed to practitioners and theologians, but most particularly to couples in crisis. The pain of their frustrated desire for a child includes emotional and spiritual suffering. The ministry of conscience formation properly begins with a focus on their desire for a child. Some Catholic moral theologians have focused on the attitude toward the generation of a child which underlies *in vitro* fertilization. This paper will explore the characteristics of upright desire for children with reference to the United States Conference of Catholic Bishops (hereafter USCCB) publication, *Life Giving Love in an Age of Technology* (hereafter LGL 2009). It starts with a brief overview of the crisis of frustrated desire experienced by the infertile couple and moves to discriminate between an ethically upright desire for a child and those attitudes which deform that desire and lead to immoral choices of artificial reproductive technology.

A staggering 1.3 million patients in the United States receive professional advice or treatments for infertility every year, and this number may represent only half of those struggling with difficulty in conceiving. Secular commentators explain that reaction to a diagnosis of infertility may include grief and a sense of loss, depression, anger, and loss of self-esteem. This can also include destabilizing stress within the marriage, a loss of personal confidence, a feeling of having lost control over one's projected future. There can be tension with friends and family members, especially those who either are pregnant or who have children already. Patients receiving pharmacological treatment may, in addition, find themselves dealing with psychological side effects ranging from anxiety, irritability, and interrupted sleep to mood swings and depression. Patients face financial worries. Those who begin fertility clinic appointments must cope with treatment failures, and this may be particularly hard for Americans because our culturally reinforced work ethic presupposes that rewards will come if you just keep on goal, work hard, and don't give up. In fact, stopping treatment can strain relationships, although gradually patients who are unsuccessful at the clinic will transition from wanting children "of their own" to either being childless or considering adoption (Miller 2009, pp. 1-3).

Religious commentators explain that the diagnosis of infertility can occasion a spiritual crisis as couples rethink their relationship with God. Perhaps they have been living chastely before marriage and trustingly following the Church's teaching on birth control after marriage. They may now feel that God is not treating them fairly. Or perhaps they were guilty of abortion or sexual misconduct or have tried *in vitro* fertilization (hereafter IVF) or other assisted reproductive technology (hereafter ART) and now suspect that God is punishing them. In either case their relationship with God is shaken. Their faith support group may be eroding, their marriage is being tested, and their relationship with other couples and with their own family may be strained. Infertility is experienced as a crisis of self, a failure to achieve, a feeling of inferiority to the fertile. Because children represent continuation, it can feel like a loss of the ability to do anything eternal, long-lasting, and transcendent, to reach out into the next generation, to contribute to the family and society. Couples have to rethink their spiritual life. Why is God holding back his blessings? (Ryan 2003, pp. 71-73, 150-67).

Married couples, almost without exception, start with the desire for their children to come into the world as the fruit of their marriage. They desire to be blessed by God with the gift of new life, to share in the creative work of God, to form a family and to join in parenting their child. They want the child they conceive to be the fruit of their most intense, most personal act of self-gift. Their attitude of generosity with one another spills over into the desire to procreate. Yet some of these same couples, as they cope with a diagnosis of infertility, may well abandon that nexus of values which gives rise to their desire for children.

Pastoral outreach to couples suffering from infertility takes many forms, and holistic care is essential (Mindling 2009). Recognition that early discussion of infertility prepares couples to begin thinking about this challenge as something they may have to face has led for calls to include this material in marriage preparation programs or for the preparation of specialized teams modeled on the resources and training provided for the Project Rachel program for post-abortion counseling (Zimmerman 2009). Websites like that of the USCCB's Secretariat of Pro-Life Activities and manuals such as the one produced by the Family Life Institute (Bozza 2000), and other similar organizations and support groups too numerous to itemize here, are providing pastoral, practical, and theological resources as well as support groups.

One facet of this much more all-encompassing ministry is moral guidance. The compassionate and accurate formation of conscience for couples who literally face decisions of life and death compels us to reach out in solidarity and to stand with them in defense of the dignity of each spouse, of their marriage and conjugal love, and of the gift of human life at its most precious and fragile beginnings. To this end the USCCB published *Life-Giving Love in an Age of Technology* (LGL) on the heels of the statement by the Congregation for the Doctrine of the Faith, *Dignitas Personae* (hereafter DP) and in keeping with the document it reaffirmed, updated and clarified, *Donum Vitae* (hereafter DV).

THE SUFFERING OF UNFULFILLED DESIRE

The mere fact that a couple is childless does not mean that the couple carries the cross of infertility. Couples could enter marriage after childbearing age, or enter into a union which is known and accepted by both parties to be sterile. Antecedent and even permanent sterility is not an impediment to marriage (1983, Code of Canon Law, c. 1084, §3). The suffering of infertility, properly understood, has to do with unanticipated sterility. The cross experienced by the couple is occasioned by the frustration of a desire for children, by unexpected childlessness, by failure or repeated failure to carry a child to term, or especially by the absence of conception/pregnancy and birth after a long period of engaging in acts thought to be fertile.

Much of the literature in ethics on this topic appropriately focuses on the moral evaluation of particular acts or procedures available to the infertile couple to overcome this frustration. The experience of the couple, however, and the moment most opportune for catechesis or counseling, begins not with treatments or therapies, but with the crisis brought on by the frustration of desire for a child. The crucial, initial moral question concerns the perspective of the moral agent(s) in their desire for a child. It is precisely a frustrated desire which produces anxiety and suffering and the exploration of alternatives for action. Couples may have been trying to conceive for a year before they determine to seek professional advice, visit a fertility clinic, let alone speak with a priest. During all this time their desire and frustration have been intensifying, and the connection of this desire with the values from which it springs may be shifting.

For this reason, it is crucial in the ministry of the formation of conscience of such couples to help them come to a better understanding of the natural and graced desire for children in the teachings of the Church. They can be helped to reflect on their initial hope for a child when they first married, when such desire was strongly linked to the sacrament of matrimony, to their hope to engage in fruitful conjugal acts, to their own personal dignity and sense of self, to the vocation of parenthood they had heard and wanted to answer, and to the sanctity of life of their hoped for child. Pastorally we start by compassionate and empathetic listening as the couple tells us of their great desire for a child and the web of values in which this desire is enmeshed. With a view to the formation of conscience, we also listen attentively and help the couple discern how their desire for a child, now frustrated by infertility, risks being detached from those goods.

Upright Desire

Gaudium et Spes (hereafter GS) speaks of children as a gift, the language used in the very title of the Congregation for the Doctrine of the Faith's document *Donum Vitae* (*The Gift of Life*): "Marriage and conjugal love are by their nature ordained toward the procreation and education of children. Children are really the supreme gift of marriage and contribute in the highest degree to their parents' welfare" (GS, no. 50). The Council document goes on to explain that spouses *transmit* this gift by cooperating with the creative *act of God*. The desire for a child therefore is a desire to cooperate with the creative act of God. It is a desire to receive a gift even as it is a desire to participate in the very transmission of that gift in a marvelous interaction with the Creator of life. It is a desire inherent in the very nature of their love for each other and in their marriage itself.

Grisez's comments on *Gaudium et Spes*, no. 50, are illuminating in making the point that marriage is a basic good, not an instrumental good. "This formulation avoids the suggestion that marriage and conjugal love are means to the end of offspring, and points instead to the view that having and bringing up children normally belongs to the full unfolding of marriage and conjugal love themselves" (Grisez 1993, p. 565). This same idea appears in *Humanae Vitae*: "husband and wife through that mutual gift of themselves which is specific and exclusive to them alone, develop that communion of persons in which they perfect each other, so that they may cooperate with God in the generation and rearing of new lives" (*Humanae Vitae*, no. 8; hereafter HV). This cooperation shapes the life of the parents and fulfills them as a couple.

> For while children, as distinct persons, are good in themselves and should be loved for their own sakes, procreating and raising children, as activities in which the husband and wife cooperate, not only benefit the children but fulfill the couple. Insofar as it fulfills the couple, parenthood—having a family—is not an extrinsic end to which one flesh unity is instrumental, but a realization of its potentiality (Grisez 1993, pp. 567-568).

In sum, the desire for a child is a desire for a gift and also a desire for the fulfillment of the marriage, for fulfillment as a couple. Marriage and the expression of conjugal love are not means to get a child (that would render marriage as a mere means measured as a good to the extent that is effective or fertile). The child is desired as a gift, good in itself and not as a mere means (instrumental good) judged as a good only if and to the extent it fulfills the parents. *Humanae Vitae* helps us to see that the desire for children is an essential characteristic of spousal love. Intentionally rendering conjugal love sterile contradicts its essence. The desire for a child is part of the unrestrained love of the spouses, part of open-endedness of their conjugal love for one another. Conjugal love "is not confined wholly to the loving interchange of husband and wife; it also contrives to go beyond this to bring new life into being" (HV no. 8).

Donum Vitae explains the desire for children as natural and intimately linked to and expressive of the spouses' natural and supernatural vocation to parenthood. "On the part of the spouses, the desire for a child is natural: it expresses the vocation to fatherhood and motherhood inscribed in conjugal love. This desire can be even stronger if the couple is affected by sterility which appears incurable" (DV, II, B, 8). It is not about what the couple *wants* but about what the couple *is*, what their vocation prompts them to desire, what their very conjugal love seeks as a fulfillment. The *Catechism of the Catholic Church* summarizes:

> Called to give life, spouses share in the creative power and fatherhood of God. Married couples should regard it as their proper mission to transmit human life and to educate their children; they should realize that they are thereby cooperating with the love of God the Creator and are, in a certain sense, its interpreters. They will fulfill this duty with a sense of human and Christian responsibility (CCC, no. 2367, notes omitted).

Life-Giving Love was not written as a theological treatise, but it accurately describes the desire for children as an openness which emerges from the intensity of conjugal love. "I want to have children with you," means, it explains, "I love you so much that I want our married love to be open to children we can love and care for together" (LGL, p. 1).

Desire for a child, notes Ronheimer, is a *legitimate* desire if the statement "if only we had a child," means, "if only we could *receive* a child. … By this is expressed the fact that the goodness of the coming into being of a new baby is not measured by the fact that a *desire* of the parents is fulfilled, rather by the fact that the new human life has *come about* as the fruit of reciprocal love" (Ronheimer 2010, p. 158). In other words, legitimate desire for a child is a desire for a gift, a desire which entails recognition that there is no right or entitlement to a child. Legitimate desire for a child includes the recognition that the desire may not be fulfilled. Furthermore, legitimate desire for a child recognizes that the child, even if not explicitly desired or even undesired, is a valuable life. The witness of those couples who have faced the challenge and blessing of problem pregnancies and difficult pre-natal diagnoses attests to the full impact of what it means to desire and accept the child as a precious and invaluable gift (see Nugent 2008; see also Mayer-Whittington 2007).

The 10th General Assembly of the Pontifical Academy for Life contrasts *legitimate* desire for a child with what they label as *arrogant* desire. They also point out that the initial desire for a child may well start out as healthy and positive but later become distorted and domineering:

> Sterility in the case of spouses who wish to find "in their child a confirmation and completion of their reciprocal self-giving" (DV, II, A, 1) can undoubtedly be a real reason for great suffering and

> also a source for them of further problems. There can be no doubt that such a real desire is in itself more than legitimate and a positive sign of a conjugal love that wants to grow and be expressed in all its forms. It should be stressed, however, that a more than understandable and licit "desire for a child" can never be transformed into an arrogant "right to a child" and, moreover, a "right to a child *at all costs*." No person can claim the right to the existence of another; otherwise the latter would be placed on a lower level of value than the one who claims such a right. In reality, a child can never be understood as an "object of desire" to be obtained at any cost (Pontifical Academy for Life 2004).

The Pontifical Academy is echoing *Donum Vitae*:

> [The child] cannot be desired or conceived as the product of an intervention of medical or biological techniques; that would be equivalent to reducing him to an object of scientific technology. No one may subject the coming of a child into the world to conditions of technical efficiency which are to be evaluated according to standards of control and dominion (DV, II, B, 4c).

Note the same analysis in *Dignitas Personae*:

> The Church recognizes the legitimacy of the desire for a child and understands the suffering of couples struggling with problems of fertility. Such a desire, however, should not override the dignity of every human life to the point of absolute supremacy. The desire for a child cannot justify the "production" of offspring, just as the desire not to have a child cannot justify the abandonment or destruction of a child once he or she has been conceived (DP, no. 16).

To put this succinctly, "to manufacture the child is to make him subordinate to his manufacturers" (Haas 1990, p. 111).

Reflection on the desire for a child by an adoptive parent is insightful for instructing couples suffering from infertility on the subject of legitimate desire. The Church has long been involved in adoption (see Destro 1997). Tollefsen, paralleling John Paul II, provides a rich analysis of the upright desire which should be present in prospective *adoptive* parents (Tollefsen 2010, pp.75-85; cf. John Paul II 2000, *Address to Adoptive Families*). He believes that by reflecting on the love of God manifest in creating us and inviting us to join in the loving communion of persons which is the Trinity, we can gain insight into what God expects of such parents in their desire to adopt. God creates us not because he needs us; rather, creation of the universe and of human beings in his image and likeness is an entirely gratuitous action which flows from the abundance of his love. God's offer to us to enter into the interpersonal family life of love of the Trinity is likewise an expression of his generosity and not reflective of any need for fulfillment on God's part. Accordingly, couples should not have an attitude toward children as the way to satisfy themselves or meet what they judge to be their need. Such a self-focus devalues parenthood as a vocation, perverts it into a self-centered and self-serving activity that one performs for self-satisfaction or a misguided notion of personal fulfillment. This is not to say that having a family is not fulfilling, but rather that it is wrong to view the family merely as a means to one's fulfillment. Tollefsen cautions that such a flawed perspective is only a short step from the mistaken conclusion that one has a right to fulfillment and hence a right to a child, and that one ought not be blamed for arrogantly demanding that right be met and all obstacles (my health, my infertility or that of my sexual partner) be overcome by any means available. He contrasts desire for a child "out of abundance" which imitates God's attitude in creating us with desire "out of need." This latter misunderstands the proper relationship of parent and child and even misconstrues the generosity of God in giving the gift of marriage as well as the gift of children:

> Adoptive parents perpetuate this misunderstanding when they adopt primarily "out of need." They should not look at their prospective adopted children from a standpoint of what they do not have, but of what, it is to be hoped, they do have: a flourishing, loving marriage. By adopting as an expression and outpouring of their mutual love, they mirror God more adequately than if they adopted to complete or to satisfy themselves. At the same time, it should be noted, what I [have] called adoption out of abundance should not be mistaken for anything condescending, nor its initial condition be thought of as one of self-sufficiency. For our starting point—mutual love of spouses and the desire to share that love more abundantly with children—is itself a gift, and not something for which we are self-sufficiently responsible (Tollefsen 2010, p. 80).

Furthermore, legitimate desire for children is connected to and entails respect for one's own dignity. Sexuality "is not something simply biological, but concerns the innermost being of the human person as such pertains to the innermost being of the person" (CCC, no. 2361).

Life-Giving Love does not elaborate on the challenges that some reproductive technologies pose to the personal dignity of the individual spouse (LGL, p. 18). Commentators on the booming fertility industry, however, point out many ways that reproductive technology puts woman at risk (see Anderson, 2004). Reflecting on the anthropology implicit in ART, it is clear that these technologies replace the personal dimension of sexual expression with a technique that is neither conjugal, nor personal, nor interpersonal. One need only think of the terminology: "harvesting" egg cells, "selection" of the healthiest embryos for implantation, "test tube" babies or "technology." The language should be unmasked. Egg or sperm *donors* are actually paid venders, *clinics* are all too often labs producing, freezing, and transferring embryos. Fertility *treatments* using heterologous eggs do not make a woman fertile but only a carrier of another woman's child. Commercialization of child-bearing raises questions of exploitation and manipulation of parents, particularly women (see Ryan 2001, p. 49). Much of ART takes what is intimately personal, marital and spiritual—one's capacity to share in the creative activity of God with one's spouse by a marital act of interpersonal self-donation and reception of the gift of the other—and substitutes for it technologies of engineered conception done without intercourse, and with neither parent in the room. This replacement of what is deeply human and personal with the technological cannot but depersonalize both fatherhood and motherhood. It leads to a diminishment of the role of the person in conjugal sexual communication, of the spirituality of each person as a creature loved by a personal God and invited to share in his power and life, of the marital covenant which is expressed and deepened in acts of life giving and love communicating, and of one's awareness and appreciation of one's own body and gender (see Melina 2005, pp. 114-26).

It is not surprising then that women in the midst of fertility protocols feel isolated from their own bodies and even from their spouses, and perceive that the clinical procedures are done more to their reproductive organs, their gametes, or their endocrine systems than to themselves as sexual persons. The pressure to produce, keep trying, never to give up can force the woman to step back from her body emotionally and focus on cycles, costs, and outcomes in a way that promotes body/person dualism. Some feminists have pointed out that instead of "liberating women" by providing them a freedom from the complications of conception, the experience of many women is that this only entangles their agency and "life process" in a maze of experts and "technologists" and holds out a specter of conception dominated by technicians and where the woman's role is redundant (Ryan 2001, pp. 45-46).

The Church, by contrast, insists that the profoundly personal and interpersonal context for engendering human life be respected as part of the perfection of procreation. The coming to be of a person with full human dignity should be the direct consequence of personal action respectful of the full human dignity of each spouse, joined in an action fully respectful of its marital dignity (John Paul II, 2004, *Address to Pontifical Academy for Life*, no. 2). *Donum Vitae* explicitly uses the language of perfection: "From the moral point of view procreation is deprived of its proper perfection when it is not desired as the fruit of the conjugal act, that is to say of the specific act of the spouses' union" (DV, II, B, 4a). Haas correctly explains that the totality of the marital act includes its physical, emotional, and spiritual dimensions, and that it is this totality that constitutes the dignity of the marital act. Although conception can indeed take place without the physicality of conjugal coitus, such a mode of conception is less than fully human, it is deprived of its human perfection (because it lacks the physical dimension), and it therefore falls short of the dignity of the fully human marital act. In other words, the coming to be apart from marital intercourse dehumanizes and depersonalizes the event (Haas 1990, p. 113). Respect for the dignity of the spouses and their activity is respect for their contribution to the proper perfection of procreation (Cataldo 2009, p. 105).

Furthermore, if the desire for a child has lost its mooring in the dignity and sanctity of marriage, such desire has become illegitimate. By their marriage vows spouses have reciprocally and irreplaceably capacitated one another for marital intercourse, something they can do only with each other (see May 2008, p. 70). Conjugal intercourse expresses and symbolizes, by the spouses becoming one flesh, the *unitive* meaning of their marriage and simultaneously—because a truly conjugal act is not intentionally impeded—the *procreative* meaning of their marriage (May 2008, p.70; see also Cataldo 2009, p. 105). It is obvious that spouses violate the dignity of their marriage by giving themselves to third parties (violating the unitive dimension). It is equally obvious that they violate the dignity of their marriage if, despite their vows to use their procreative powers only with one another, they participate in acts to generate children with third parties (May 2008, p. 81).

Life-Giving Love (LGL, p. 7) explains this as a violation of the integrity of the marital relationship, i.e., the exclusive relationship of the spouses. The *Catechism of the Catholic Church* explains that it is a violation of justice which infringes on the child's rights as well as the spouse's rights

> Techniques that entail the dissociation of husband and wife, by the intrusion of a person other than the couple (donation of sperm or ovum, surrogate uterus), are gravely immoral. These techniques (heterologous artificial insemination and fertilization) infringe the child's right to be born of a father and mother known to him and bound to each other by marriage. They betray the spouses' "right to become a father and a mother only through each other" (reference to DV, II, 1; CCC, no. 2376).

The choice made by a married couple to seek heterologous artificial reproductive technology entails a decision "not to be fully the mother and father of their child, because they have delegated part of their role to others" (LGL, p. 6). In effect, they have redefined their marriage, saying to one another and to society that when it comes to fertility, theirs is not necessarily an exclusive and faithful relationship because they will welcome the use of organs and gametes from third parties in producing a child. This contradicts the divinely established reality of marriage as an exclusive and faithful covenant of life and love (GS, no. 48). Furthermore, God cannot bless with fertility the act by which they uniquely express their conjugal love because they have chosen to substitute this act with a technological act, one involving third parties.

The witness of the marriage as a faithful and exclusive community of persons in the world, a dimension of the sacramentality of their marriage, is dimmed by the choice of ART. Nor is the impact on the social unit of the family to be underestimated. ART allows for procreation by the unmarried, the homosexual, and the single. For us who correctly see the family as the primary building block of society and the locus for handing on values and faith, immoral reproductive technology poses a serious and immediate threat beyond its impact on the couple and their child (Ryan 2001, pp. 46-47).

Legitimate desire for a child is rooted in respect for the dignity and sanctity of life. "The desire for a child cannot justify the 'production' of offspring, just as the desire not to have a child cannot justify the abandonment or destruction of a child once he or she has been conceived" (DP, no. 16). All life is a gift from God, and to say that a child is a gift is to recognize that it is received, that the recipient has no right to it, and that it was not merited.

In a rich summary of the teachings of *Evangelium Vitae* on the idea of the gift of life, Peter Cataldo identifies "several qualities of human life that are inextricably bound up with the fact that life is a gift from God" including these five: (1) "God shares something of himself in giving life to man; (2) God is the Lord of life; (3) life is sacred and inviolable; (4) the gift of life is a commandment; and (5) life is not a mere object of manipulation" (Cataldo 2009, p. 103). In giving us the gift of life, God has chosen to give us something we cannot deserve, our very existence. Life, as God's gift, does not belong to us for God retains dominion over life. The life we have involves the creative act of God, the Lord of life, and in fact is both sacred and inviolable because of his Lordship and because we are created in his image. Life, since it is not subject to the dominion of man, has a truth of its own, a direction and purpose not subject to the manipulation of man. The gift of life can be termed an "embodied obligation" because "in giving life to man, God *demands* that he love, respect, and promote life. The gift thus becomes a commandment, and the commandment is itself a gift" (Cataldo 2009, pp.103-04).

The theology of the child as *gift* was discussed above in connection with the distinction between couple's legitimate or arrogant desire for a child. This same theology grounds the foundational moral principle that demands that no reproductive method be used that entails disregard for life at its earliest stages. There can be no legitimate desire for a child if a choice is made to use a technology that will destroy one's own offspring as part of the process of producing an offspring.

Life-Giving Love decries technologies that exercise "quality control," i.e., pre-implantation or post-implantation genetic screening to determine who lives and who dies. It decries multiple implantations followed by "selective reduction" (targeted abortions) to eliminate the extra or unwanted children. It decries cryogenic preservation of "excess" or "spare" embryos and their absurd fate to be abandoned, subject to experimental purposes, or "wasted." It decries the manufacture of cloned human beings whose worth is measured by the traits they share with their donor. Underlying these last-mentioned procedures are attitudes (flawed desires) of profound injustice common to the worst ethnic or racial prejudice, which judge that only those lives that have value to us have any value at all. Such an attitude contradicts the fundamental demand of justice, the recognition of the respect that should be given to all human life (LGL, pp. 11-12).

This teaching applies to artificial reproductive technology, and particularly to IVF procedures. *Dignitas Personae* affirms that the human embryo, from the first moment of his or her existence has the dignity of a human person. It also notes that every *in vitro* procedure treats the human embryo as a mere mass of cells to be used or selected or even thrown away. For each "success," IVF procedures kill many embryos. The loss of embryos is sometimes seen as an undesired collateral effect that may be reduced in time. But in many other cases, the destruction of embryos is foreseen and intended because discarded embryos are defective, lack desired traits, or are deemed to be superfluous. These are abortions. They are the outcome of arrogant desire. Because these abortions are linked to procedures that separate conception from marital intercourse, they simultaneously embody a convergence of disrespect for the spouses, the marriage, and the offspring (DP, nos. 5, 14, 15-16, and n. 27).

> The blithe acceptance of the enormous number of abortions involved in the process of *in vitro* fertilization vividly illustrates how the replacement of the conjugal act by a technical procedure—in addition to being in contradiction with the respect that is due to procreation as something that cannot be reduced to mere reproduction—leads to a weakening of the respect owed to every human being. Recognition of such respect is, on the other hand, promoted by the intimacy of husband and wife nourished by married love (DP, no. 16).

FROM DESIRE TO CHOICE

Certainly there are marital acts that are filled with hope and the legitimate desire that a new life come to be, even as there are acts that remain open to life without that desire being explicit. Likewise, choices are made to facilitate or increase the likelihood that these acts will be fertile by removing blockages, enabling the sexual act to be complete, or taking advantage of the cycle of fertility. All these can embody the legitimate desire for a child as a gift because they facilitate the conjugal act, the very expression of the love the couple desires to be crowned with the gift of a child. As *Donum Vitae* affirms:

> The human person must be accepted in his parents' act of union and love; the generation of a child must therefore be the fruit of that mutual giving which is realized in the conjugal act wherein the spouses cooperate as servants and not as masters in the work of the creator who is love" (DV, II, B, nos. 4, 7).

It is also true, however, that there are acts, even ones involving only the biological material of the married couple, which cannot but express an arrogant attitude toward the coming to be of a child. These sorts of actions can be identified by reflection on what facilitates and expresses openness to the gift of a child and what facilitates and expresses a technological process by which a child is sought as an instrumental good for the fulfillment of the father and mother. It is not the case that all marital acts embody the right desire for a child. So the distinction is not merely between assisting and substituting the marital act. Rather, it is found in the difference between acts that embody upright desiring and acts that cannot embody upright desiring. A couple who engages in acts that express the unitive and procreative meaning of their conjugal love can indeed hope for a child as the crowning gift of their marriage and conjugal love. A couple who engages in acts that substitute for the marital act can only wish that the substituted act be successful in the production of the object of their desire. While they may well hope that the child who comes about will be happy and that their marriage be fulfilled by the cooperative experience of raising the child, in the choice of a technology, they can only be hopeful that it be a success in producing what they want. The *Catechism of the Catholic Church* teaches that techniques which dissociate the sexual act from the procreative act are flawed. They express a relationship of domination of the parents over the child. The act which gives rise to a child is no longer the conjugal act by which the spouses give themselves to one another. In this case procreation is no longer willed as the fruit of the conjugal act. It is rather a technical act (CCC, no. 2377; cf., DV, II, B, nos. 4-5).

William E. May explains the difference between "making babies" and receiving the gift of a child:

> The marital act is *not* an act of making or producing. It is not a transitive act issuing from spouses and terminating in some object

> distinct from them. It is something that they 'do.' In it they do not "make" love or "make" babies. They *give* love to each other by giving themselves bodily to each other, and they open themselves to the gift of human life. The life begotten through their one-flesh union is not the product of their art, but 'a gift supervening on and giving permanent embodiment to' the marital act itself (May 2008, p. 73).

This is why, in *Life-Giving Love,* the bishops explain that children "are not parents' possessions to manufacture, manipulate, or design," instead, "children deserve to be 'begotten, not made" (LGL, p. 19). This phrase is familiar to us from the Creed, where we speak of Christ in these very terms. May uses this language to draw out the parallel between the child begotten of the conjugal love of parents with the relationship of God the Father to his only begotten Son. The Father does not make the Son, the Son is not subordinate in dignity to the Father, but is rather begotten by an act of personal love. Children are not products inferior to producers but rather equal in personal dignity with their mothers and fathers. "That dignity is respected when their life is 'begotten' in an act of self-giving spousal union, in an act of conjugal love. It is not respected when that life is 'made' as the end product of a series of transitive acts of making" (May 2008, p. 88).

Objections & Responses

Life-Giving Love explains the Church's clear teaching that "children have a right to be conceived by the act that expresses and embodies their parents' self-giving love" (LGL, pp. 8-9; see also DV, II, B, no. 8). But some theologians claim that it is sometimes licit to substitute a technological procedure for the conjugal act. They argue that conception need not be the fruit of a *particular* conjugal act, but only the fruit of an *overall* marital relationship. Only an outdated and impersonal "act-centered" moral theology could hold otherwise, they claim. In their view, one can separate the procreative act from the marital act in a given instance. They use the example of artificial insemination, a procedure by which a woman is injected with her husband's sperm (AFH). The authors reason that "though procreation in AFH would not be the result of one act of marital coitus, it would be the fruit of an overall *marital relational act* (sic) that expresses and facilitates the just love, commitment, care, concern and dignity of the couple shared with a new human being, their child" (Salzman and Lawler 2008, p. 248). In short, they propose that as long as the totality of the marriage embodies the proper attitude toward the gift of human life, an occasional use of artificial means to bring about conception without a sexual act could be morally legitimate (see Cahill 1990, p. 142; Ryan 2001, p. 52).

A similar "totality" argument was raised, and is still heard, in the birth control debates from those who deny that each and every marital act must remain open to the transmission of life. In *Humanae Vitae* (1968), the totality argument for the occasional use of artificial contraception is identified (no. 3) and rejected (no. 14) as a serious error (McInerny 1993, pp. 329-41). In line with this and in relationship to individual procreative acts, *Donum Vitae* (DV, II, B, nos. 4c, 8) teaches that children have a right "to be the fruit of the specific act of the conjugal love of his parents." Particular acts of homologous artificial fertilization are rejected by name (DV, II, B, 6; DP, no. 12). The totality argument is not compatible with Church teaching. In addition, such an approach would seem to open the door to occasional lying in the context of a truth telling relationship, occasional infidelity in the context of an otherwise faithful marriage, etc.

Although a couple who conceives a child by the use of artificial means may later, even very quickly, have a proper attitude toward the gift of that child as equal in dignity to his or her parents, the attitude unavoidably embodied in the choice of a particular act of artificial means entails choosing to *produce* this child through a technological substitute for conjugal intercourse. The underlying volitional stance by the spouses toward the child's conception coming about in this way is the attitude of a producer to a product. They are not engaging in conjugal love in the hope of receiving the gift of human life to crown their marital embrace; neither are they collaborating with the Creator as the two become one flesh. Grisez correctly observes that the child *coming to be* in this way cannot fulfill the "one-flesh unity" of the couple since it is not the fruit of a marital act, hence neither can the child's *coming to be* be willed by them as such. Their relationship to the child is biological: the elements used in the process stem from the parents, but the child cannot be hoped for as the gift crowning the conjugal expression of the marriage in the mutual self-giving of spousal intercourse because the choice was to make the child by a technical process (Grisez 1997, p. 247). Despite an overriding intention to establish a relationship with their offspring that respects his or her dignity and equality as a person, the couple has chosen to produce this child in a way that subjects their child to an injustice by denying the child the right to conception within the conjugal act (DV, III).

A variant on the "totality" objection posits that if bringing about human life by technological means is wrong because children have a right to be conceived by their parents in conjugal acts, how can adoption not be entangled in evil because it does not link parenthood to specific marital acts. And if adoption is morally acceptable, even to be encouraged, then surely there is nothing wrong with trying to have a child with a process like artificial insemination of the intended mother with the sperm of the intended father. In response, Grisez correctly explains that adoptive parents act with the view to establish community with an already-existing child. The choice to adopt does not entail any inevitable treatment of the child as inferior in dignity to the parents nor willing of the child to become a "product." Adoption, while it could be done in a way which embodies an attitude toward the child as an object whose worth is measured by the desire for fulfillment of the parents, need not be undertaken with such an attitude. Adoption can, and hopefully routinely is, undertaken to invite an existing child into the community of love of a family (see John Paul II 2000, *Address to Adoptive Families*).

> In seeking to produce a child by technical means, however, people cannot be acting for the sake of community with that child, since there is, as yet, no one with whom to initiate community. Hence in seeking to produce a child, a couple must be acting for their own fulfillment as parents, and since the child to be produced is, as such, extrinsic to that, it is inevitable that he or she *initially* be sought as an instrumental good, not loved for his or her own sake (Grisez 1993, p. 248, emphasis mine).

In sum, the legitimate desire for a child has been seen to embody an understanding of the child as gift. Only in the conjugal act is this desire fully respectful of the child and of the conjugal acts by which the child is engendered. In *Life-Giving Love* the bishops recognize that the desire to share life with a son or daughter is natural and positive and strong. Fertility is not just a biological function but a gift from God to husbands and wives who share the responsibility to bring children into the world in ways that do justice to the full dignity of the child. The desire for a child must itself be legitimate, and the means chosen to act on that desire must also embody that same respectful attitude toward the child. The conscience of the couple suffering from infertility must be formed to make this distinction in their hope for a child and in the processes which embody that longing.

Addendum: The Sterile Couple

Catechesis on legitimate desire, particularly the attitude that a child is a gift, entails an openness to the possibility that some couples must accept unintended childlessness. Some couples understand from the beginning that their marriage will likely be childless due to their age or physical condition. For others, the desire for children remains unfulfilled. Perhaps the marriage has not been blessed with children despite the efforts of the couple to take advantage of all that science and medicine have to offer them that is respectful of Church teaching. Perhaps morally upright assistance was not available, affordable, or effective in their particular case. The Church does not cease to applaud, encourage and support the efforts of the scientific community to address infertility in ways consistent with Church teaching. The Church also speaks to those who bear the cross of permanent infertility:

> The community of believers is called to shed light upon and support the suffering of those who are unable to fulfill their legitimate aspiration to motherhood and fatherhood. Spouses who find themselves in this sad situation are called to find in it an opportunity for sharing in a particular way in the Lord's Cross, the source of spiritual fruitfulness. Sterile couples must not forget that "even when procreation is not possible, conjugal life does not for this reason lose its value. Physical sterility in fact can be for spouses the occasion for other important services to the life of the human person, for example, adoption, various forms of educational work, and assistance to other families and to poor or handicapped children" (*DV*, 1987, II, B, 8, quoting *Familiaris Consortio*, no. 14).

Echoing this sentiment, the Pontifical Academy for Life (PAL) explains that conjugal fecundity is a broader concept than biological fertility: "Spousal love, as a practical expression of God's love for humankind, is always called to love, serve, defend and promote human life [reference omitted] in all its dimensions, even when, in actual fact, it cannot in a biological sense generate it" (PAL, 2004). Pope John Paul II speaks of a procreative love realized in adoption:

> Adopting children, regarding and treating them as one's own children, means recognizing that the relationship between parents and children is not measured only by genetic standards. Procreative love

> is first and foremost *a gift of self*. There is a form of "procreation" which occurs through acceptance, concern and devotion. The resulting relationship is so intimate and enduring that it is in no way inferior to one based on a biological connection (John Paul II 2000, *Address to Adoptive Families*, no. 4).

Adoption is mentioned specifically in *Life-Giving Love* as a wonderful way to build a family, imitate God who has made us his sons and daughters by adoption (Gal 4:5), benefit a child in need, and contribute to building a culture of life. It is praised as giving a great witness to charity, especially when a child suffers from disabilities or illness (EV, no. 63). It can even be done from afar.

> Among the various forms of adoption, consideration should be given to adoption-at-a-distance, preferable in cases where the only reason for giving up the child is the extreme poverty of the child's family. Through this type of adoption, parents are given the help needed to support and raise their children, without their being uprooted from their natural environment (EV, no. 93).

Not to be overlooked are other ways of expressing generativity such as work for justice, concern for children's welfare, and the whole array of service to others (Ashley 2006, pp. 66-67).

Inevitably the question of embryo adoption surfaces within this discussion. The debates on the morality of embryo adoption would take us too far afield. Suffice for our purposes to cite *Dignitas Personae*:

> The proposal that these embryos could be put at the disposal of infertile couples as a *treatment for infertility* is not ethically acceptable for the same reasons which make artificial heterologous procreation illicit as well as any form of surrogate motherhood (DV II, A, nos. 1-3); this practice would also lead to other problems of a medical, psychological and legal nature. It has also been proposed, solely in order to allow human beings to be born who are otherwise condemned to destruction, that there could be a form of "*prenatal adoption*." This proposal, praiseworthy with regard to the intention of respecting and defending human life, presents however various problems not dissimilar to those mentioned above (DP, no. 19).

Accordingly, *Life-Giving Love* contents itself to point out that the Church's teaching authority has acknowledged the moral concerns associated with embryo adoption, and so does not urge such adoption. Suffice to say here that the questions of the legitimate desire for children and what has been said above about adoption are particularly relevant to this question.

CONCLUSIONS

"I Don't: The Case Against Marriage" (Bennett 2010) presents the current nightmare that 41% of American births occurred outside marriage in 2008, that the number of unmarried-but-cohabiting partners is up 1000% since 1970, that the median age of those who are marrying is 28 for men and 26 for women, the oldest ever. The dignity of marriage and parenting is under fire culturally. Assisted reproductive technology (ART) may be the poisoned fruit of this disregard for marriage. It certainly contributes to it. Effective ministry to the infertile couple is part of the promotion of marriage, the dignity of the spouses, and the sanctity of life. It faces a culture reluctant to hear Church teaching on this subject.

Will the nightmare described by the Pontifical Academy for Life come to pass, a future where ART is the preferred method for generating new life?

> We refer here to the progressive emergence of a new mentality, according to which recourse to ART constitutes a preferential route—compared to the "natural" route—to bring a child into this world, because it is possible through these techniques to exercise a more effective "control" over the quality of the conceived child in line with the wishes of those who ask for such a child (Pontifical Academy for Life 2004).

Ministry to infertile couples is a ministry of hope. The formation of conscience for those struggling with infertility is an evangelization of the heart, a purification of our very desires. Perhaps by a focus on the natural and graced desire for children and its rootedness in a matrix of values, this ministry may bring compassion and clarity to those making decisions. It is an evangelization of culture promoting and celebrating life-giving love in an age of technology.

SOURCES CONSULTED

Anderson, Marie, John Bruchalski. 2004. "Assisted Reproductive Technologies are Anti-Woman." *Respect Life Program*. United States Conference of Catholic Bishops. www.usccb.org/prolife/programs/rlp/04anderson.shtml.

Bozza, Steven. 2000. *Begotten, Not Made: Pastoral Care for Couples Experiencing Infertility: Priest Manual.* Manassas, VA: Family Life Institute.

Bennet, Jessica, Jesse Ellison. 2010. "I Don't: The Case Against Marriage." *Newsweek.* June 21, 2010: 42-45.

Cataldo, Peter. 2009. "Reproductive Technologies." In *Catholic Health Care Ethics: A Manual for Practitioners*. Second Edition. Edward J. Furton et al. Eds. Philadelphia: National Catholic Bioethics Center: 103-110.

Catechism of the Catholic Church. 1997. Updated according to the *Editio Typica*. The Holy See online. www.vatican.va/archive/catechism/ccc_toc.htm.

Congregation for the Doctrine of the Faith. 1987. *Donum Vitae.* The Holy See online. www.vatican.va/roman_curia/congregations/cfaith/documents/rc_con_cfaith_doc_19870222_respect-for-human-life_en.html.

———. 2008. *Dignitas Personae.* The Holy See online. www.vatican.va/roman_curia/congregations/cfaith/documents/rc_con_cfaith_doc_20081208_dignitas-personae_en.html.

Destro, Brenda. 1997. "Celebrating the Good Message of Adoption." *Respect Life Program*. United States Conference of Catholic Bishops. www.nccbuscc.org/prolife/programs/rlp//97rlpdes.shtml.

Grisez, Germain. 1993. *Living a Christian Life*. Vol. II, *The Way of the Lord Jesus*. Quincy, IL: Franciscan Press.

———. 1997. *Difficult Moral Questions.* Vol. III, *The Way of the Lord Jesus.* Quincy, IL: Franciscan Press.

Haas, John M. 1990. "The Natural and the Human in Procreation." In *Gift of Life: Catholic Scholars Respond to the Vatican Instruction.* Washington, DC: Georgetown University Press.

John Paul II. 1981. *Familiaris Consortio.* Apostolic Exhortation. The Holy See online.www.vatican.va/holy_father/john_paul_ii/apost_exhortations/documents/hf_jp-ii_exh_19811122_familiaris-consortio_en.html.

———. 1995. *Evangelium Vitae.* Encyclical Letter. The Holy See online. www.vatican.va/holy_father/john_paul_ii/encyclicals/documents/hf_jp-ii_enc_25031995_evangelium-vitae_en.html.

———. 2000. "*Address of the Holy Father John Paul II to the Meeting of the Adoptive Families Organized by the Missionaries of Charity.*" The Holy See online. www.vatican.va/holy_father/john_paul_ii/speeches/2000/jul-sep/documents/hf_jp-ii_spe_20000905_adozioni_en.html.

———. 2004. "*Address to the Participants in the Plenary Assembly of the Pontifical Academy for Life.*" The Pontifical Academy for Life. www.

academiavita.org/template.jsp?sez=AssembleaGenerale&pag=2004/comfin&lang=english).

Mindling, J. Daniel. 2009. "Addressing Infertility with Compassion and Clarity." *Respect Life Program*. United States Conference of Catholic Bishops. www.usccb.org/prolife/programs/rlp/2009/mindlingpamphlet.pdf.

Moraczewski, Albert S. 2009. "The Human Person and the Church's Teaching Authority." In *Catholic Health Care Ethics: A Manual For Practitioners*. Second Edition. Edward J. Furton, et al. Editors. Philadelphia: National Catholic Bioethics Center: 3-8.

May, William E. 2008. *Catholic Bioethics and the Gift of Human Life*. Second Edition. Huntington IN: Our Sunday Visitor, Inc.

Mayer-Whittington, Nancy. 2007. *For the Love of Angela*. Indianapolis: Saint Catherine of Siena Press.

McInerny, Ralph. 1993. "*Humanae Vitae* and the Principle of Totality." In Janet Smith. Editor. *Why Humanae Vitae Was Right: A Reader*. San Francisco: Ignatius Press: 329-341.

Melina, Livio. 2005. "The intrinsic logic of interventions in the field of human artificial procreation: ethical aspects." *Proceedings of the Tenth Assembly of the Pontifical Academy for Life*. Juan de Dios Vial Correa. Editor. Vatican City: Libreria Editrice Vaticana: 114-126.

Miller, Michael. Ed. 2009. "The Psychological Impact of Infertility and Its Treatment." *Harvard Mental Health Letter* 25: 1-3.

Nugent, Madeline. 2008. *My Child My Gift: A Positive Response to Serious Prenatal Diagnosis*. New York: New City Press.

Paul VI. 1968. *Humanae Vitae*. Encyclical Letter. The Holy See online. www.vatican.va/holy_father/paul_vi/encyclicals/documents/hf_p-vi_enc_25071968 humanae-vitae_en.html.

Pontifical Academy for Life. 2004. *Final Communiqué on "The Dignity of Human Procreation and Reproductive Technologies: Anthropological and Ethical Insights."* The Holy See online. www.vatican.va/roman_curia/pontifical_academies/acdlife/documents/rc_pont-acd_life_doc_20040316_x-gen-assembly-final_en.html

Ronheimer, Martin. 2010. *Ethics of Procreation & The Defense of Human Life: Contraception, Artificial Fertilization, and Abortion*. Washington, DC: The Catholic University of America Press.

Ryan, Maura A. 2001. *Ethics and Economics of Assisted Reproduction: The Cost of Longing*. Washington, DC: Georgetown University Press.

Salzman, Todd A., Michael G. Lawler. 2008. *The Sexual Person: Toward a Renewed Catholic Anthropology*. Washington, DC: Georgetown University Press.

Tollefsen, Christopher. 2010."Divine, Human, and Embryo Adoption: Some Criticisms of *Dignitas Personae*." *National Catholic Bioethics Quarterly* 10.1: 75–85.

United States Conference of Catholic Bishops. 2009. *Life-Giving Love in an Age of Technology*.

Washington, DC: United States Conference of Catholic Bishops. www.usccb.org/lifegivinglovedocument.pdf.

Vatican Council II. 1965. *Gaudium et Spes*. The Holy See online. www.vatican.va/archive/hist_councils/ii_vatican_council/documents/vat-ii_cons_19651207_gaudium-et-spes_en.html.

Zimmerman, Julie Irwin. 2009. "Science and the Path to Parenthood." *America* (July 6-13):13-15.

17

Adoption Works Well

A Synthesis of the Literature

PATRICK F. FAGAN, PHD

Senior Fellow & Director, Marriage & Religion Research Institute (MARRI), Family Research Council

ABSTRACT

Adopted children greatly benefit from adoption. They experience a dramatic improvement in their socioeconomic status and are often found to be in materially advantaged homes with supportive, educated adoptive parents who are very interested and supportive of their children's development in all dimensions. The majority live in small families, with all the extra advantages it brings. The earlier the child is adopted the better he does in every outcome measured: attachment to mother; height and weight; IQ; educational achievement; in family, peer and social relationships; and in adult relationships. The birth mother does better as well. The later the adoption, the greater the lags in comparative development, especially in language development and attachment. The more children have been exposed to drugs, or to neglect or abuse, the greater the chance of lesser adjustments. In all cases, however, the adopted child does better than the child who remains in the same situation from which the adopted child came, or from which he/she was rescued. Girls tend to do slightly better than boys. The more flexible the parents and the more time they give the child, the more he thrives. Adoption is a powerful form of healing for children and adults.

INTRODUCTION

Adopted children greatly benefit from adoption. They experience a dramatic improvement in their socioeconomic status and are often found to be in materially advantaged homes with supportive, educated adoptive parents who are very interested in their child's development from all dimensions (Maughan, Collishaw and Pickles 1998, p. 682). The majority of adopted children live in small families, with all the extra advantages that brings them (Maughan et al. 1998, p. 673).

A number of major research projects, literature overviews and meta-analyses attest to the benefits of adoption. Here, a sample will be discussed.

Nicholas Zill and colleagues, using the National Survey of Child Health (Zill, Caoiro and Bloom 1994), compared four groups: adopted children, children of unmarried mothers being raised by the mother, children of intact families and children being raised by their grandparents. They found that adopted children enjoy a quality of home environment superior to all the other groups. Adopted children have superior access to health care compared to all the other groups. They enjoy health similar to that of children of intact families and, interestingly, are superior to the other two groups, in that respect. Adopted children also do better in educational attainment than single-parent children and children raised by their grandparents.

When compared with those adopted later, born outside of marriage and raised by the single mother, or raised in an intact family, children who are adopted in infancy repeat grades less often than any other group. They see mental health professionals less than all other groups (with the exception of children of intact families), have better health status than all other groups, have better standing in their school classes than all other groups (with the exception of children raised in intact families), and have fewer behavioral problems than all other groups (with the exception of children raised in intact families). On health measures, Zill found that adopted children and children of intact families share similarly high scores, and both those groups score significantly higher than children raised by single parents (Zill 1985).

At about the same time that the Zill team was conducting its research, another team, using a different large national data set, found that teens who were adopted at birth were more likely than children born into intact families to live with two parents in a middle class family. They scored higher than their middle class counterparts on indicators of school performance, social competency, optimism and volunteerism. They were less depressed than children of single parents and less involved in alcohol abuse, vandalism, group fighting, police trouble, weapon use and theft. They scored higher than children of single parents on self-esteem, confidence in their own judgment, self-directedness, positive view of others, and on feelings of security within their families (Benson, Shorma and Roehlkepartain 1994).

Using a Dutch meta-analysis, an adoption catch-up model was tested on more than 270 studies that included more than 230,000 adopted and non-adopted children and their parents. Although their catch-up with current peers was incomplete in some areas of development—in particular, physical growth and attachment—adopted children largely outperformed their peers. Those adopted before 12 months of age had an even more complete catch-up than later adoptions in terms of height, attachment, and school achievement. Interestingly, in most outcomes, international adoptions did not lead to lower rates of catch-up than domestic adoptions (van IJzendoorn and Juffer 2006, pp. 1228-1245).

In the United Kingdom a major national sample study of adults who were adopted before their first birthday were compared at age 23 and again at age 33 to a birth comparison group of non-adopted adults of the same age from similar birth circumstances and to the general population of the same age. Adopted women, in particular, showed positive adjustment across all domains studied and *were often doing better than the general population comparisons*. While generally doing as well as the general population comparison group, adopted men experienced more employment-related difficulties, and their social supports were more restricted than men in the general population. However, compared with their birth comparison group, both adopted men and women at age 33 were doing much better socially and economically (Johnson 1998, p. 50).

Finally, in a thirty year follow up on the Texas Adoption Project, the outcomes for both the adopted and biological offspring of the adoptive parents were generally positive on educational, occupational, and marital outcomes, as well as adult problems and personality, though some outcomes for the adopted offspring were somewhat less so (Loehlin, Horn and Ernst 2007, pp. 463-476). Compared to foster parenting, adoption provides higher levels of emotional security, a stronger sense of belonging and a more enduring psychological base in life (Triseliotis 2000, p. 31).

Birth mothers who give up their children for adoption also do better: they have higher educational aspirations, are more likely to finish school, and are less likely to live in poverty or receive public assistance than mothers who keep their children (Bachrach 1986, pp. 243-253; see also Bachrach 1983, pp. 171-179). They delay marriage longer and are more likely to eventually marry; they are more likely to be employed 12 months after the birth and less likely to repeat an out-of-wedlock birth. In addition, these birth mothers are no more likely to suffer negative psychological consequences, such as depression, than are mothers who rear children as single parents (McLaughlin, Manninen and Winges 1988).

With results such as these, adoption is a tremendous gift and advantage for the vast majority of children who experience it. This great good is not achieved, however, without its own special efforts, stresses and even sufferings, as will be seen in the following parsing of the efforts and benefits to parents and children.

PARENTS AND FAMILY ADJUSTMENT

Ninety percent of adopting Americans view adoption positively, although half said that it was not quite as good as having one's own child. This held for both domestic and international adoptions (see Johnson 2002, p. 40). More than a decade after the adoption, most feel a great sense of gratitude, and less than 15 percent express any regret (Fisher 2003, pp. 335-361). A common negative is that the adoption tends to restrict the family's social networks (McDonald, Propp and Murphy 2001, p. 81). These stresses and negatives are proportionally lessened the younger the child at the time of adoption, and the closer geographically the parents are to social support from others (McDonald et al. 2001, p. 88).

Married adoptive parents report more positive adjustment than non-married parents (McDonald et al. 2001, pp. 86-88) and the more the parents themselves collaborate well and put the children's interests first in portraying the adoption to the child, the more the children will thrive (Grotevant, Dumbar, Kohler and Lash Esau 2000). Parents who did not feel close to their adopted children cite reasons such as learning difficulties, conduct problems, emotional "phoniness," and rejecting behavior demonstrated by their children (Rees and Selwyn

2009, p. 563). All these difficulties tend to arise when children are adopted, not at infancy, but later in childhood. The older the child at adoption and the greater their special needs, the greater the need for flexibility by the adopting parents in their manner of parenting. In order that a good connection and firm attachment form between them and their new child, adoptive parents have to exhibit high levels of consistency, flexibility, and involvement with the child, while also having easy relationships with others in the community (Clark, Thigpen and Yates 2006, p. 190).

The more adopted children there are in a home the more likely the adoption will be positive and stable (McDonald et al. 2001, p. 80), though the more children overall, the less positive the adjustment (McDonald et al. 2001, p. 89). Neither the presence of biological children in an adoptive family, nor the order of adoption have much, if any, influence on the adjustment of the adopted children and their parents, at least in situations involving early adoption (Brodzinsky and Brodzinsky 1992, p. 73). Given all these attributes and capacities adoptive parents tend to have, it is no wonder they are less likely to divorce (National Committee for Adoption 1985).

The Adopting Mother: Attachment & Child Adjustment

According to attachment theory, children form secure attachments to caregivers who are sensitive, responsive, and predictable. This holds in adoption where the mother's attachment security and attachment capacity are found to be very important to the success of the adoption, even more so, the younger the child placed with her for adoption (Feeny, Passmore and Peterson 2007, p. 136). The sensitivity of mothers during interactions with their children is a consistent predictor of their adopted children's developmental outcomes (Vermeer and Bakermans-Kranenburg 2008, pp. 263-273).

At birth, all babies learn to recognize different people and develop their own foundational capacity to form attachments. By about six months most babies already show a preference for one person. By nine months, their primary attachment bond to this person (usually the birth mother) is well advanced, and their ability to differentiate between familiar people and unfamiliar strangers has developed. By 12 to 14 months, their bond to their primary attachment figure is usually well established (Bowlby 2007, pp. 307-319). Thus the social and cognitive advantages of children with a secure attachment history will be very important for their later social competence, especially with peers and intimate friends, but also will be a very important aspect of their psychological functioning (Thompson 2008, pp. 295-296). This being the normal pattern for biological children with their biological mother, the same attachment process is just as critical for successful adoption outcomes.

With adopted children taken into the family later than infancy some level of disagreements and strain between mother and the adopted child will occur. Despite these difficulties, these children have the great benefit of having an adoptive mother because such mothers spend more time with their children than do mothers in all the other family structures, including intact families (Lansford, Ceballo, Abbey and Stewart 2001, p. 849). Even though patterns of negative interaction are most often traced to mother-child interactions (in such cases, leaving the father more frequently with the warmer and more supportive communication with their children), (Rueter, Keyes, Iacono and McGue 2009, p. 63), nonetheless it is the mother's total time with the infant or child that predicts the adaptation of the child (Huston and Aronson 2005, p. 476). Thus a previously unidentified attribute, the frequency with which a parent thinks of the child when he is away, can be understood as being a significant variable in explaining the level of satisfaction with and the success of the adoption (Huston and Aronson 2005, p. 476). By contrast, avoidant or anxious attachment styles by the mother increase the sense of social and family loneliness for the child (Feeny et al. 2007, p. 140).

The Adoptee's Sense of Attachment

As with so many other adopted child outcomes, problems with attachment are frequently related to the age of adoption: adoptees placed before twelve months of age show secure attachments as often as non-adopted children, while those adopted after 12 months of age show significantly less secure attachments than non-adopted children. Although adopted children come into the family with disorganized attachments after deprivation and neglect, nonetheless they show an impressive, although incomplete, catch-up after some time in their placement in adoption (van den Dries, Juffer, van IJzendoorn and Bakermans-Kranenburg 2009, p. 417).

Interestingly, although adopted children sometimes say that they felt different from their adoptive family while growing up, this is not necessarily a negative feeling, nor does it mean that the adopted child felt that he or she did not belong in the adoptive family (Howe 2001, p. 229). In the vast majority of these cases attachment is present even if accompanied by feelings of difference. Even when attachment problems are present, adoption still proves to be in the best interest of the child, as foster children have more disorganized attachments when compared to adoptees or children reared by their biological parents or in institutional care (van den Dries et al. 2009, p. 415).

Parent-child communication further evidences the fact that adoption is in the best interest of the child. A study of 450 adolescents found that adoptive children report more positive communication with their parents than biological children do, and even more positive relationships with their parents than their peers (Lanz, Lafrate, Rosnati and Scabini 1999, p. 789). However, there are exceptions to this high level of communication, due mainly to parent-child conflict during adolescence (Rueter, Keyes, Iacono and McGue 2009, pp. 62-63).

PHYSICAL HEALTH AND GROWTH

The large Dutch meta-analysis mentioned earlier found that when adopted children are placed in a new family, be it in their first, second or later years, they tend to lag very significantly behind in height and weight compared to their non-adopted peers of the same age. Though they do not totally catch up, they do close the gap with their general peers and greatly outperform their non-adopted birth peers. Children adopted before twelve months of age close the gap the most. This also holds for international adoptions (van IJzendoorn and Juffer 2006, pp. 1228-1245).

This meta-finding can be seen also in the results of a California study of 83 African-American adoptive families where the one-third of newly adopted children who were rated as less than "very healthy" at the time of adoption, later had improved very significantly (Smith-McKeever 2006, p. 834). There is one health anomaly worth noting: adopted girls of international adoptions, more especially those who are most growth impaired—and thus being most likely to close this health gap—are also most likely to develop precocious menarche, on average at 10.5 years of age. Such precocious puberty is very rare for boys (Johnson 2002, pp. 46-47).

The power of adoption to restore health can be seen in a special study of children through six years of age who were exposed to cocaine *in utero*. Compared to their non-adopted drug exposed peers who were raised by their birth mothers, the adopted children generally functioned within the normal range. They were almost identical in most outcomes to non-drug-exposed adopted children (Johnson 2002, p. 48).

EDUCATIONAL OUTCOMES FOR ADOPTED CHILDREN

Adopted children do well at school. In a 1981 study only seven percent of children adopted in infancy repeated a grade, while 12 percent of children living with both biological parents repeated a grade (Zill 1995). Adoption increases a child's ability to learn, and the earlier a child is placed for adoption the more beneficial it is for their overall development (Ply and Vijverberg 2003, p. 637). Both the Zill and Benson studies cited above recount findings similar to these. Although adopted children's IQ tends to correlate with their biological mothers' background factors, e.g. the natural mothers' education level, the earlier a child is placed in an adoptive home, the higher their later IQ score (Scarr and Weinberg 1983, p. 263). The adopting family influences their cognitive abilities and "the IQ correlations of adopted siblings are as high as those of biological siblings reared together" (Scarr and Weinberg 1983, p. 263).

Language Acquisition

The age at which children are adopted directly affects their language development. The earlier that children are adopted, the better the development. The later the adoption, the greater the lag in language development and the more severe the problems (Glennen and Masters 2002, p. 420). Adoption also shows its power of healing in the area of language, but the later the adoption, the slower the process: those adopted up to one year of age reached average English language developmental standards within two years of adoption, though the rate of catch-up slowed with the older the age of adoption. Thereafter those adopted later experienced an increasingly greater lag in language development and more severe problems in learning language. For instance, those adopted at 25 to 30 months of age were eight to ten months delayed a year into their adoption (Glennen and Masters 2002, p. 420). Consequentially, later-adopted children need special education for their learning problems twice as frequently as non-adopted children do (van IJzendoorn and Juffer 2005, p. 329).

Education Attainment

Many general studies show that when the academic performance of adopted and non-adopted children are compared, the findings are mixed:

- the non-adopted adolescents have fewer academic learning problems and reported significantly better grades than do the adopted (Burrow, Tubman and Finley 2004, p. 273).
- teachers rate adopted children as scoring lower than non-adopted children in originality, independent learning, school involvement, productive involvement with peers, and school achievement (Brodzinsky 1993, p. 157).
- adopted children need significantly more special treatment in their learning than do non-adopted children (van IJzendoorn, Juffer and Poelhuis 2005, p. 310).
- adopted children are repeatedly found to perform better than their siblings or birth peers in tests of reading, mathematics, and general ability, retaining this advantage in grade attainment and later in adult qualifications (van IJzendoorn et al. 2005, p. 309; Maughan et al. 1998, pp. 677-678).
- adopted children never fall significantly below the general population performance, and
- adopted boys did better than the general population in reading, primarily attributable to parental interest in their education (Maughan et al. 1998, pp. 675-676).

Overall Educational Achievement

Later adoptees are able to profit substantially from the positive change of environment offered by adoption and subsequent upbringing in educationally stimulating adoptive families (van IJzendoorn and Juffer 2005, p. 327). A Swedish longitudinal study (Johnson 2002, pp. 49-50), followed four groups of children from gestation through young adulthood (adopted children, long-term foster care children, children originally registered for adoption by birth mothers who changed their minds, and classmates living with their biological parents). At 11 years of age adopted girls had lower math scores but otherwise did not differ. Adopted boys had a higher rate of problem behavior, as rated by teachers, compared to their non-adopted classmates. At 15 years, adopted boys and girls both had a tendency for lower mean grades than classmates. Foster children and those adolescents living with their birth mothers, however, were more problematic. At 18 years, military records revealed that IQ scores of adopted boys and control group were the same. Again, young men who remained with their birth mothers or were in long-term foster care scored significantly lower than the control groups on most IQ subtests (Johnson 2002, pp. 49-50).

Repeating a strong, almost immutable pattern, another study found that children adopted in their first year of life do not show any delays in school performance, whereas children adopted after their first birthday lag behind (van IJzendoorn and Juffer 2005, p. 328).

In international studies adopted children were referred to special education twice as often as non-adopted children, in each country studied. It was also found, however, that adoptive parents are more aware of available services and more alert to potential problems than non-adoptive parents, thus being more inclined to refer their children to special education (van IJzendoorn and Juffer 2005, p. 328).

Educational Effects of Abuse & Neglect

Adopted children who were exposed to abuse and neglect lagged farther behind in school achievement than did adopted children without such backgrounds; although their IQ scores did not show a corresponding difference (van IJzendoorn and Juffer 2005, p. 328).

Adopted children exposed to drugs *in utero*, despite attaining good grades as frequently as non-exposed children and doing as well in speech and language, did have more problems with hyperactivity, repeated a grade more frequently, or needed classes for the behaviorally or emotionally disturbed (Johnson 2002, p. 49). Not surprisingly, having more special needs generated by problems such as these is associated with poorer adjustment (McDonald et al. 2001, p. 86) and leads to weaker or even negative outcomes.

PSYCHOLOGICAL ADJUSTMENT

Although studies show that there are no significant differences in psychological adjustment or physical health between adopted and non-adopted adolescents (Burrow, Tubman and Finley 2004, p. 267), adopted children exhibit lower self-esteem than children from intact families and may not be much different from children of separated or divorced families (Lanz, Lafrate, Rosnati and Scabini 1999, p. 785). Some adoptive parents experience problems including depression and unhappiness. Behavioral problems present the greatest challenge by far, especially among children who were older at the time of adoption, or who have special needs (Wright and Flynn 2006, p. 499). At the same time, the 1988 National Interview Survey of Child Health found that adopted children see mental health providers less than all other groups except children from intact families (Zill 1985), thus attesting to the general good mental health of adopted children.

Aggressive & Anti-Social Behavior

Adopted children are about twice as likely to display aggressive antisocial behavior than are non-adopted children, but the closer they are to the adoptive parents and the higher the mother's educational status, the less the aggression (Grotevant, van Dulmen, Dunbar, Nelson-Christinedaughter, Christensen, Fan and Miller 2006, p. 113). Conversely, the more the maltreatment the child has suffered, the greater the aggression (Grotevant et al. 2006, p. 113).

In the face of such difficulties, the healing power of adoption and the role of the adoptive mother can be seen. The more the mother has easy access to memories of her own childhood and the more secure her own attachment capacity, the lower the levels of aggression these abused children exhibit (Steele, Hodges, Kaniuk, Hillman and Henderson 2003, p. 193). On the other hand, a mother's unresolved mourning in her own life can exacerbate the emotional worries of maltreated adopted children (Steele et al. 2003, p. 194). Thus the parent's emotional and attachment capacities have much influence on the outcomes of adoptees who have special emotional needs because of prior neglect, physical or sexual abuse. The Swedish four-group, longitudinal study quoted above, in looking at 23-year-olds, found no differences in alcohol-related problems or criminal activities for adoptees compared to controls, although boys in long-term foster care were likely to have more problems (Dana 2002, pp. 49-50).

Longing to Know their Birth Mother

A common psychological issue for adopted children is the desire to reunite, at some stage, with their birth mother. Because this area of research deals almost totally in subjective appraisals of feelings and perceptions of one's own and others' feelings, many of the findings are quite complex and seemingly contradictory (Howe 2001, p. 230). Threading through the data, the following is an effort to make sense of these ambiguous findings.

About 70 percent of adult adoptees express feeling moderate to significant degrees of uncertainty and ambiguous loss regarding their birth parents. One study showed that 70 percent of adoptees studied were experiencing such feelings, though, of course, the other 30 percent of the participants expressed security and no apparent loss (Powell and Afifi 2005, p. 138). Adoptees desiring more biological background information, frequently express stronger emotions of anger, frustration, and a sense of powerlessness over their lack of access to this key aspect of their selves. However, these feelings may be affected more by searchers' inability to re-connect with their biological ties than with any adoption outcome per se (March and Miall 2000, p. 360).

Adoptees with significant degrees of uncertainty and ambiguous feelings of loss usually claim that disapproval, or fear of disapproval, from family members contributes to their avoidance and secrecy about the adoption. Conversely, those adoptees who do not express such loss said they experience, instead, acceptance and openness in communicating with their adoptive families. The most frequent reason they cite for their security is "the love and closeness of the adoptive family" (Powell and Afifi 2005, p. 138).

A modeling exercise carried out on a broad array of data found that whether or not adopted people felt loved by their adoptive mother was also predictive of who searched and who did not. Whereas 23 percent of those who searched said that they had not felt loved by their adoptive mother, or at least had not felt certain of her love, only nine percent of non-searchers reported similar feelings of rejection. However, from these data, it is worth noting that of those 77 percent who searched, the overwhelming majority did feel loved by their adoptive mother (Howe 2001, p. 230).

From the United Kingdom we learn that adopted women are twice as likely as men to search for their birth relatives (Howe 2001, pp. 225-226). When adopted children finally make contact with their birth mother the likelihood of frequent contact with her parallels strikingly the age at which the adoption took place: the earlier the adoption, the much more likely is frequent contact. Also, the older the child at adoption, the more likely the adopted person will not make contact with the birth mother (Howe 2001, pp. 226-227). Thus, it would seem that the earlier the adoption, the greater the capacity of attachment to the birth mother, at least for females.

Social Adjustment

A mix of complex factors relating to early experience, the adjustment of the child within the family and the community, and societal attitudes about adoption, all influence adoptive identity development and illustrate the difficulties for the adopted child of combining a sense of self with other spheres of identity (Dunbar, Grotevant, Kohler and Lash Esau, 2000, p. 385).

Adoptees' Adjustment to Their New Home

Quite a few studies, some already quoted, illustrate that adopted children are no different from other children in myriads of ways. This includes differences in problem behaviors for children aged zero to four years, and in pro-social and problem behaviors in children aged six to eleven years and those aged twelve to eighteen (Borders, Black and Pasley 1998, p. 240). Special needs adoptees, those who experienced a combination of neglect, abuse, and multiple changes in caretaking before being placed in adoption, are significantly more likely to experience adjustment difficulties, including adoption disruption (Brodzinsky 1993, p. 159). Older adopted children also have more difficult adjustments to their adoptive homes (McDonald, Propp and Murphy 2001, p. 86).

Child's Adjustment

Adopted children begin to understand the meaning and implications of being adopted when they are five to seven years of age, resulting in increased sensitivity or ambivalence about adoption. Some attempt to put adoption out of their mind or avoid things that remind them of their adoption (Brodzinsky 1993, pp. 161-162). A child's ability to adjust can be affected by how they view their own adoption, though the mere fact of being a boy increases the likelihood of maladjustment to adoption (Brooks and Barth, 1999, p. 96). For instance, though not necessarily carrying a negative connotation, 68 per cent of adoptees say they 'feel different' from their adoptive family (Howe and Feast 2001, p. 355).

Differences in racial or ethnic backgrounds between adoptees and the families have relatively little impact on their socialization. In one study, according to the adoptive mothers, most adopted children do not experience serious negative reactions from peers or adults regarding their skin color or origin. Though in the study 30 percent of adopted children received some negative reactions, only seven percent had many such experiences (Juffer, Stams and van IJzendoorn 2004, p. 703).

Adolescent Adjustment by Age at Adoption

As in so many other outcomes, age at adoption seems to be the biggest reason for the differences between adopted and non-adopted adolescents: the older the child when adopted, the greater the differences from those adopted earlier. For instance, the Benson study, noted earlier, states that "the most interesting result from this study was the remarkable lack of differences . . . between youth adopted at ages 2-5 years and those adopted at ages 6-10 years" (Sharma, McGue and Benson 1996, p. 101). This impact of the age-at-adoption difference can be seen in a study of teenage attachment problems:

> If the child had arrived at 1 year of age or earlier and had been 6 months or less in an orphanage or foster home, 6 percent showed attachment problems. In the group where the child had arrived after 1 year of age and had been in an orphanage or foster home for more than 6 months, 23 percent showed attachment problems." (Cederblad, Höök, Irhammar and Mercke 1999, p. 1244)

The earlier the child is adopted the more he or she thrives.

Adult Adoptee Adjustment

Adult relationships make up another significant aspect of an adopted child's life, and in these relationships, the positive impact of adoption continues.

Adult adopted women tend to be emotionally stable and less likely to report high levels of psychological distress than women in their birth comparison group (Collishaw, Maughan and Pickles 1998, p. 61). Women gain much higher levels of social support from multiple sources, including friends and their parents, in comparison to a control non-adopted birth group. Adopted men, by contrast with their control group, were least likely to turn to a friend for help with personal problems and had increased rates of dependence and higher levels of unemployment (Collishaw et al. 1998, p. 63).

Regarding romantic relationships, in 1998, a study showed that adopted women, on average, began their first romantic relationship at 22.1 years of age, while their birth comparison group began at 20.5 years and the general population at 21.7 years (Collishaw et al. 1998, p. 61). A similar but more pronounced delay happens in childbearing, with adopted women delaying by two years, compared to the general population, and by three years, compared to their birth comparison group (Collishaw et al. 1998, p. 61).

CONCLUSION

Adoption is a remarkable practice by generous people who give of their affection, attention, time and resources to help young children have a better chance in life. Though not without difficulty for some, compared to what life was offering them, adoption makes an enormous positive difference in all dimensions of the lives of all involved. For the overwhelming number of those who adopt and are adopted, adoption works very well. The accumulating research teaches what Henderson (2002) puts well:

> Every adoption represents both gains and losses, and that adoption is a multigenerational and ongoing process which only begins with the final adoption, and which permanently affects the lives of all involved. We know that the story of an adoption does not "end" the day the adoptive parents and their new child walk out of court as a legal family. The adoption does not "end" the day that the birthparent becomes legally childless, or the parent of one less child. The adoption experience for the adoptee only begins with the adoption process itself, and likely never really "ends." (Henderson 2002, p. 134)

SOURCES CONSULTED

Borders D., L. K. Black, K. Pasley. 1998. "Children and Their Parents at Greater Risk for Negative Outcomes?" *Family Relations* 47:237-241.

Bowlby, R. 2007. "Babies and Toddlers in Non-parental Daycare Can Avoid Stress and Anxiety if They Develop a Lasting Secondary Attachment Bond with One Carer Who is Consistently Accessible to Them." *Attachment & Human Development* 9:307-319.

Brodzinsky, D. M. 1993. "Long-Term Outcomes in Adoption." *The Future of Children. Adoption* 3:153-166.

Brodzinsky, D. M., A. B. Brodzinsky. 1992. "The Impact of Family Structure on the Adjustment of Adopted Children." *Child Welfare* 71:69-76.

Brooks, D., R. Barth. 1999. "Adult Transracial and Inracial Adoptees: Effects of Race, Gender, Adoptive Family Structure, and Placement History on Adjustment Outcomes." *American Journal of Orthopsychiatry* 69:96.

Burrow, A. L., J. G. Tubman, G. E. Finley. 2004. "Adolescent Adjustment in a Nationally Collected Sample: Identifying Group Differences by Adoption Status, Adoption Subtype, Developmental Stage and Gender." *Journal of Adolescence* 27:267-282.

Cederblad, M., B. Höök, M. Irhammar, A. M. Mercke. 1999. "Mental Health in International Adoptees as Teenagers and Young Adults. An Epidemiological Study." *Journal of Child Psychology and Psychiatry* 40:1239-1248.

Clark, P., S. Thigpen, A. M. Yates. 2006. "Integrating the Older/Special Needs Adoptive Child into the Family." *Journal of Marital and Family Therapy* 32:181–194.

Collishaw, S., B. Maughan, A. Pickles. 1998. "Infant Adoption: Psychosocial Outcomes in Adulthood." *Social Psychiatry and Psychiatric Epidemiology* 33:57-65.

Dana, E. J. 2002. "Adoption and the Effect on Children's Development." *Early Human Development* 68:39–54.

Dunbar, N., H. D. Grotevant, J. K. Kohler, A. M. Lash Esau. 2000. "Adoptive Identity: How Contexts within and beyond the Family Shape Developmental Pathways." *Family Relations* 49:385.

Feeney, J. A., N. L. Passmore, C. C. Peterson. 2007. "Adoption, Attachment, and Relationship Concerns: A Study of Adult Adoptees." *Personal Relationship* 14:129-147.

Fisher, A. 2003. "Still Not Quite as Good as Having Your Own? Toward a Sociology of Adoption." *Annual Review Sociology* 29:335–361.

Glennen, S., M. G. Masters. 2002. "Typical and Atypical Language Development in Infants and Toddlers Adopted from Eastern Europe." *American Journal of Speech-Language Pathology* 11:17-33.

Grotevant, H. D., M. H. van Dulmen, N. Dunbar, J. Nelson-Christinedaughter, M. Christensen, X. Fan, B. C. Miller. 2006. "Antisocial Behavior of Adoptees and Nonadoptees: Prediction from Early History and Adolescent Relationships." *Journal of Research on Adolescence* 16:105-131.

Howe, D. 2001."Age at Placement, Adoption Experience and Adult Adopted People's Contact with their Adoptive and Birth Mothers: An Attachment Perspective." *Attachment and Human Development* 3:222–237.

Howe, D., J. Feast. 2001. "The Long-term Outcome of Reunions Between Adult Adopted People and their Birth Mothers." *British Journal of Social Work* 31:351-368.

Huston, A. C., S. R. Aronson. 2005."Mothers' Time with Infant and Time in Employment as Predictors of Mother-Child Relationships and Children's Early Development." *Child Development* 76:476-477.

Johnson, D. E. 2002."Adoption and the Effect on Children's Development." *Early Human Development* 68:39–54.

Juffer, F., G. Stams, M. Van IJzendoorn. 2004."Adopted Children's Problem Behavior Is Significantly Related to their Ego Resiliency, Ego Control, and Sociometric Status." *Journal of Child Psychology and Psychiatry* 45:697-706.

Lansford, J. E., R. Ceballo, A. Abbey, A. J. Stewart. 2001. "Does Family Structure Matter? A Comparison of Adoptive, Two-Parent Biological, Single-Mother, Stepfather, and Stepmother Households." *Journal of Marriage and Family* 63:840-851.

Lanz, M., R. Lafrate, R. Rosnati, E. Scabini. 1999. "Parent-Child Communication and Adolescent Self-Esteem in Separated, Intercountry Adoptive and Intact Non-Adoptive Families." *Journal of Adolescence* 22:785-794.

Loehlin, J. C., J. M. Horn, J. L. Ernst. 2007. "Genetic and Environmental Influences on Adult Life Outcomes: Evidence from the Texas Adoption Project." *Behavior Genetics* 37:463-476.

McLaughlin, S. D., D. L. Manninen, L. D. Winges. 1988. "Do Adolescents Who Relinquish Their Children Fare Better or Worse Than Those Who Raise Them?" *Family Planning Perspectives* 20:25-32.

March, K., C. Miall. 2000. "Adoption as a Family Form." *Family Relations* 49:359-362.

Maughan, B., S. Collishaw, A. Pickles. 1998."School Achievement and Adult Qualifications among Adoptees: A Longitudinal Study." *Journal of Child Psychology and Psychiatry* 39: 669-685

McDonald, T., J. Propp, K. Murphy. 2001. "The Postadoption Experience: Child, Parent, and Family Predictors of Family Adjustment to Adoption." *Child Welfare League of America* 80:71-94.

National Committee for Adoption. 1985. *Unmarried Parents Today.* Cited in Pat Fagan, 1996. "Promoting Adoption Reform: Congress Can Give

Children another Chance." The Heritage Foundation. www.heritage.org/research/reports/1996/05/bg1080nbsp-promoting-adoption-reform; accessed December 2010.

Plug, E., W. Vijverberg. 2003."Schooling, Family Background, and Adoption: Is It Nature or Is It Nurture?" *Journal of Political Economy* 111:611-640.

Powell, K. A., T. D. Afifi. 2005. "Uncertainty Management and Adoptees' Ambiguous Loss of their Birth Parents." *Journal of Social and Personal Relationships* 22:129-153.

Rees, C. A., J. Selwyn. 2009."Non-Infant Adoption from Care: Lessons for Safeguarding Children." *Child: Care, Health & Development* 35:561-567.

Rueter, M. A., M. A. Keyes, W. G. Iacono, M. McGue. 2009. "Family Interactions in Adoptive Compared to Nonadoptive Families." *Journal of Family Psychology* 23:58-66.

Scarr, S., R. A. Weinberg. 1983."The Minnesota Adoption Studies: Genetic Differences and Malleability." *Child Development* 54:260-267.

Sharma, A. R., M. K. McGue, P. L. Benson. 1996. "The Emotional and Behavioral Adjustment of United States Adopted Adolescents: Part II. Age at Adoption." *Children and Youth Services Review* 18:101.

Smith-McKeever, C. 2006."Adoption Satisfaction among African-American Families Adopting African-American Children." *Children and Youth Services Review* 28:825-840.

Steele, M., J. Hodges, J. Kaniuk, S. Hillman, K. Henderson. 2003."Attachment Representations and Adoption: Associations between Maternal States of Mind and Emotion Narratives in Previously Maltreated Children." *Journal of Child Psychotherapy* 29:187-205.

Thompson, R. A. 2008. "Measure Twice, Cut Once: Attachment Theory and the NICHD Study of Early Child Care and Youth Development." *Attachment and Human Development* 3:295-296.

Triseliotis, J. 2000. "Long-term Foster Care or Adoption? The Evidence Examined." *Child and Family Social Work* 7:23-33.

van den Dries, L., J. Femmie, M. H. van IJzendoorn, M. J. Bakermans-Kranenburg. 2009."Fostering Security? A Meta-analysis of Attachment in Adopted Children." *Children and Youth Services Review* 31:410-421.

van IJzendoorn, M. H., J. Femmie. 2005."Adoption is a Successful Natural Intervention Enhancing Adopted Children's IQ and School Performance." *Current Directions in Psychological Science* 14:326-330.

van IJzendoorn, M. H., F. Juffer. 2006."The Emanuel Miller Memorial Lecture 2006: Adoption as Intervention. Meta-analytic Evidence for Massive

Catch-Up and Plasticity in Physical, Socio-emotional, and Cognitive Development." *Journal of Child Psychology and Psychiatry* 47:1228-1245.

van IJzendoorn, M. H., J. Femmie, C. W. Klein Poelhuis. 2005. "Adoption and Cognitive Development: A Meta-Analytic Comparison of Adopted and Nonadopted Children's IQ and School Performance." *Psychological Bulletin* 131:301-316.

Vermeer, H. J., M. Bakermans-Kranenburg. 2008. "Attachment to Mother and Nonmaternal Care: Bridging the Gap." *Attachment and Human Development* 10(3):263-273.

Wright, L., C. Flynn. 2006. "Adolescent Adoption: Success Despite Challenges." *Children and Youth Services Review* 28:487-510.

Zill, N. 1985. "Behavior and Learning Problems Among Adopted Children: Findings from a U.S. National Survey of Child Health." Washington, DC: Child Trends Inc., paper presented to the Society for Research in Child Development, April 27, 1985. Cited in Pat Fagan, 1996. "Promoting Adoption Reform: Congress Can Give Children another Chance." The Heritage Foundation. www.heritage.org/research/reports/1996/05/bg1080nbsp-promoting-adoption-reform; accessed December 2010.

Zill, N. 1995. Adopted Children in the United States: A Profile Based on the National Survey of Child Health. Testimony before the House Ways and Means Subcommittee on Human Resources, May 1995. Cited in Pat Fagan, 1996. "Promoting Adoption Reform: Congress Can Give Children another Chance." The Heritage Foundation. www.heritage.org/research/reports/1996/05/bg1080nbsp-promoting-adoption-reform; accessed December 2010.

Zill, N., M. J. Caoiro, B. Bloom. 1994. "Health of Our Nation's Children." *Vital and Health Statistics*, Series 10, No. 191, U.S. Public Health Service. Hyattsville, MD: Department of Health and Human Services, DHHS Publication No. (PHS) 95-1519.

PANEL III

THE EFFECT OF CULTURE & THE ARTS ON GOD'S PLAN FOR MARRIED LOVE

18

Changing Human Behavior

How Culture, Contraception, and Religion Combined in the Early 20th Century to Create the Modern Sexual Revolution

THERESA NOTARE, PHD

Assistant Director, Natural Family Planning Program, United States Conference of Catholic Bishops

ABSTRACT

The modern sexual revolution offers an example of how human behavior radically changed in the modern period (late nineteenth century to current day), due to a conflation of personal and global influences.

Although most people believe that the sexual revolution began in the 1960s, its genesis was much further back, in the late 19th and early 20th centuries. Its tenets have to do with the nature of human sexuality and its expression in human relationships. The history of the modern sexual revolution is multifaceted and enmeshed in a web of interrelated movements. No single element was responsible for the sexual revolution. It takes in popular or social elements as well as religious, philosophical, academic, scientific, medical, psychological, economic, political, and legal elements, and even gender history.

Some of the messages of the modern sexual revolution represent real advances for humanity. Other elements both expose and feed the dark side of humanity. Due to the breadth and complexity of the subject, only a few snapshots are examined in this article: (1) the emergence of the topic of human sexuality as an appropriate subject for public discourse; (2) the role of academia in rethinking sexual activity and marriage; and (3) the popular movement to rethink marriage and sex. These topics alone reveal the potent concoction that fed the modern sexual revolution, where truth and goodwill were mixed with misinformation and lies.

INTRODUCTION

Human beings are complex creatures—mortal and bound to the earth, yet also able to transcend the material world, reaching for heaven itself. Human behavior is equally complex—at various times, easily or not very easily influenced. Strong elements that potentially influence human behavior can arise from familiar, personal sources, such as trusted friends or beloved family members. More potent and global influences also affect a person's behavior. Those forces can be grouped under the headings of religious beliefs and culture. What happens when personal and global forces intersect or combine in one subject? Change. Indeed, a radical change in human behavior may result.

The modern sexual revolution offers an example of how human behavior radically changed in the modern period (late nineteenth century to current day), due to a conflation of personal and global influences, some of which will be discussed here.

Although most people believe that the sexual revolution began in the 1960s, its genesis was much earlier, in the late 19th and early 20th centuries. Its tenets had to do with the nature of human sexuality and its expression in human relationships. At first, only a handful of messages emerged, but they rapidly shifted and spread. From the beginning, core ideas of the modern sexual revolution have seriously misled and even hurt people. This is because among the false ideas of the modern sexual revolution are specific elements that touch human needs and goods.

The history of the modern sexual revolution is multifaceted and enmeshed in a web of interrelationships. This point cannot be overemphasized. No single element is responsible for the sexual revolution. It takes in popular or social elements as well as religious, philosophical, academic, scientific, medical, psychological, economic, political, legal elements, and even gender history. Some of its elements represent real advances for humanity. Other elements both expose and feed the dark side of humanity. Due to the breadth and complexity of the topic, only a few snapshots can be examined in this article. I have decided to focus on three little known aspects of its history: (1) the emergence of the topic of human sexuality as an appropriate subject for public discourse; (2) the role of academia in rethinking sexual activity and marriage; and (3) the popular movement to rethink marriage and sex. These examples reveal the potent concoction that fed the modern sexual revolution, where truth and goodwill were mixed with misinformation and lies.

Before the three points above are examined, a definition of the modern sexual revolution is provided. After discussion of the three points, brief mention will be made of the contributing role of birth control methods and activists. By way of conclusion, a short discussion of the influence of organized religion will also be offered. This history is focused on the United States and England because those two countries would take a world-wide lead in the promotion of the modern sexual revolution.

DEFINING THE MODERN SEXUAL REVOLUTION

The modern interest in all things sexual is the outcome of multiple and diverse trends that emerged in the late nineteenth century. These trends have been identified as the beginnings of the modern sexual revolution in the West. Historians debate this time frame.[1] Some place the beginning of this revolution in the 1920s. The majority find its roots in the late nineteenth century.[2] A minority of historians claim that there is no "modern sexual revolution." They posit a cyclical pattern of sexual permissiveness followed by restrictive beliefs and behaviors, back to permissiveness, and so forth (see Taylor 1953 and Stone 1977).

How historians define the modern sexual revolution explains the disparities in date.[3] If the modern sexual revolution is defined by an increase in non-marital sexual activity after a period of widespread restrictions in a given population, other time periods would qualify, and the cyclical pattern would be supported. Defining the sexual revolution as only the shift in emphasis from sex for procreation to sex for personal pleasure, is also problematic. In pre-Christian societies (e.g., the Roman Empire, early medieval Germanic and other European tribes), a system of polygamy, concubinage, and/or slavery allowed great sexual license for the male head of a household.[4] If the definition includes an acceptance of non-heterosexual intercourse, again, other time periods can be used as examples of acceptance.[5] If the modern sexual revolution represents the shift from a male controlled sexuality to that of a female controlled sexuality, the argument could be made that the revolution has not yet begun.[6]

The above considerations invite a deeper question not often asked by historians: "What does sexual activity mean in a particular age, and when does that meaning change so radically that it constitutes a revolution?"[7] A definition of the modern sexual revolution must take this fundamental question into consideration.

Due to the dominant influence of Christian beliefs in the West, it is useful and even necessary to examine the modern sexual revolution in light of Christian beliefs about men, women, human sexuality and marriage. A brief review of these beliefs follows.

Rooted in both Hebrew and Christian scriptures, a clear anthropology can be identified in the Christian belief system. The first two chapters of Genesis are foundational to this anthropology. Genesis begins by noting the equal dignity of both men and women. Chapter One reveals that the Creator made humanity "in His image." (Gen 1:27) The text explains that men and women were made to be in relationship with one another. "God blessed them, saying to them: 'Be fruitful and multiply.'" (Gen 1:28) Procreation, was therefore seen as a gift of God that entails a serious responsibility, indeed, a command for humanity. Christians would, in fact, emphasize procreation as a primary function of human sexuality.

The second chapter of Genesis describes the kind of union that should exist between a man and a woman. It is worth quoting at length.

> The Lord God said:
> "It is not good for the man to be alone.
> I will make a suitable partner for him." ....
>
> So the Lord God cast a deep sleep

upon the man,
and while he was asleep,
he took out one of his ribs,
and closed up its place with flesh.

The Lord God then built up into a woman
the rib that he had taken from the man.
When he brought her to the man, the man said:

"This one, at last, is bone of my bones
and flesh of my flesh;
This one shall be called 'woman,'
for out of 'her man' this one has been taken."

That is why a man leaves
his father and mother
and clings to his wife,
and the two of them
become one body. (Gen 2:18, 21-24)

Using language that mirrors God's sacred covenant with Israel, the author of Genesis underscores the complementarity and unity between a man and a woman in marriage. Together the two Genesis accounts yield a moral standard that has shaped Western civilization for millennia: men and women, being created in the image of God and having a sexual capacity which is both potentially procreative and bonding, can live out their sexuality fully within the sacred covenant of marriage. This is the design for life and love ordained by God.

Notwithstanding the admonitions in Genesis, customs incompatible with the exclusivity and permanence of the marriage bond arose among the Jews. When asked "May a man divorce his wife?," Jesus restores the original unity and permanence of marriage:

> Have you not read that from the beginning the Creator "made them male and female" and said, "For this reason a man shall leave his father and mother and be joined to his wife, and the two shall become one flesh"? So they are no longer two, but one flesh. Therefore, what God has joined together, no human being must separate. (Mt 19:4-7)

Many other passages of Hebrew Scripture and of the New Testament offer insights into the Christian understanding of human sexuality and marriage, but that subject has been treated comprehensively by others (see for example Olsen 2001, pp. 1-100; see also Schillebeeckx1976, pp.7-229). For our purposes, the quotations from Genesis and the Gospel of Matthew are by themselves adequate to convey the foundational beliefs that have influenced the culture of Christians wherever they have lived. These beliefs flourished and endured especially in the West.

In summary, we can say that Christian beliefs assert that sexual activity, as created by God, is good and exists as a gift and responsibility for the bonding of a man to a woman (the permanent "one flesh" union of husband and wife) and for the procreation and nurture of children. Sexual activity is designed to be an integral part of marriage, which is exclusive, faithful and permanent. Taken as a whole, and despite the innovations of the Reformation[8] or the details of culturally specific courting and marriage customs over the centuries, these beliefs have served as the standard by which the West has measured sexual and marriage morality since the time of Christ.

With Christian beliefs as the standard, the modern sexual revolution can be defined by the following characteristics: a "qualitatively more positive evaluation of sex as a human activity" (Smith 1978, p. 426); an acceptance of non-reproductive sexual activity typically facilitated by birth control methods or sterilization; a substantial sustained increase in non-marital coitus; a willingness to expand definitions of human sexuality and sexual activity;[9] a multi-faceted questioning of the truth of the Judeo-Christian understanding of sexuality and sexual activity, often accompanied by either a partial or complete rejection of it; and an on-going attempt to separate sexual activity from the social institutions of marriage, cultural and religious moral structures. Each of these elements can be found in the early history of the modern sexual revolution.

THE SILENCE IS BROKEN

The first piece in the puzzle that comprises the modern sexual revolution is the movement of the subject of sex from an *inappropriate* to an *appropriate* topic for public discussion. That change came from good sources—Christian social reformers, feminists, socialists, and physicians—who would form the Social Purity and later Social Hygiene movements. Historians agree that public discussion regarding human sexuality was possible only because of these reformers. They identified a major social problem, sought to create a solution which, in turn, moved sex from the shadows into the public square. Their story follows.

The Problem

During the 19th century, public attention became almost obsessively focused on the issue of prostitution with its accompanying problem of venereal disease. This focus was related to a major characteristic of the period that also came under severe public scrutiny: the "double standard."

Victorians understood male sexuality as explosive and brutish, whereas the feminine ideal was calm, pure (like the angels), and delicate. As one historian has noted, Victorian men "saw themselves as patriarchal and authoritarian because they suppressed a sexual nature that was aggressive, even potentially brutal. ... they saw woman as innocent, dependent, good, and generous because she was—ideally—sexless" (Kennedy 1970, p. 63). This is not an extreme historical interpretation. Victorian women were expected to maintain virginity and ignorance of human sexuality. Men, on the other hand, were generally expected to experiment sexually before marriage. This double standard was partly based on medical opinion that male biology required regular sexual release while female biology did not.

In this world view, women were to be worshiped, cared for, and respected by men, who were expected to assume a protective and supportive role. Growing out of a resurgence of interest in all things medieval (especially chivalry), and possibly developing in reaction to the significant political and social upheavals of the late eighteenth century, these notions placed women on a pedestal, crowned motherhood as the apex of femininity, separated the spheres of men and women, and named the home as woman's sacred domain. With marriage and the family as the great edifice that contained and directed the expression of human sexuality, the contemporary Henry James could admit what most believed, that only in marriage could men's "baser nature," i.e., their sexuality, be adequately contained. The purpose of wedlock, James maintained, "is to educate us out of our animal beginnings" (James 1870, p. 364).

Within this precise division of male and female, flavored with medical support for male sexual license, the double standard relied upon prostitution. Indeed, many Victorians viewed prostitution as a "necessary evil." In essence, it permitted one segment of the female population to meet the needs of men's more primeval nature, and, these "needs" were great. Prostitution flourished in both England and the United States.

Prostitution, a most ancient practice, received a type of new life in the Industrial Age. As men and women flocked to the factories, many far from their families, the new urban environment proved conducive to the growth of sexual trade (see D'Emilio and Freedman 1988, p. 132). Prostitution was not systematically prohibited by law in England and the United States. It just existed. No matter the size of the city or town, Victorian society maintained what they referred to as the "underworld."

Prostitution was typically organized around saloons, pubs, dinner clubs and "houses of assignation" (or brothels). Working-class men could buy a girl a drink in saloons or pubs and use a back room to pay for her other pleasures. Dinner clubs catered to upper-class men where "ladies" trained in music and card games easily sold their affections. Wealthy men might purchase a town house to maintain an exclusive mistress. Whatever form prostitution took, its brothels were plenteous and its range of sexual services satisfying men's tastes in virgins, same sex encounters, or with children, were provided. As one reform-minded investigator reported in 1869, England's seaports alone had more than 1,500 prostitutes under the age of fifteen and about a third of them under age thirteen (see Tannahill 1992, p. 374). This sordid picture eventually did not go unchallenged.

The Solution

At first, pioneering Christian women offered the solution to this problem. From as early as the 1830s in the United States, they sought to "rescue" women from prostitution. The same activity occurred in England, although a bit later, in the 1860s. Soon, these activities revealed other root causes of prostitution, namely, poverty, labor issues, and gender inequality. These new insights brought diverse people to the issue which, in turn, caused the formation of the Social Purity movement. The name "social purity" was derived from their central tactic—to promote chastity, especially among men. Two examples from these diverse groups—feminists and physicians—can provide insight into the all-embracing character of this movement.

Early Feminists

The early feminists had two aspirations when they started their work: equal citizenship and acceptance into the professions (e.g., medicine, the academy). Their fundamental desire was to have a better world in which women could take their rightful place. To that end, early feminists harshly critiqued the Victorian double-standard, unbridled male sexuality, marriage practices in general, and the burdens of motherhood. They were not, however, opposed to marriage and motherhood. In fact, they continued to promote a middle-class reverence for both. Like the majority of their contemporaries, they were also against the emerging movement to promote "preventive checks" (birth control). Early feminists viewed contraception as encouraging male sexual abuse of women. They believed that if women were to accept contraception, they too would fall into the same abusive behavior resulting in a general lowering of morality (see Bolt 1993, p. 134; see also, Bland 1986, p. 129). Feminists wanted a true reform of society and this had to happen at the level of the most basic unit, the male/female relationship. Thus, marriage, sex, and motherhood had to be reformed based upon egalitarian ideals.

Early in their history as "the suffrage struggle intensified," feminists began "to insist that the campaign for women's citizenship and the demand for legislation to curb male immorality were interlinked" (see Mort 1985, p. 219). After all, the double standard revealed man's mistreatment of woman. It abused the female prostitute, disrespected and harmed the wife and, in turn, the family. The double standard created a dangerous myth that insisted "male need" had to be immediately "satisfied" by women. That fostered slavery in marriage, hence the severe feminist critique of accepted marriage behaviors that insisted a "wife's duties" included satisfying her husband's sexual demands with no regard to her feelings or desires. This "grave social crime," as American feminist and social purity leader Elizabeth Blackwell named it, became a common accusation among early feminists (see D'Emilio and Freedman 1988, p. 154).

Feminists argued that the double standard supported a false classification of a different type of woman in society—the fallen woman. What was needed was male self-mastery, not indulgence. To ensure a just relationship between men and women, feminists called for chastity for men outside of marriage and sexual restraint within marriage.

In England, it would be feminists, led by women such as Christabel Pankhurst and Josephine Butler, who made male immorality their target. They issued fierce denunciations of the double standard and called for chastity reform. Pankhurst was a particularly strong advocate for male chastity. She wrote pamphlets and gave lectures arguing "that sexuality had been given in trust for the perpetuation of the race but men chose to squander it in degeneracy and debauchery" (quoted by Mort 1985, p. 218). Watchful that such behavior was not encouraged by the British government, Josephine Butler zealously fought unjust gender-based laws. One set of problematic laws, the British Contagious Diseases Acts (CDA; 1864, 1866, and 1869) were particularly discriminatory against women. The CDAs targeted female prostitutes. They required "compulsory examination" of only women "suspected of working as prostitutes" (Jeffreys 1985, p. 7). Nothing was done to criminalize the men who used the prostitutes. Women who were picked up by police as possible prostitutes did not have recourse to a judge or jury. They were immediately incarcerated and physically examined. Butler fiercely argued that the CDAs violated a woman's civil rights and did nothing to punish the male clients (Jeffreys 1985, p. 7).

Early feminists sought to change how men and women related to each other, especially in marriage and sex. They believed that such a reform would "satisfy both personal and social aspirations" (Leach 1989, p. xii). Concepts such as a woman's "right to herself," meaning a woman's control of her own person, were interfaced with an emphasis on the "equilibrium" or "symmetry" between the sexes. Symmetry between the sexes was a feminist appropriation of a health movement concept, especially promoted by American feminists (c. 1830-1840). Nineteenth century health movements placed an emphasis on the balance, or "symmetry," of the created order. All of nature had to exist in its purity, each part fully existing in interrelationship with the other, without excess, domination or restriction. "Health" was equated with balance or symmetry, while illness and disease, with their absence. This was applied to the human body, the person, and society. It meant that all elements connected with the human were subject to the principle of "symmetrical action," where the "positive and negative forces," as one feminist said, "must come to a perfect state of equilibrium in all social and governmental arrangements as well as in the mental and physical organizations of individuals" (Leach 1989, p. 35).[10] The relevance of these principles to marriage and sex was ground-breaking.

Feminists argued that if equilibrium were left to develop freely, men and women would "begin to develop the character of the other" (Leach 1989, p. 34).[11] Men would integrate feminine nurturing characteristics and virtues like tenderness and purity. Women, for their part, would acquire male traits like "abstract thinking" and "courage" (Leach 1989, see pp. 34 and 97 respectively). Significantly this was thought to lead to evolutionary progress, because more perfect children would be born due to the "perfect equilibrium of forces" (Leach 1989 p. 34).

In any case, the early feminists' broader platform of gender equality and harmony between the sexes formed part of their contribution to nineteenth century aspirations for a better world. Ending male promiscuity was part of that world. When speaking on "Marriage Reform" at the International Council of Women (Washington 1888), American feminist Lucinda B. Chandler summed up this feminist belief commonly held on both sides of the Atlantic:

> It is the riot of carnalism, which the license of marriage claims to sanctify, that perpetuates the lustful, selfish propensities in force and fury .... Women as well as men must eliminate from marriage the features of prostitution, for when prostitution ceases inside of marriage it will disappear outside. (Quoted by Jeffreys 1985, p. 23.)

Physicians

The involvement of more physicians into the Social Purity movement resulted in a shift in focus that highlighted the public health concerns of venereal disease. One American physician in particular almost single-handedly moved his colleagues to act. His name is Prince Albert Morrow, MD (1846-1913).

Morrow, a doctor of dermatology,[12] understood that venereal disease was more than a medical problem because it was so tied to human beliefs and behavior. In 1904, he wrote that it might appear that the prevention of venereal diseases

> ... lies exclusively within the province of the medical profession. But experience has shown that this class of diseases cannot be dealt with as a purely sanitary problem. ... In their essential nature they are not merely diseases of the human body, but diseases of the social organism. (Morrow 1906, in D'Emilio and Freedman 1988, p. 205.)

Morrow typically blamed "masculine unchastity" and the double standard for the problem; but he also identified the obstacles that the medical community created.

In the nineteenth and early twentieth centuries, venereal disease was considered shameful. Patients did not easily seek medical attention. When some patients did seek help they were turned away not infrequently by hospital staff because the disease was seen as vulgar or obscene. Physicians, too, viewed the subject with a combination of reservation and moral disgust. Often, doctors would not record the infection in order to protect the patient's reputation. In fact, regardless of the patient's class or position in society, if the infected person were married, the physician typically did not alert the spouse.[13] Morrow knew this and brought it to public attention in a 1904 paper he delivered to colleagues (Morrow 1906). He pleaded with his colleagues to organize a systematic public effort to end venereal disease. The following year he founded the Society of Sanitary and Moral Prophylaxis in New York City. Almost immediately, other groups were formed across the nation forming the American Social Hygiene movement. These groups had a simple goal: "to wipe out the ignorance and the prejudices that allowed venereal disease to infect the nation" (D'Emilio and Freedman 1988, p. 205).

The American Social Hygiene reformers attempted to reach their goal through aggressive educational campaigns. Their insistence on frank, clear education put them at odds with obscenity laws and those who continued to cling to Victorian etiquette on these matters. Nevertheless, they "spoke before local medical associations, state conferences of charities ... and professional associations" (D'Emilio and Freedman 1988, p. 205). They also effectively collaborated with other groups such as the Women's Christian Temperance Union (WCTU), the Young Men's Christian Association (YMCA), state boards of health, superintendents of public schools, and teachers' organizations.

Accomplishments

The Social Purity movement was an international effort. Before 1900 the Social Purity movement had two primary goals—to end prostitution and the abuse of girls. The necessary sub-goal was the elimination of the double standard. After 1900, sex education, social hygiene and eugenic concerns would become prominent. Throughout its history, energetic educational campaigns were waged. Schedules of speaking engagements by purity leaders were published weekly in local papers, pamphlets were handed out on street corners, booklets and books readily published and sold, and calls for education in human sexuality were issued. The general public could not escape the topic of social purity even in the smallest towns and villages. Due to the work of these reformers, prostitution was largely made illegal in both the United States and England.[14] Venereal disease was classified as a public health concern by both nations, and government policies were implemented.[15] Physicians and the general public were better educated about human sexuality and venereal disease. Most significantly, the topic of human sexuality had moved firmly into the public square. For good or ill, academics would fortify this last point.

THE ACADEMIC STUDY OF HUMAN SEXUALITY

The late 19th and early 20th centuries saw human sexuality as a worthy subject to study and even reform. Sociologists led and, from the start, quickly attacked Christian beliefs about sex and marriage.

The first serious blow to Judeo-Christian morality was struck by Ireland's William Edward Hartpole Lecky (1838-1903). His 1869 text, the History of European Morals, revealed his agenda—he was out to expose the hypocrisy of what he believed was an arbitrary and restrictive moral code. He carefully analyzed moral codes of generations past and, to his thinking, demonstrated that "virtue is first formed by circumstances, and men afterwards make it the model upon which their theories are framed" (Lecky 1955, p. 150, quoted by O'Neill 1967, p. 93). In his scheme, Christianity was identified as the cause of prostitution and "other antisocial practices" because of its severe and unnatural teachings that all sexual activity outside of marriage is criminal (O'Neill 1967, pp. 94-95). Habit and custom, according to Lecky, were the defining forces of a society's morality (O'Neill 1967, p. 94). Although Lecky was not out to destroy the family and he did believe that monogamy was the "best domestic institution and the one most conducive to happiness," he advocated that it should be one structure of many available in society (O'Neill 1967, p. 96). He therefore thought that society should not condemn non-marital sexual activity.

Lecky's work influenced other intellectuals. It had an effect on those who supported liberal divorce laws, Free Love, and trial and companionate marriage. Great Britain's leading radical individualist, philosopher, and liberal political theorist in the late 19th century, Herbert Spencer (1820-1903), was one such person. In his 1876 text, Principles of Sociology, Spencer "came out firmly on the side of free divorce" (O'Neill 1967, p. 97). He wrote that marriage was divided into a "union by law" and a "union by affection." He saw no problem in dissolving the legal bond when the natural bond of affection ceased. In the United States, Lester Frank Ward (1841-1913), a self-trained sociologist and Freethinker, concurred. He saw Christianity as "nothing less than a 'calamity,' particularly as it led to the degradation of women into a species of property" (quoted by O'Neill 1967, p. 98). Although he, too, saw monogamy as best for men and women, and, like Lecky and Spencer, did not want to do away with the family, he saw no problem with sex outside of marriage. He, therefore, had great sympathy for the prostitute who he saw as supplying a need that was in great demand. Ward eventually served as the first president of the American Sociological Association and wielded great influence in his discipline. These three men are representative of the early sociologists. They had intellectual clout, which gave respectability to alternative forms of sexual behavior, easy divorce, and (although unintentionally) challenged the very nature of marriage. The work of the early sociologists enabled the development of more radical philosophies by others, notably the sexologists—a mixed group of physicians, scientists, and intellectuals. The most influential and representative of the sexologists is England's Henry Havelock Ellis (1859-1939). Many historians, in fact, refer to him as the father of the modern sexual revolution.[16]

Trained in medicine, Ellis and his colleagues contributed to the scientific classification of the variety of sexual behaviors. He was the leading proponent of the existence of the female sexual drive. What was radical in Ellis' thinking was his perception that human sexual behavior was neither right nor wrong but existed on a continuum from normal to what he termed, "apparently" abnormal. He could do this because he maintained that "normal" was completely man-made and determined by the combined sensibilities of a people as is evidenced in their culture. As he applied this framework to human sexuality, he popularized a number of radical ideas. For example, Ellis believed that men and women were, among other things, "polysexual." He therefore advocated for more flexible unions which could "accommodate ... committed unions ... flexible enough to allow outside emotional and sexual involvement." He promoted non-marital sexual behavior and "trial marriage" where couples lived together without legal benefits and practiced birth control. Ellis also believed in the family, yet was in favor of divorce law reform. He wanted to do away with restrictive regulations of all sexual acts which he perceived as "entirely private" (O'Neill 1967, p. 123).

Although the sexologists were a minority, they exerted great influence on others. They wrote not only serious academic texts, but popular articles and essays. They mingled with, and some were part of, other social movements of the early twentieth century, notably socialists, neo-Malthusians, and advocates of birth control and eugenics. They identified the changes in perspectives on human sexuality which they hoped to establish, and they did something utterly modern—they strategized to achieve long term goals. By 1928 they formed themselves into the World League for Sexual Reform. The specific planks of their mission combined both reasonable and radical solutions to problems related to human sexuality. Among the reasonable positions were the "protection of unmarried mothers and the illegitimate child," the "prevention of venereal disease and prostitution," and the "improvement of sex education among the general public." Their radical positions included the reform of marriage and divorce laws, the promotion of birth control, and the legalization of abortion (Weeks 1981, p. 185).

The sexologists disbanded as an international league by the 1930s. Individually they continued their activism, planting ideas of change regarding the nature and role of human sexuality in the collective mind of Western society. Their professional academic work also lent credence to an even smaller radical minority, the Free Lovers, who had been experimenting with alternative sexual beliefs from the late eighteenth century.[17]

RETHINKING SEXUAL ACTIVITY AND MARRIAGE

Generally speaking, Free Lovers were opposed to governmental and religious institutional interference in sexual matters. They were for the "women's question" (i.e., "feminism") and pro-voluntary parenthood (although this last point did not necessarily mean contraceptive use). Highly critical of marriage, Free Lovers were not interested in its reform, but in its demise. Their significance is two-fold. In the period from the late 19th century to 1929, they contributed to the positive shift in marital expectations regarding spousal companionship as well as to a more positive view of sexual intercourse within marriage. This shift placed a high value on a loving relationship which included the sexual satisfaction of both husband and wife. Secondly, and despite the early struggles against this, the long term effect of their rhetoric paved the way for widespread non-marital sexual behavior that is a hallmark of the modern sexual revolution.[18]

In their basic beliefs, Free Lovers maintained that sexual intercourse should be the result of the mutual love between a man and a woman, not the legal contract of marriage. They did not believe that society, government or church should restrict sexual love. Consequently, they stood against legal marriage and any law that restricted sexual behavior. They supported sex between the unmarried, so long as love bound the couple. They were not against monogamy per se. They opposed marriage imposed by the state and the church. They attacked the institution of marriage, naming it a type of slavery. Like the Freethinkers and anarchists, they insisted that marriage "inhibited individual growth" and "deprived married persons of some liberties" (O'Neill 1967, p. 91). They also saw marriage as imposing a type of prostitution on the woman who often had to perform her wifely duties regardless of the presence of desire or love. In their view, the male/female sexual relationship had to be freely based on love and desire. Thus a monogamous relationship received their full blessing only if love prevailed.

This view of the sexual relationship was not a mere romanticization by the Free Lovers. It was firmly rooted in a clear political philosophy that combined individualism, anarchism, socialism, and varying degrees of feminist theory. The emphasis was firmly on the individual's right to make personal sexual decisions without interference from culture, state, or church. By the late nineteenth century, Free Lovers would also promote the feminist concept of "self-ownership" as part of the sexual rights of free individuals.

In order to promote their philosophy, proponents of Free Love formed communities, gave lectures, published articles, journals, books, and pamphlets and even wrote plays. They opposed any law that regulated sexual behavior, including laws regulating age of consent, cohabitation, adultery, divorce, rights of individuals within marriage, birth control, abortion, prostitution, obscenity, and homosexuality.[19] Free Lovers advocated for sex education and the freedom to speak about sexual issues in the public square. Needless to say, for most of their history, Free Lovers were opposed by the majority of society, denounced in the press, and often jailed on obscenity charges,[20] at least until such personalities as socialist Edward Carpenter and writers H. G. Wells and Bernard Shaw joined their ranks.

The foundational beliefs of the Free Lovers remained consistent until the turn of the century. Once Havelock Ellis suggested, however, that variety in sexual partners "might serve as fuel for the passions" and that "psychological, or emotional, fidelity was more significant than sexual fidelity," the Free Love radicals in turn of the century bohemian circles would add their own interpretation. They "did not believe that a coupled relationship, whether in marriage or not, demanded sexual exclusivity" (D'Emilio and Freedman 1988, p. 230). The age of multiple sexual partners was born.

Effects

Although the Free Love radicals were a distinct minority in their day, they too planted deep seeds in Western culture that bore fruit by 1900. In the years before World War I people "described and understood themselves to be undergoing significant changes in morals" (McGovern 1968, p. 316). A provocative source that reveals the shift in perspectives on sexuality is the marriage manual. Marriage manuals were a type of educational literature for engaged and married couples whose content touched upon many facets of married life including human sexuality. They were very popular in the 19th and early 20th centuries, produced and read by respectable people (in other words, they were "mainstream"). By the late 19th to early 20th centuries, their content clearly shifts from a "rights and duty" mentality where procreation is the reason for conjugal relations to a more positive view of non-procreative sexual intercourse and sexual pleasure in marriage. Quotes from three marriage manuals illustrate this point.

> 1897: Whatever may be the object of sexual intercourse, whether intended as a love embrace merely, or as a generative act, it is very clear that it should be as pleasurable as possible to both parties. (Quoted by Gordon 1971, p. 58.[21])

> 1912: The Great power which controls us does not intend that misery in sex relations and mating shall be our lot. No other state but that of happy and joyous sex relations can keep the world moving and progressing. (Quoted by Gordon 1971, p. 60.[22])

> 1922: ... the union of true lovers apart from marriage is [not] impure. ... such lovers make a very serious mistake .... [and] society is utterly right in condemning such unions. ... But impure is not the word to apply to them. They are clean and beautiful compared to the bodily intimacies of those who marry without love. (Quoted by Gordon, p. 64.[23])

This shift in perspective does not necessarily prove an increase in non-marital sexual behavior in the majority of the population, but it certainly constitutes a new direction in attitudes about sex. The role of the Free Lovers in this scheme prepared the general public for a major change in sexual standards, change that—when combined with the contributions of the sexologists, social purity and social hygiene leaders, as well as other sexual liberals—contributed to the modern sexual revolution. These ideologies marked a turning point of which some contemporaries were quite aware. "The present age is a critical one," said George Santayana in 1913, the "civilization characteristic of Christendom has not yet disappeared, yet another civilization has begun to take its place" (quoted by May 1959, p. v).

A WORD ABOUT CONTRACEPTION

It should not be surprising that birth control existed and was practiced throughout the period we have been discussing. The desire to manage human fertility is part of the human experience. The motivation can be noble or base. The methods can be moral or immoral. Given the period's shift in emphasis on the good of sexual pleasure *separate from* its procreative good and the willingness to take morality out of the sexual equation, the modern sexual revolution could not help but foster, and eventually rely on, the development of artificial methods of birth control. Contraception thus became the instrument by which sexual pleasure could be set free, or so people thought.

From the late 19th century through the 1930s, periodic abstinence and coitus interruptus would remain among the top four most popular methods of birth control, the others being condoms, and douching with some type of spermicide. What people of the period termed as "appliances"– vaginal pessaries such as sponges, cervical caps, diaphragms, and intrauterine stem pessaries ("IUDs")—existed but did not gain in popularity until later in the 1930s. With regard to the diaphragm and cervical cap, it should be noted that their popularity grew due to the direct and unrelenting advocacy of Margaret Sanger and

England's Marie Stopes. It should also be noted that all of the appliances were extremely uncomfortable and carried significant risk of infection. Understandably, most physicians condemned them in the early years. In addition, birth control appliances were not regulated until the 1930s. Before then, unscrupulous manufacturers advertised them in magazines, newspapers and catalogues throughout the period, mostly under the category of "feminine hygiene."

What changed this haphazard and dangerous situation was the ingenuity of birth control activists. Margaret Sanger and Marie Stopes both had the intelligence to understand that if contraception could be brought under the control of physicians it would be viewed as respectable and even as part of health care. In addition, immediately after World War I, Sanger purposefully changed her rhetoric from a focus on personal benefits of contraceptive use to that of the social benefits. She promoted contraceptive use as the one factor that would eliminate poverty and war. This captured the attention of many people who increasingly viewed large families as related to poverty. The physicians and scientists that Sanger recruited would promote these messages, also focusing on the "collective eugenic, racial, and population control advantages of contraception." (Borell 1987, p. 54) In essence, Sanger used biologists "to judge the practice of contraception as biologically sound; physicians, to provide birth control counseling; and laboratory researchers, to improve available contraceptive methods" (Borell 1987, pp. 54-55). In this way she appealed to a broader more conservative segment of the society. As we know, she achieved her goals.

CONCLUSION

In 1901, H. G. Wells made an uncanny prediction. He said that by the year 2000, moral standards would be "shifting and uncertain," that "monogamy, would dissolve and sexual standards would alter greatly." Traditional moral codes would "remain nominally operative in sentiment and practice, while being practically disregarded" (Wells 1901, pp. 73-74). The various cultural elements just reviewed enabled Wells to make his prediction at such an early date.

The Social Purity and Social Hygiene reformers brought the subject of sex into the public square through education and activism. The academic rethinking of sexual behavior and marriage provided a foundation for popular messaging and legitimized radical experimentation in behavior. These efforts supported each other and influenced the expression of the reformers' ideas in literature, art, music, theater, and entertainment to create the modern sexual revolution. Contraception played a supporting role as it became the instrument to live out the new perspective on sex and marriage. One final concession was needed to ensure the spread of the modern sexual revolution: the blessing of religion. That blessing was given on August 7, 1930, when the prestigious gathering of the Anglican bishops at Lambeth Palace promulgated Resolution #15. It stated that although abstinence was the primary method of family planning for Christians,

> in those cases where there is such a clearly-felt moral obligation to limit or avoid parenthood, and where there is a morally sound reason for avoiding complete abstinence, the Conference agrees that other methods may be used,
>
> [Carried by 193 votes; 67 dissenting; 46 bishops did not vote; *Lambeth Conference* 1930.]

The effect of the pronouncement was nothing less than an ideological shock wave that would penetrate all aspects of modern life. Indeed, a high ranking liberal Anglican Churchman wrote, "For good or evil," Resolution #15 "will modify profoundly the whole future of mankind" (Inge 1930, p. 702). And it did. Almost immediately, opportunists grabbed their seats on the ride into the future, as one advertisement proclaimed: "Have no more moral scruples. At the Lambeth Congress one hundred and ninety-three Bishops voted in favor of suitable methods of birth control" (Pope 1930, p. 731). The nascent modern sexual revolution was now baptized and reborn.

END NOTES

1. The topic of the dating of the modern sexual revolution is complex and cannot be fully treated here. For a brief but useful summary see D'Emilio and Freedman, 1988, p. xiii. An endnote provides a list of relevant secondary sources up to the 1980s. (Ibid., note 3, p. 361).

   Although focused on the sexual revolution in the United States, another useful source that provides a substantive discussion of the topic is Smith's "The Dating of the American Sexual Revolution: Evidence and Interpretation," 1978, pp. 426-438. Smith notes that in the broadest sense, the late nineteenth century laid the intellectual basis for a more positive understanding of marital intercourse. In addition, that period saw an increase in public discussion of a variety of sexual issues (e.g., divorce, venereal disease, prostitution, etc.). In the sphere of personal behavior, according to Smith, there was a rise in pre-marital coitus in the 1920s, at least among white middle-class women in the United States.

2. Smith speaks of the sexual revolution as happening in "waves." He concludes that the first wave of the sexual revolution occurred in the last third of the nineteenth century and only in certain strata of Anglo-Saxon society. He arrives at his conclusion through a method of analysis based on an examination of the timing of first childbirths to marriage records. Where there are discrepancies between the first birth date and that of the normal length of pregnancy, Smith presumes premarital intercourse. He corroborates his method with that of illegitimacy rates, and data from early sexual behavior surveys as well as marriage manuals and other writings of the period (see Smith 1978, p. 435).

   For a thorough discussion of the nineteenth century roots of the modern sexual revolution see Kennedy 1970, pp. 36-71; see also Foucault 1978.

3. The complexities of this topic include the approach the historian brings to the subject. Jeffrey Weeks neatly categorizes two major orientations: those who follow a naturalist approach and those who take a meta-theoretical approach. The naturalist describes, classifies, and categorizes sexual behavior and beliefs. The strength of this approach lies in the objective, disinterested attempt to allow the sources to speak for themselves. Its weakness lies in the fact that it does not attempt to explain the motivations or changes in sexual mores.

   The meta-theoretical approach utilizes a "screen" such as neo-Freudian theory, or feminist philosophy, to interpret behavior and beliefs. Its strength lies in the fact that it has the potential to provide significant insight while its weakness is that fact is often sacrificed for the theoretical construct (see Weeks, 1981, pp. 1-3).

   To Weeks' insights, can be added a third approach not acknowledged by most historians. The majority of historians, including Weeks, share a perspective in favor of modern Western sexual liberties based on masculine sexuality—pleasure focused, relationship free, and non-procreative. This bias supports few social restrictions on human sexuality in public discourse and private behavior. Any belief system or person to the contrary is critiqued unfavorably. It is rare to find an historian who acknowledges this perspective. An unusual exception is feminist historian, Sheila Jeffreys. Jeffreys identifies the bias in the example of histories of the early feminists. She observes that "When historians have mentioned the work of ... feminist campaigners in the area of sexuality they have represented them as prudes and puritans, criticizing them for not embracing the goal of sexual freedom or women's sexual pleasure." Jeffreys argues that to understand the work of the early feminists in the area of sexuality, the bias of historians who have viewed them as "backward and retrogressive" must be shed (Jeffreys 1985, p. 1).

4. Olsen quotes the chronicler Fredegarius who in commenting on the culture of Germanic tribes "declared he did not have the space to name all the concubines of King Dagobert (629-39), who also had three wives, and labeled his son Clovis II (639-57) 'fornicator and exploiter of women'" (Olsen 2001, p. 164).
5. For example, in ancient Crete "homosexuality was ... officially supported as a population control tactic" (see McLaren 1994, p. 13).
6. Feminist historians take this position, and are hypercritical of standard definitions of the modern sexual revolution. Sheila Jeffreys maintains that the history of sexuality must include a critical examination of the "power relationships" between men and women (see Jeffreys 1985, pp. 2-5).
7. Typically, many authors who write on sexual history (including the modern sexual revolution) do not provide a clear definition of human sexuality. As Jeffrey Weeks notes, there is in fact, a certain assumption on the part of the historian "that sex is a definable and universal experience, like the desire for food, with the minority or unorthodox forms filtering off into distributaries" (see Weeks 1981, p. 1). Why define what the reader already knows? This, of course, is inadequate if an understanding is to be gained about the subject in each time period. For an engaging discussion of the issue of sexuality and the historian, see the first chapter of Weeks 1981, pp. 1-18.

   Curiously, and despite his dense analysis, Weeks does not define the meaning of sexual activity in the modern period. He also neglects to identify his deeper assumption, that the modern notions of sexuality and sexual freedom are superior and preferable to earlier expressions.
8. With regard to the removal of marriage from the list of Christian sacraments for most Protestant denominations, all Protestant reformers continued to condemn the practice of contraception and sex outside of marriage. The issue of divorce is more complicated and beyond the scope of this study; however it can be said that most reformers placed restrictions on it, allowing divorce and remarriage (at least for the innocent person) in cases of adultery, desertion and cruelty.
9. This expansion includes an acceptance of same sex attraction and what in the past was labeled 'deviant' sexual behavior. For example, in the late twentieth century many international non-governmental organizations attached to the United Nations have promoted the idea that there are five genders: heterosexual, homosexual, lesbian, bisexual, and transgender. This can be read in the official documentation of U.N. meetings, especially those treating world population rates, development, and women's concerns.
10. Leach quotes Mary Hibbard, *New Northwest* (November 7, 1873).
11. Leach quotes Antoinette Brown Blackwell, *The Sexes Throughout Nature* (New York: G. P. Putnam, 1875).

12. During this period dermatology included venereal disease in its discipline.
13. Morrow summarized these points in a 1904 talk he gave to the Medical Society of the County of New York (see Morrow, 1906, quoted by D'Emilio and Freedman 1988, p. 205).
14. British law went about the process a bit back-handedly. The Criminal Law Amendment Act of 1885 made "procuring and brothel-keeping" illegal, not the exchange of money for sexual services. After this period, organized prostitution became a crime. In the United States, parts of the country continued to have legalized prostitution in certain sections of cities, such as New Orleans (1870-1874) and San Francisco (1911-1913). (See Tannahill 1992, p. 367.)
15. For example, in England, the Royal Commission on Venereal Disease was established in 1913. Its 1916 report compelled the government to accept and implement their main recommendations: "State backed pathology laboratories were established; free supplies of salvarsan [the medicine used at the time to treat VD] were given to doctors; and local authorities were encouraged to set up free special clinics in general hospitals" (Weeks 1981, p. 215). In the United States, after World War I individual states began to enact "mandatory reporting laws" and required "blood tests before marriage." The U.S. Public Health Service also created the Division of Venereal Diseases (see D'Emilio and Freedman 1986, p. 213).
16. In his own day, he and two others—Iwan Bloch and August Forel—were named the founding fathers of sexology at the1929 Sex Reform Congress in London.
17. The Free Love philosophy can be traced to French and British Jacobins of the late 18th century. Among the more prominent British advocates are the poet William Blake (1757-1827) and the early feminist, Mary Wollstonecraft (1759-1797). It was, however, American John Humphrey Noyes (1811-1886), a utopian and socialist, who coined the term "Free Love" in the mid-nineteenth century. Mid-nineteenth century adherents aggressively organized themselves and took on a public campaign bordering on proselytism to promote their philosophy. Free Love thus became a "movement" in this period.
18. Free Lovers did not promote promiscuity intentionally. Early Free Lovers were concerned that selfishness and excess would distort their utopian philosophy, as eventually it did. As early as the turn of the century, some Free Lovers were advocating multiple sexual partners and sexual experimentation, without the presence of love.
19. Although Free Lovers opposed laws regulating homosexuality, they did not promote it. They, like most Victorians, viewed homosexuality as an "unnatural act" and therefore were philosophically against it.

20. Free Lovers were targeted when the U.S. Congress and twenty-four states passed the Comstock Laws in 1873.
21. Gordon quotes, R. T. Trall, MD, *Sexual Physiology and Hygiene* (New York: Fowler and Wells, 1897), p. 295.
22. Gordon quotes William Lee Howard, *Facts for the Married* (New York: E. J. Clode, 1912), p. xii.
23. Gordon quotes A. Herbert Gray, *Men, Women, and God* (New York: Association Press, n.d.; first published in 1922), p. .

SOURCES CONSULTED

Bland, Lucy. 1986. "Marriage Laid Bare: Middle-Class Women and Marital Sex 1880s-1914." In Lewis, Jane. Ed. *Labour and Love, Women's Experience of Home and Family 1850-1940*. Oxford: Basil Blackwell, Ltd.

Bolt, Christine. 1993. *The Women's Movements in the United States and Britain from the 1790s to the 1920s*. New York: Harvester Wheatsheaf.

Borell, Merriley. 1987. "Biologists and the Promotion of Birth Control Research 1918-1938." *Journal of the History of Biology* 20:54.

D'Emilio, John and Estelle B. Freedman. 1988. *Intimate Matters: A History of Sexuality in America*. New York: Harper and Row.

Foucault, Michel. 1978. *The History of Sexuality, Volume I: An Introduction*. Trans. by Robert Hurley. New York: Pantheon Books.

Gordon, Michael. 1971. "From an Unfortunate Necessity to a Cult of Mutual Orgasm: Sex in American Marital Education Literature 1830-1940." In Henslin, James M. Ed. *Studies in the Sociology of Sex*. New York: Meredith Corporation.

Inge, W. R. December 1930. "Birth Control and the Moral Law." *The Atlantic Monthly*, 146:697-703.

James, Henry. March 1870. "Is Marriage Holy?" *Atlantic Monthly*, 364. In Kennedy, 1970, p. 62.

Jeffreys, Sheila. 1985. *The Spinster and Her Enemies. Feminism and Sexuality 1880-1930*. Boston: Pandora Press.

Kennedy, David M. 1970. *Birth Control in America: The Career of Margaret Sanger*. New Haven: Yale University Press.

The Lambeth Conference 1930. Encyclical Letter from the Bishops with Resolutions and Reports. London: Society for Promoting Christian Knowledge, 1930.

Leach, William. 1989. *True Love and Perfect Union, The Feminist Reform of Sex and Society*, 2nd ed. Middletown, CT: Wesleyan University Press.

Lecky, William Edward Hartpole. 1955. *History of European Morals: From Augustus to Charlemagne.* New York. In O'Neill, William L. *Divorce in the Progressive Era.* New Haven: Yale University Press, 1967.

Lewis, Jane. Ed. 1986. *Labour and Love, Women's Experience of Home and Family 1850-1940.* Oxford: Basil Blackwell, Ltd.

McGovern, James R. September 1968. "The American Woman's Pre-World War I Freedom in Manners and Morals." *The Journal of American History* 55:316.

McLaren, Angus. 1994. *A History of Contraception, From Antiquity to the Present Day.* Oxford: Blackwell, 1990; reprint 1994.

May, Henry R. 1959. *The End of American Innocence, A Study of the First Years of Our Own Time 1912-1917.* Chicago: Quadrangle Books.

Morrow, Prince A. 1906. "A Plea for the Organization of a Society of Sanitary and Moral Prophylaxis," in *Transactions of the American Society of Sanitary and Moral Prophylaxis.* Quoted by John D'Emilio and Estelle B. Freedman, *Intimate Matters: A History of Sexuality in America.* New York: Harper and Row, 1988.

Mort, Frank. 1985. "Purity, feminism and the state: sexuality and moral politics, 1880-1914," in Langan, Mary and Bill Schwarz. Eds. *Crises in the British State 1880-1930.* London: Hutchinson and Co., Ltd.

The New American Bible. Nashville: Thomas Nelson Publishers, 1987.

O'Neill, William L. 1967. *Divorce in the Progressive Era.* New Haven: Yale University Press.

Olsen, Glenn W. 2001. Ed. *Christian Marriage.* New York: Crossroads.

Pope, Hugh. December 1930. "The Lambeth Report—Resolution 15." *Blackfriars* 11:725-740.

Schillebeeckx, Edward. 1976. *Marriage: Human Reality and Saving Mystery.* London: Sheed and Ward.

Smith, Daniel Scott. 1978. "The Dating of the American Sexual Revolution: Evidence and Interpretation." In Gordon, Michael. Ed. *The American Family in Social-Historical Perspective.* 2d. Ed. New York: St. Martin's Press, 1978:426-438.

Stone, Lawrence. 1977. *The Family, Sex and Marriage in England 1500-1800.* London: Weidenfeld and Nicolson.

Tannahill, Reay. 1992. *Sex in History.* Revised and updated edition. New York: Scarborough House Publishers.

Taylor, Gordon Rattray. 1953. *Sex in History.* London: Thames and Hudson.

Weeks, Jeffrey. 1981. *Sex, Politics and Society. The Regulation of Sexuality Since 1800*. London: Longman Group UK, Ltd.

Wells, H. G. 1901. "Anticipations: An Experiment in Prophecy—II." *North American Review* 173:73-74.

19

Freaks, Fertility, & Cultural Fiasco

DANIEL MCINERNY, PHD

Associate Professor of Philosophy, Great Texts Program, Baylor University[1]

ABSTRACT

"The movies are onto the search, but they screw it up." Such is the assessment of Binx Bolling, the hero of Walker Percy's 1961 novel, *The Moviegoer*, and such, also, will be the assessment of this essay. In the past four years, including perhaps especially this year 2010, there has been a surge of popular Hollywood films having to do with human fertility: *Bella* (2006), *Juno* (2007), *Waitress* (2007), *Knocked Up* (2007), *Baby Mama* (2008), *Away We Go* (2009), *The Back-Up Plan* (2010), *The Switch* (2010), *Life As We Know It* (2010), *Babies* (2010), *The Kids Are All Right* (2010), *Due Date* (2010). The films on this list take on a range of issues involving human fertility, among them: unwanted teen pregnancy, unwanted adult pregnancy, abortion, adoption, contraception, In vitro fertilization, surrogacy, and parenting. Broadly speaking, however, they can all be understood as attempts to make sense out of human fertility within the chaos of post-modern American culture. In their often crude, exploitative, morally offensive ways, these films pursue the human quest for meaning, for hope over despair, for a life of authenticity as opposed to one driven by hypocrisy and self-deception. In such terms, these movies are very much onto the search. But in this paper, I point out the ways in which they very badly screw it up. My interest is to praise the moral instinct manifest in these films, but

1 At the time of the conference, Daniel Mcinerny was Associate Professor of Philosophy, Great Texts Program, Baylor University. Dr. Mcinerny is now CEO of Trojan Tub Entertainment.

also to indicate how that instinct is deranged by the social structures, attitudes, and choices portrayed in them. In doing so, I will say something about how these films reflect a deep malady in our culture, the horizon against which all of our questions and concerns about human fertility arise.

> Where then was I, and how far from the delights of Your house, in that sixteenth year of my life in this world, when the madness of lust—needing no licence from human shamelessness, receiving no licence from Your laws—took complete control of me, and I surrendered wholly to it?
>
> St. Augustine, *Confessions*

> The Self since the time of Descartes has been stranded, split off from everything else in the Cosmos, a mind which professes to understand bodies and galaxies but is by the very act of understanding marooned in the Cosmos, within which it has no connection. It therefore needs to exercise every option in order to reassure itself that it is not a ghost but is rather a self among other selves. One such option is a sexual encounter.
>
> Walker Percy, *Lost in the Cosmos*

"The movies are onto the search, but they screw it up." Such is the assessment of Binx Bolling, the hero of Walker Percy's 1961 novel, *The Moviegoer*, and such, also, will be the assessment of this paper. In the past four years, including perhaps especially this year 2010, there has been a surge of popular Hollywood films having to do with human fertility: *Bella* (2006), *Juno* (2007), *Waitress* (2007), *Knocked Up* (2007), *Baby Mama* (2008), *Away We Go* (2009), *The Back-Up Plan* (2010), *The Switch* (2010), *Life As We Know It* (2010), *Babies* (2010), *The Kids Are All Right* (2010), *Due Date* (2010)—that's twelve films, a list that I do not claim to be exhaustive, and one which does not include explorations of fertility themes in recent television, such as on MTV's reality show, *16 and Pregnant*, the acclaimed teen-melodrama *Glee*, and *Desperate Housewives*. The films on this list take on a range of issues involving human fertility, among them: unwanted teen pregnancy, unwanted adult pregnancy, abortion, adoption, contraception, In vitro fertilization, surrogacy, and parenting. Broadly speaking, however, they can all be understood as attempts to make sense out of human fertility within the chaos of post-modern American culture. In their often crude, exploitative, morally offensive ways, these films are onto what Binx Bolling calls the search. What is the search? In the terms of Percy's novel, one may think of it as a quest for meaning, a quest for hope over despair, for a life of authenticity as opposed to one driven by hypocrisy and self-deception. In such terms, these movies are very much onto the search. But in what follows I would like to point out the ways in which they, very badly, screw it up. In doing so, I do not mean to engage in customary, conservative bashing of the immorality of Hollywood films. My interest is more to praise the moral instinct manifest in these films, while also indicating how that instinct is deranged by the social structures, attitudes, and choices portrayed in them. In doing so, I will say something about how these films reflect a deep malady in our culture, the horizon against which all of our questions and concerns about human fertility arise.

FLANNERY O'CONNOR ON THE FREAK

Consider one of the most intriguing protagonists from the films on our list, Juno, the eponymous heroine of Diablo Cody's Oscar-winning original screenplay, directed by Jason Reitman. Juno (Ellen Page) is a sixteen year-old student at Dancing Elk High School somewhere in Minnesota, who becomes pregnant after a liaison with her friend Paulie Bleeker (Michael Cera). After first considering an abortion, she decides to carry the child to term in order to give the baby up for adoption. Early in the film, a jock named Steve Rendazo and his posse pass by Juno's locker in the hallway at school. Juno drops some papers. Steve Rendazo makes a cutting remark and exchanges high-fives with his buds. As they pass, we are privileged to overhear Juno's interior monologue:

> JUNO V.O.
>
> The funny thing is that Steve Rendazo secretly wants me. Jocks like him always want freaky girls. Girls with horn-rimmed glasses and vegan footwear and Goth makeup. Girls who play the cello and wear Converse All-Stars and want to be children's librarians when they grow up. Oh yeah, jocks eat that shit up....They just won't admit it, because they're supposed to be into perfect cheerleaders like Leah. Who, incidentally, is into teachers (Cody 2007, p. 11).

Juno is a self-described "freaky girl." The shooting script introduces her as "an artfully bedraggled burnout kid" (Cody 2007, p. 1). Her fashion selections underscore the point. Ellen Page herself suggested to *Juno*'s costume designer, Monique Prudhomme, that her character wear flannel shirts and sweater vests (*Entertainment Weekly*, December 5, 2007). Juno's taste in music, revealed, first of all, in the posters that wallpaper her bedroom, gravitates toward the era of classic punk: The Damned, The Germs, The Stooges, Television, Richard Hell—music probably some thirty years behind the tastes of most of her compatriots.

I want to take my cue from Juno here and explore this idea of the "freak." But, in using this word, I need to be clear that I am not simply trying to deride, or express my moral repugnance at, Juno and other protagonists from the movies on our list—though I do find them in substantial ways morally repugnant. My point, rather, is to claim that a character like Juno has something to teach us precisely because she is a freak, understanding that term in all its moral richness. No one has mined the riches of the character of the freak more than the Catholic novelist and short story writer, Flannery O'Connor. In the essays collected by Sally and Robert Fitzgerald in *Mystery and Manners*, O'Connor discusses the literary character of the freak, or what she alternatively calls the "grotesque," in a way that can both illuminate and serve as a contrast to the sense of the freak operative in our list of films.

The freak is "a figure for our essential displacement." So O'Connor argues in her essay, "Some Aspects of the Grotesque in Southern Fiction" (O'Connor 1997a, p. 45). We may ask: "Displaced from what?" For O'Connor, the freak is displaced from the ordered universe of Christian theology; he is that lonely, alienated figure that Walker Percy describes as being "lost in the cosmos." In their literary essays, both O'Connor and Percy contrast the world in which their characters operate from the medieval world, where everything, including human beings, occupied the place assigned to it by God in the harmony of Creation. O'Connor writes:

> I am often told that the model of balance for the novelist should be Dante, who divided the territory up pretty evenly between hell, purgatory, and paradise. There can be no objection to this, but also there can be no reason to assume that the result of doing it in these times will give us the balanced picture that it gave in Dante's. Dante lived in the thirteenth century, when that balance was achieved in the faith of his age. We live now in an age which doubts both fact and value, which is swept this way and that by momentary convictions. Instead of reflecting a balance from the world around him,

> the novelist now has to achieve one from the felt balance inside himself (O'Connor 1997a, p. 49).

Percy is more historically precise than O'Connor when he argues that the contemporary world is a break not only from the Middle Ages, but from the modernity of the last several hundred years:

> To state the matter as plainly as possible, I would echo a writer like [Romano] Guardini who says simply that the modern world has ended, the world, that is, of the past two or three hundred years, which we think of as having been informed by the optimism of the scientific revolution, rational humanism, and that Western cultural entity which until this century it has been more or less accurate to describe as Christendom (Percy 1991a, p. 208).

O'Connor's freak, therefore, is a denizen of an unbalanced world in which the hierarchal universe of Christian theology that serves as the backdrop to Dante's *Commedia* has been dismantled, first, by modern science and its attenuated version of rationality, and second, by the post-modern distrust of even this attenuated reason. Both fact and value have been called into doubt. But in this cultural condition, Percy spies an opportunity for the novelist: "When one age ends and the traditional cultural symbols no longer work, man is exposed in all his nakedness, which is uncomfortable for man but revealing for those of us who want to take a good look at him; which is to say, at ourselves" (Percy 1991a, p. 218).

Set loose upon this metaphysically barren landscape, "shucked like an oyster and beheld in all his nakedness," as Percy says (Percy 1991a, p. 218), the freak must come to grips with the mystery of freedom. Without the old cultural signposts to direct him, the freak must forge a path of his own. In her preface to the second edition of her novel, *Wise Blood*, O'Connor speaks of the mystery of free will as an arena of conflict between a choice to obey an authority outside oneself, above all, Christ, and a choice to cast off all authority in a brazen exaltation of the self. The protagonist of *Wise Blood*, Hazel Motes, is "a Christian *malgré lui*," (O'Connor 1997b, p. 114). The founder of the Church Without Christ, he wants to rid himself of the authority of Christ forever, but he cannot bring himself to do so:

> That belief in Christ is to some a matter of life and death has been a stumbling block for readers who would prefer to think it a matter of no great consequence. For them, Hazel Motes' integrity lies

> in his trying with such vigor to get rid of the ragged figure who moves from tree to tree in the back of his mind. For the author, his integrity lies in his not being able to. Does one's integrity ever lie in what he is not able to do? I think that usually it does, for free will does not mean one will, but many wills conflicting in one man (O'Connor 1997b, pp. 114-15).

From this description of Hazel Motes we can see that O'Connor's freaks are not typified primarily by their bizarre or even vicious behavior. Certainly, they do bizarre and vicious things. With a twisted sense of asceticism, Hazel Motes wraps himself in barbed wire and puts stones and cut glass in his shoes; the serial killer nicknamed The Misfit in the story, "A Good Man Is Hard to Find," murders an entire family, including three children, one of them a baby; and Helga, the lady Ph.D. with a wooden leg and a taste for Heidegger in the story, "Good Country People," tries to seduce a Bible salesman—who ends up running off with her wooden leg. But, if such behavior were all that made for a freak, O'Connor's writing would not possess the depth that it does. What is distinctive about O'Connor's freaks is that they are still engaged in that conflict of wills that helps make up the mystery of free will. Their integrity lies in what, despite their best efforts, they are not able to do. "I think it safe to say," O'Connor observes, "that while the South is hardly Christ-centered, it is most certainly Christ-haunted" (O'Connor 1997a, p. 44). Time and again in her stories, she presents us with freaks desperate to tear every thought of Christ from their hearts—and failing.

O'Connor's self-described aim as a writer of fiction is "the action of grace in territory held largely by the devil" (O'Connor 1997b, p. 118). The challenge of such a program, she admits, is first of all that of showing a modern audience, holding for the most part that freedom is found in sin, that the territory they frequent is indeed in the devil's hands. Percy articulates the same challenge when he says that one of the most important tasks for the contemporary novelist is to name that "death in life" so characteristic of our relentlessly and paradoxically life-affirming age (Percy 1991b, p. 162). In order to show sin as grotesque, as death in life, to a world that sees it as freedom, affirmation, and fulfillment, O'Connor chose as her strategy the way of distortion and violence. But the point of the freak is not just to image the distortion and destruction of sin. The freak is also meant to serve as a conduit of grace. "I suppose the reasons for the use of so much violence in modern fiction will differ with each writer who uses it, but in my own stories I have found that violence is strangely capable of returning my characters to reality and preparing them to accept their moments of grace" (O'Connor 1997b, p. 112).

In its concentration on the action of grace, O'Connor's writing exemplifies a form of realism she calls "the realism of distances." In her novels and stories, the eccentricity and savage nature of the freak, apparently so distant from the life of grace, turns out to be the very means by which grace is brought near and offered. The freak turns out to be a prophet. O'Connor is really speaking of her own work when she says the following about "our present grotesque characters":

> They seem to carry an invisible burden; their fanaticism is a reproach, not merely an eccentricity. I believe that they come about from the prophetic vision peculiar to any novelist whose concerns I have been describing. In the novelist's case, prophecy is a matter of seeing near things with their extensions of meaning and thus of seeing far things close up. The prophet is a realist of distances, and it is this kind of realism that you find in the best modern instances of the grotesque (O'Connor 1997a, p. 44).

THE FREAK IN RECENT FERTILITY-THEMED FILMS

Let us now return to the freak-protagonists of our list of fertility-themed films, and see how they compare with O'Connor's uses of the grotesque in the pursuit of the realism of distances. Like Hazel Motes, The Misfit, and Helga, in these films we find protagonists, whatever the intentions of the filmmakers, who figure our essential displacement from a Christian understanding of the world. They are set within a metaphysically barren landscape, whether it be the hallways of Dancing Elk High School or the offices and apartments of independent, career-obsessed urbanites. The more conventional surroundings of our cinematic freaks should not blind us to the fact that these folks are misfits just as much as The Misfit. O'Connor remarks that she does not view her characters as any more freakish than ordinary fallen man usually is (O'Connor 1997a, p. 43). This idea that the freak is present to some degree in all of us is reflected, obliquely, in the topsy-turvydom of the high school sexual combat in *Juno*. Steve Rendazo, the jock, is more interested in freaky girls than cheerleaders, while pretty Leah, the cheerleader, is more interested in geeky, middle-aged teachers than jocks.

The film *Bella* aside, which was produced and written by Catholics, and prominently features an intact Catholic family, these films do not present us with Christian social worlds. After Juno tells them about her pregnancy and her plans to give the baby up for adoption, Juno's stepmother, Bren, says to Mac, Juno's father, "Somebody else is going to find a precious blessing from Jesus in this garbage dump of a situation. I friggin' hope" (Cody 2007, p. 30). But this is only after Bren has asked Juno if she's thought of the "alternative" to bringing the baby to term—an alternative that Bren, presumably, would not be against Juno pursuing. Beyond this reference to the baby as "a precious blessing from Jesus," Christian faith and Christian culture play no role in Juno's story. Not that any other religious faith fills the gap. For Juno, as well as the other freak-protagonists in our list of films, the world is pretty well drained of religious significance. However they choose to deal with their problems, it is not by leaning upon God for help.

Still, they do have to deal with their problems. Our company of freaks must find a way to get along, and so, they too, like O'Connor's freaks, must come to terms with the mystery of human freedom. At least at the beginnings of their stories, we often find them exalting in a freedom without substantial authority, commitment or limit. Juno and her friends pursue their sexual misadventures with a certain anxiety about parental interference, but outside of instruction in Health class about the proper use of birth control, they are not troubled by their parents and teachers with actual formation in the true meaning and use of human sexuality. When we first encounter Ben, the twenty-something slacker of Judd Apatow's *Knocked Up*, we find him passing his days living off the compensation received from an injury, smoking pot and hanging out with his friends, and idly attempting to develop a pornographic website. His world is that of Pinocchio's Pleasureland, with the added attractions of sex, drugs, and 21st-century technology. But although it is not quite a fertility-themed film, the most illuminating image of unbridled freedom in recent films is found in *Up in the Air* (2009), written and directed by Jason Reitman and starring George Clooney. Nominated for six Academy Awards, and winner of the Golden Globe for Best Screenplay, *Up in the Air* is the story of Ryan Bingham, a corporate downsizer who spends most days of the year in airports and hotels, crisscrossing the country in order to fire employees on behalf of employers without the guts to do the dirty work. His professed goal is to join the exclusive group of people who have earned ten million frequent flyer miles with American Airlines. What's interesting is that Bingham enjoys his rootless existence. He even gives talks to corporate groups on the virtues of living life without baggage. Here is part of his schtick:

> A SPOTLIGHT reveals RYAN BINGHAM standing at a podium.
>
> RYAN
>
> How much does your life weigh?
>
> Ryan pauses to let us consider this.
>
> RYAN (Cont'd)
>
> Imagine for a second that you're carrying a backpack ... I want you to <u>feel</u> the straps on your shoulders ... You feel them?
>
> (gives us a beat)
>
> Now, I want you to pack it with <u>all</u> the stuff you have in your life. Start with the little things. The stuff in drawers and on shelves. The collectables and knick-knacks. Feel the weight as it adds up. Now, start adding the larger stuff. Your clothes, table top appliances, lamps, linens, your TV. That backpack should be getting pretty heavy at this point—Go bigger. Your couch, your bed, your kitchen table. Stuff it all in ... Your car, get it in there ... Your home, whether you have a studio apartment or a two storey house, I want you to stuff it into that backpack.
>
> Ryan takes a beat to let the weight sink in.
>
> RYAN (Cont'd)
>
> Now try to walk.
>
> We hear people around us chuckling. Ryan smiles. Reveal:
>
> INT. HOTEL CONFERENCE ROOM—AFTERNOON

> The kind that shifts between lower-income corporate retreats and lower-income weddings.
>
> We look around the room. The few dozen people seem to be visualizing as told. Some are taking notes.
>
> RYAN (Cont'd)
>
> Kind of hard, isn't it? This is what we do to ourselves on a daily basis. We weigh ourselves down so that we can't even move. And make no mistake—Moving is living (Reitman 2008, p. 1).

This is the opening scene of the movie, and make no mistake, in the course of the story, the one thing that Ryan Bingham is going to learn is that there is much more to living than moving. But in Ryan Bingham before his transformation we have an idealized version of a certain kind of post-modern freak: the person who desires to live, not just without stuff, but without the communities within which stuff accumulates. It's not just the kitchen appliances that go into the backpack, but the kitchen and the entire house, too. So what happens in the end to the backpack?

> RYAN (Cont'd)
>
> Now I'm going to set your backpack on fire. What do you want to take out of it? Photos? Photos are for people who can't remember. Drink some gingko and let the photos burn. In fact let everything burn and imagine waking up tomorrow with nothing.
>
> (a beat of emphasis)
>
> It's kind of exhilarating, isn't it? That is how I approach every day. (Reitman 2008, p. 2)

Who is this person who revels in having no place in the world? Who, as we see as his story unfolds, only connects with other people through casual sexual encounters?

In his *Politics* Aristotle speaks of the *polis* as the highest and best of human communities. It is the natural habitat for rational beings; the "place" which organizes our participation in family and other social relationships. As Aristotle famously attests, to flourish outside the community of the *polis* is to be either a beast or a god. It is to live in a place either too high or too low for human beings. From Aristotle's point of view, any human attempt to live outside the community of the *polis* would be madness. It would be a futile attempt to strip oneself of human nature itself. Yet this is just what we find in Ryan Bingham, burner of backpacks (backpacks, notice, full of *things*, not people). His is the attempt to live the life of a god, "up in the air," exercising his powers for his pleasure alone—which ends up bringing him right down to the level of the beasts.

The kind of freedom first embraced by Ryan Bingham, Juno, Ben Stone, and the rest of the protagonists on our list of fertility-themed films is freedom understood as autonomy, or what Charles Taylor calls "self-determining freedom" (Taylor 1992, esp. chapters IV and VI). In an increasingly secular world, freedom is forced to determine both what the self is and what the self is to become. Yet, self-determining freedom has a dangerous after-effect. On the one hand, self-determining freedom promises mastery of nature through instrumental reason embodied, above all, in technology. But on the other hand, the very pursuit of mastery, as Romano Guardini observes in the text Percy alludes to, leads to

> ... man's loss of his objective sense of belonging to existence. With the breakdown of the old world picture, man came to feel now only that he had been placed in a life of strange contradictions but also that his very existence was threatened. Modern man awoke to that anxiety which menaces him to this day, an anxiety never found in the medieval world (Guardini 1998, p. 34).

When we first encounter certain of the freaks in our list of films, they are in thrall to the allures of self-determining freedom. But at least by the first turning point in these films, when the protagonists are forced to come to terms with some consequence of their actions—such as a pregnancy resulting from a one-night stand—we find them suffering from the anxiety of which Guardini speaks. For now, "placed in a life of strange contradictions," they have to show the mettle of their freedom. They have to prove themselves to have the power of a god—and they are terrified by the prospect.

Terrified, yes. But are they "haunted" in the way that O'Connor's freaks are? Do they manifest that strange form of integrity that consists in what they are *not* able to do? The short answer is assuredly no. None of our cinematic freaks desperately fail to rid themselves of "the ragged figure who moves from tree to tree in the back of [Hazel

Motes's] mind." These films do not portray Christ-centered cultures, nor do they portray Christ-haunted ones. And yet, it would be wrong to deny that these characters are haunted in some sense. There is something that produces the anxiety they feel, that keeps them from the headlong pursuit of self-determining freedom. What makes our list of fertility-themed films so interesting is that they are all negative comments upon the ideal of self-determining freedom. In their different ways, our protagonists recognize that self-determining freedom cannot lead to fulfillment. Perhaps, then, we should say that what our freaks are haunted by is the specter of self-determining freedom—a ghost-life unbound by authority and commitment, yet lonely, rootless, and full of anxiety. But it is also true that they are haunted, in a more positive sense, by the hope for something more—for a freedom that does not lay upon their shoulders the burden of a divinity. That hope, however, is not in any explicit way the hope of Christ, or any religious promise. Our freaks may be prophets of a kind, but what they prophesy in their eccentricity and vileness does not appear to be the life of grace. So, what is it that they "see"? What "far things" do they seek to bring close up?

THE FREAK, FERTILITY AND AUTHENTICITY

However we might philosophically characterize the ghost that haunts our freak protagonists, on a literal level the ghost takes the form of a baby. All the films on our list have as their central conflict the difficulties encountered by someone who was not expecting a baby, or who is struggling to have one, adopt one, or raise one. If I have to hazard a guess as to why there have been so many fertility-themed films and television shows in recent years, a trend that shows as yet no signs of letting up, I would say it is because, four decades into it, we have finally come to recognize the serious drawbacks of the sexual revolution—as well as the obsessed careerism that has followed in its wake. If these films are telling us anything, it is that human fertility, even in an age of contraception and abortion, gives the lie to the ideal of self-determining freedom.

The freak laboring under the illusion of self-determining freedom suffers what Percy calls an "ontological impoverishment" (Percy 1991a, p. 214). Outside of the self, there isn't much for such a person that counts as *real*, as substantial to a fulfilling life. This condition creates both alienation and anxiety, from which there are few sources of relief.

One kind of relief, as Percy notes, is a sexual encounter, because amid such ontological impoverishment, "genital sexuality [comes] to be seen as the only, the "real," the basic form of human intercourse" (Percy 1991a, p. 215). "I think kids get bored and have intercourse," Juno's step-mom Bren tries to explain to her husband, Mac (Cody 2007, p. 30). Another, and more twisted, source of relief from ontological impoverishment—one that O'Connor's work explores—is violence. Like sex, violence produces at least a momentary *ek-stasis*, a transcendence of the prison of the self, one that apes both sexual and spiritual ecstasy. Yet I would like to propose that our list of films suggests another form of relief from the ontological impoverishment of the freak: *the miracle of the baby*. Time and again in these films, it is the prospect of a baby that jolts the protagonist out of his complacency. The brute fact of another, tiny person alive and growing in a womb is powerful enough to cut through all the ideology and social pressure generated by the proponents of sexual self-determination. In this, as in other ways, *Juno* is especially illuminating.

In the parking lot of the Women's Choice clinic, Juno runs into her classmate, Su-Chin, protesting what is going on inside the clinic. Su-Chin attempts to dissuade Juno from getting an abortion by calling out to her—

> SU-CHIN
>
> Your baby probably has a beating heart, you know. It can feel pain.
>
> And it has fingernails (Cody 2007, p. 19).

Fingernails. The theme returns a few moments later as Juno waits her turn inside the clinic:

> She takes a seat in the WAITING ROOM and rifles through a pile of old magazines. The magazine selection is lots of "mommy mags" and health related periodicals. She selects an issue of *Family Digest* and gingerly flips through for a few moments.
>
> Then she looks over and notices the FINGERNAILS of a nearby teen, who looks as nervous as she does. The girl bites her thumbnail and spits it onto the floor.

Juno looks away, but immediately notices another waiting woman, who absently scratches her arm with long fake nails.

Suddenly, she sees fingernails EVERYWHERE. The receptionist clicks her nails on the front desk. Another woman blows on her fresh manicure. Everyone seems to be fidgeting with their fingers somehow. Juno suddenly looks terror-stricken...

CUT TO:

PUNK RECEPTIONIST

Excuse me, Miss MacGoof?

There's no answer. We see that Juno's chair is EMPTY (Cody 2007, p. 20).

A little later, Juno describes the moment to Leah this way—

JUNO

I couldn't do it, Leah! It smelled like a dentist in there. They had

these really horrible magazines, with, like, spritz cookie recipes and bad fiction and water stains, like someone read them in the tub. And the receptionist tried to give me these weird condoms that looked like grape suckers, and she told me about her boyfriend's pie balls, and Su-Chin Kuah was there, and she told me the baby had fingernails. Fingernails! (Cody 2007, p. 21)

So what's happening here? Why does Juno decide *not* to abort her child? Clearly, because she recognizes that the fingernails of the human beings surrounding her in the squalid clinic are also attributes of the child in her womb, and so she sees that what she bears is no "sea monkey," as she jokes about it, but a human person that cannot casually be dispensed with.

What I am calling the miracle of the baby is manifested in different ways in our list of films. In *Waitress,* it occurs, as in *Bella, Juno* and *Knocked Up,* through an unwanted pregnancy. When Jenna (Keri Russell) finds out that she is pregnant by her abusive husband, she is set on a course of events in which she eventually decides to leave her husband and embark on a new life with her new-born baby daughter.

In this case, the unwanted pregnancy works a miracle of sorts by forcing Jenna finally to confront the difficulties in her life. The miracle of the baby occurs in *Knocked Up* when Ben discovers that Alison, the girl he slept with after getting drunk with her at a bar, is pregnant and he decides to support her in any way he can. Analogous to the fingernails scene in *Juno* is the scene in *Knocked Up* when Ben's Dad, on hearing of Alison's pregnancy, encourages his son to think of the event as the best thing that will ever happen to him, as Ben himself is the best thing that ever happened in his Dad's life.

In comedies such as *Baby Mama, The Back-Up Plan,* and *The Switch,* the miracle of the baby occurs first as the ardent desire for a baby by a career woman who has not yet found, or has been too busy to find, Mr. Right. But the miracle occurs on a deeper level at the end of these movies when the baby—which in all three of these comedies is conceived via IVF—is born, where the baby then serves to help reconcile the comedic-romantic conflict. In the upcoming *Life As We Know It,* similar comedy is generated by a baby who arrives via adoption, rather than by IVF.

Screenwriters speak of films having a narrative arc—a transformation, principally on the part of the film's protagonist, from one state of character to at least the beginnings of another. In the fertility-themed films on our list, the narrative arc consists, generally, in a movement from self-determining freedom to some form of commitment, a movement initiated by the prospect of a baby. Hence the films on our list, in one sense, are about growing up, and for this reason, if for nothing else, we can appreciate what they are up to. Nonetheless, it is important to ask of these films what they mean be "growing up." There is no doubt that the films are trying to persuade us that growing up means to stop living a self-indulgent life and to start living for others. After all, as I just remarked, all of these films end with a commitment of some kind—oftentimes both a commitment to a new baby and to a romantic interest. (There are, significantly, no abortions in any of the films on our list.) But we would miss the moral import of these films, I believe, if we didn't also realize that the commitments undertaken by our freak-protagonists are circumscribed within a deeper desire they hold: *the desire for authenticity.* Like Holden Caulfield in *A Catcher in the Rye,* our cinematic freaks want to escape from a world of "phoniness," hypocrisy, and self-deception. Sensing their ontological impoverishment, they want a life that is *real,* that is *authentic*—the center of which will be the realization of *who they are really meant to be.*

In his little book, *The Ethics of Authenticity,* Charles Taylor defines authenticity as the idea that

> There is a certain way of being human that is *my* way. I am called upon to live my life in this way, and not in imitation of anyone else's. But this gives a new importance to being true to myself. If I am not, I miss the point of my life, I miss what being human is for *me* (Taylor 1991, pp. 28-29).

But this should strike us as odd—for how is the aspiration to live *my* way any different from self-determining freedom? If there is no difference, then there can be no transformation among our freak-protagonists from self-determining freedom to authenticity.

Here Taylor draws a distinction. In contrast to self-determining freedom, authenticity recognizes that I cannot live any kind of meaningful life without acknowledging my dependence upon "horizons of significance"—people, institutions, nature itself—that are not the sheer creations of our choices.

A person can stake all on his exercise of self-determining freedom. Like Ryan Bingham in *Up in the Air,* he can say, "Value and meaning for me are found in earning ten million frequent flyer miles with American Airlines." But Taylor's point is that such a choice cannot make for an authentic life, because authenticity demands some *significant* standard of value against which some lives are judged to be authentic and others are not. It makes no sense to exalt choice, Taylor says, if there is no standard against which choice is meaningful. Meaning for human beings is always a function, at least in part, of "horizons of significance" existing prior to our choices.

If it is wondered why Bingham's desire to earn ten million frequent flyer miles cannot serve as a standard of value, then Taylor would answer that it *can*—after all, *anything* can be declared to be of value by *someone*—but that doesn't mean that it will be a standard of value that others will appreciate. Bingham's two sisters think that he is living an absurd life; the young woman he is mentoring at work thinks he is living an absurd life. The only person who really appreciates his freakish form of life—apart from the corporate groups who come to listen to him speak—is Alex, his frequent-flyer dopplegänger and the woman with whom he engages in an affair. Yet it is this very affair that undermines Bingham's attempt to live out his up-in-the-air existence, as he falls for Alex and seeks to turn their casual sex into a down-on-the-ground relationship. Hence Bingham demonstrates through his actions, at least, that for a form of life to be of real significance, it has to be measured against a horizon of significance that is not merely idiosyncratic. An authentic life is intrinsically communal.

All of the films on our list affirm this truth. They all end with our freak-protagonists making or renewing a commitment to others. Although she would not put it this way herself, what Juno wants more than anything else is to be a fully realized *self*. On hearing of her pregnancy, Mac says, "I thought you were the kind of girl who knew when to say when." Juno's response is, "I have no idea what kind of girl I am" (Cody 2007, p. 29). But Juno does know that what she needs in order to realize herself are certain particular *others*, others who are manifestly not creations of her powers of self-determination. Juno knows she needs parents—and not just her own parents, but parents for her child (Juno ends up successfully placing her baby with a single mother). She also knows she needs a romantic love in her life that can go the distance. This is the upshot of the conversation she has with Mac near the climax of the movie:

> JUNO
>
> Dad, it's not about that. I just need to know that it's possible for two
>
> people to stay happy together forever. Or at least for a few years.
>
> MAC
>
> It's not easy, that's for sure. Now, I may not have the best track record in the world, but I have been with your stepmother for ten years now, and I'm proud to say that we're very happy.
>
> Juno nods in agreement.
>
> MAC (CONT'D)
>
> In my opinion, the best thing you can do is to find a person who loves you for exactly what you are. Good mood, bad mood, ugly, pretty, handsome, what have you, the right person will still think

that the sun shines out your ass. That's the kind of person that's worth sticking with.

A wave of REALIZATION crosses Juno's face.

JUNO

I sort of already have. (Cody 2007, p. 90)

Taylor cautions that it "would take a great deal of effort, and probably many wrenching break-ups, to *prevent* our identity being formed by the people we love" (Taylor 1992, p. 34). Consider what we mean by "identity." It is "who" we are, "where we're coming from." As such it is the background against which our tastes and desires and opinions and aspirations make sense. "If some of the things I value most are accessible to me only in relation to the person I love, then she becomes internal to my identity" (Taylor 1992, p. 34).

THE IMPOVERISHMENT OF POST-MODERN AUTHENTICITY

But authenticity, as Taylor defends it, is tricky. It calls us out of ourselves in the attempt to free us from the Chinese handcuffs of self-determining freedom so that we can, along with other important commitments, enter into relationship with others. Yet beyond the call to *some* form of relationship, it is hard to know what precise demands Taylor's notion of authenticity places on us. Take the following example from his argument. At one point, in speaking about those who want to justify what he calls "non-standard sexual orientations," Taylor decries any attempt to justify such orientations by sheer choice—for again, choice alone does not confer worth. So where, we might ask, does the justification, if any, come from? "Asserting the value of a homosexual orientation has to be done differently," Taylor argues, more empirically, one might say, taking into account the actual nature of homo- and heterosexual experience and life. It can't just be assumed a priori, on the grounds that anything we choose is all right" (Taylor 1992, p. 38). Certainly, it is true that the justification, or lack of it, of "non-standard sexual orientations" must come from an exploration, rooted in empirical study, of the nature of human sexuality and fertility. But how, then, would the investigation go? On what grounds would we decide between the traditional Catholic family portrayed in *Bella* and the lesbian couple in *The Kids Are All Right* who produce two children with the help of an anonymous sperm donor? Are both approaches to sexuality, fertility, and the family equally authentic? If the answer is yes, then authenticity is a trivial concept. Neither of the two families in the films just mentioned would be—or should be, given their beliefs—prone to accept it. Taylor seems to count on empirical study to resolve the issue, but does not speculate as to the result. From the passage quoted above, it is plausible to infer that he thinks that "homosexual orientation" can in fact be justified "more empirically," taking into account actual experience and life. Be that as it may, what he explicitly does say only defers the collision between radically different, indeed incommensurable, interpretations of what the facts and experience relating to human sexuality, fertility, and the family really amount to.

Taylor's argument aside, the authenticity achieved by the freak-protagonists in our list of films is almost always a deeply impoverished achievement. Juno learns from her father that in order to live authentically, she must find someone who will love her exactly for who she is. Good mood, bad mood, ugly, pretty, handsome, the point is to find someone who will accept her no matter what. By the end of the film, Juno thinks that she has found such a person in Paulie Bleeker, the father of her child. In the closing moments of the film, which occur several months after Juno has had her baby and given it up for adoption, we hear her say about Paulie:

> JUNO V.O.
>
> As boyfriends go, Paulie Bleeker is totally boss. He is the cheese to my macaroni. I know people are supposed to fall in love before they reproduce, but normalcy's not really our style.

Normalcy is not really their style. Their "style" (not their *virtue*) is to be freaks who love one another despite, or rather *because of*, their freakiness (realizing, perhaps, that everyone is in a sense a freak). In our films, the romantic love that typically serves as the horizon of significance for an authentic life is based simply upon attraction, acceptance, and commitment (of ambiguous duration) to the freakiness in the other whom one has accepted. And in this, *Juno*—as well as most of the other films on our list—distorts an important truth. Yes, authenticity is a real value for human beings. After all, the ancestor of postmodern versions of authenticity is the Christian notion of divine filiation. So, even in Christian terms—*especially* in Christian terms—we need to live in such a way that we realize the very best version of our self, just as we need to be loved by others for exactly who we are. And yet, more importantly than this is the fact that we also need to be loved *for what we can and should be*. What we *can and should be* is determined by the demands of our shared human nature, on the natural level, and by God, on the supernatural level. Only a love that makes these kinds of demands upon us—which is to say, a truly *Christian* love—allows us to achieve the authenticity for which we yearn. Whatever the importance that Taylor gives in his argument to demands existing prior to our choices, his sense of these demands in nowise approaches the substance of Catholic moral theology.

Sadly, however, the Christian judgment of what we can and should be, is exactly what has been jettisoned from most of the social worlds of our films. One of the more curious consequences of the popularity of *Juno* was the way in which its story of a teenage girl deciding to endure an unwanted pregnancy was embraced by *both* pro-lifers and pro-choicers. Peter T. Chattaway's review in *Christianity Today*, for example, concluded that, while neither Juno nor her child end up in a traditional family, this "just underscores the film's implicit pro-life sensibility. Life is life, and deserves to be nurtured, even—if not especially—when everything around it is broken" (December 5, 2007). Speaking *Sed contra* was lead actress Ellen Page, who when asked point blank by the *Washington Post* whether *Juno* is pro-life, answered:

> Not in the slightest, and if you knew me and if you knew the writer and the director, no one would ever say that. It happens to be a film about a girl who has a baby and gives it to a yuppie couple. That's what the movie's about. Like, I'm really sorry to everyone that she doesn't have an abortion, but that's not what the film is about. She goes to an abortion clinic and she completely examines all the opportunities and all the choices allowed her and that's obviously the most crucial thing (February 17, 2008).

As for the screenwriter, Diablo Cody:

> You can look at it as a film that celebrates life and celebrates childbirth, or you can look at it as a film about a liberated young girl who

> makes a choice to continue being liberated. Or you can look at it as some kind of twisted love story, you know, a meditation on maturity (Fox Searchlight Pictures *Juno* Press Kit).

All of these apparently conflicting attitudes to *Juno* could be plausible readings of the film if what the film is *really* all about is *neither*, on the one hand, a celebration of life, as "pro-life" is understood in the context of America's culture wars, *nor*, on the other hand, a celebration of "choice" or "autonomy," defined as self-determining freedom. These conflicting attitudes can all be reconciled if what *Juno* is really all about is the post-modern understanding of authenticity, involving relationships with others who accept you as unconditionally as you except them—*without further demand*. As long as these criteria are accepted in the relationship, choice as to the precise nature of the relationship re-asserts itself as supreme.

By way of counterpoint, consider how many of the movies on our list end, like a classical romantic comedy, in a marriage? Not many, not even *Bella*. Most of them end with a "relationship," in the malleable, contemporary sense of that term. Juno and Paulie are last seen as boyfriend-girlfriend strumming their guitars on Paulie's front porch. Ben and Alison (*Knocked Up*) are last seen driving with their new baby to the apartment where they will live together. Jenna (*Waitress*) leaves her husband and starts a new life as a single mother. Zoe's story in *The Back-Up Plan* ends with a new baby and a new boyfriend. The twin heroines of *Baby Mama* go off with their new babies and, in one case, with her fiancé. But none of these commitments involve a deeply enriched sense of the meaning of human fertility. None of them necessarily imply a lifetime commitment. Contraception, perhaps even abortion, could well go on in all of these new relationships. In the end, our list of movies must be judged as dumbed-down versions of classical romantic comedy sanitized of the demands of virtue. They are Jane Austen without tears.

CULTURAL FIASCO

And so the culture in regard to human fertility careens ever more recklessly toward fiasco. Francis Slade has defined fiasco as the attempt to live in a world "without ends," a barren world in which nature and super-nature have been abandoned and the power of human choice is the only value. Slade cites the violent, anarchic films of Quentin

Tarantino as cinematic portrayals of this condition (Slade 2000, p. 67).

Yet it is impossible to realize a world of *utter* fiasco. We can toss nature out with a pitchfork, as Horace said, but it will always come running back. The fertility-themed films on our list have retained—could not *but* retain—a vestige of the true understanding of human fertility. At least, they manifest the truths that relationships are important, and that a baby is, in some sense, a miracle. But these are still meager crumbs from a rich feast. They are truths, but so partial and obscure that they do not distinguish between the lesbian couple with the artificially-generated children from the family who truly lives the Catholic understanding of marriage and family life.

So with post-modern authenticity becoming ever more the sole guide in questions regarding human sexuality and fertility, our culture is coming very close to fiasco. About the loss of traditional social structures related to human sexuality Roger Scruton has written:

> It is impossible for modern adolescents to regard erotic feelings as the preliminary to marriage, which they see as a condition of partial servitude, to be avoided as an unacceptable cost. Sexual release is readily available, and courtship a time-wasting impediment to pleasure. Far from being a commitment, in which the voice of future generations makes itself heard, sex is now an intrinsically adolescent experience. The transition from the virgin to the married state has disappeared, and with it the 'lyrical' experience of sex, as a yearning for another and higher form of membership, to which the hard-won consent of the other is a necessary precondition (Scruton 2000, p. 113).

This is a fair description of the culture of our fertility-based films. In all of them, little social guidance is offered to the young to help them transform their sexual desire into temperance. Families, if they exist, are deeply dysfunctional, in which parents are deemed good only insofar as they are permissive and accepting. Marriage is just one option among many (and admits of more than one definition). Sexual gratification is "readily available," and courtship, as we see in *Juno* and *The Back-Up Plan*, is something that can just as well take place after the baby is born as before.

Such cultural fiasco creates the freak, the disfigured human person determined to live either as a beast or a god, even as it makes the resources necessary for transforming the freak into an integral human being harder and harder to find.

Recall what O'Connor says of her freaks: "They seem to carry an invisible burden; their fanaticism is a reproach, not merely an eccentricity" (O'Connor 1997a, p. 44). According to my argument, the burden carried by the freaks in the recent spate of fertility-themed films is the burden, not of grace, not of a freedom that cannot wrest itself from God, but only that of realizing, in our impoverished post-modern culture, a more authentic mode of life. Their fanaticism, far from being a reproach, is an encouragement, a soothing word to the eccentric ego declaring that the kids are all right exactly as they are. Our freaks, therefore, are not the prophets we need. They make no real demands on us and do not tell us about the "far things" that we cannot see. They are no doubt onto the search, but they sadly, inevitably, screw it up.

SOURCES CONSULTED

Apatow, Judd. 2007. *Knocked Up: The Shooting Script*. New York: Newmarket Press.

Away We Go. 2009. Focus Features.

Babies. 2010. Focus Features.

Baby Mama. 2008. Universal Studios Entertainment.

Bella. 2006. Metanoia Films.

Christianity Today, December 5, 2007.

Cody, Diablo. 2007. *Juno: The Shooting Script*. New York: Newmarket Press.

Due Date. 2010. Warner Bros. Pictures.

Entertainment Weekly, December 5, 2007.

"*Juno* Press Kit." 2007. Fox Searchlight Pictures.

Guardini, Romano. 1998. *The End of the Modern World*. Wilmington, DE: ISI Books.

Life as We Know It. 2010. Warner Bros. Pictures.

O'Connor, Flannery. 1997a. *Mystery and Manners: Occasional Prose*. "Some Aspects of the Grotesque in Southern Fiction." New York: Farrar, Strauss and Giroux.

———. 1997b. *Mystery and Manners: Occasional Prose*. "On Her Own Work."

Percy, Walker. 1991a. "Diagnosing the Modern Malaise." *Signposts in a Strange Land*. New York: Farrar, Straus and Giroux.

———. 1991b. "Novel-Writing in an Apocalyptic Time." *Signposts in a Strange Land*. New York: Farrar, Straus and Giroux.

Reitman, Jason. From the novel by Walter Kirn. 2008. *Up in the Air* (unspecified draft script). SimplyScripts. www.simplyscripts.com.

Scruton, Roger. 2000. *The Intelligent Person's Guide to Modern Culture*. South Bend, IN: St. Augustine's Press.

Slade, Francis. 2000. "On the Ontological Priority of Ends and Its Relevance to the

Narrative Arts," in Alice Ramos, ed., *Beauty, Art, and the Polis*. Washington, DC: The American Maritain Association, distributed by The Catholic University of America Press.

Taylor, Charles. 1992. *The Ethics of Authenticity*. Cambridge, MA: Harvard University Press.

The Back-Up Plan. 2010. CBS Films and Escape Artists.

The Kids Are All Right. 2010. Focus Features.

The Switch. 2010. Miramax Films and Mandate Pictures.

Waitress. 2007. Fox Searchlight Pictures.

Washington Post, February 17, 2008.

APPENDIX

Science, Faith, & Human Fertility

Science Posters

ABSTRACTS

1. Kavle, Justine A. et al.
   Multi-country data on Lactational Amenorrhea Method (LAM) knowledge and practice, counseling received during routine health contacts, and challenges to implementation.
2. Lavoie, Katherine S. et al.
   Meeting clients' needs for family planning without hormones: opportunities for introducing SDM/CycleBeads.
3. Manhart, Michael D.
   First year experience with NFP instruction as a marriage requirement in the Diocese of Covington, KY.
4. Manhart, Michael D. and Manhart, Karen B.
   A profile of NFP students using a home study course.
5. Martin, Mary W.
   An algorithm for identifying and treating three groups of PCOS patients.
6. Nassaralla, Claudia L. et al.
   Characteristics of the menstrual cycle after discontinuation of oral contraceptives.
7. Owen, Christopher H.
   Natural Family Planning Archive: a valuable new resource for researchers.
8. Porucznik, Christina et al.
   Identifying the Peak Day of fertility: peri-conceptional exposure assessment.

9. Rodriguez, Dana.
Trends in family planning and NFP use among U.S. Hispanic women: 1995-2002.
10. Sinai, Irit.
The TwoDay method: a quick start approach.
11. Stanford, Joseph B. et al.
Estimating the probability of a live birth with natural procreative technology.
12. Wang, Jian, Usala, Stephen, and O'Brien-Usala, Faye et al.
The fertile and infertile phases of the menstrual cycle are signaled by cervical-vaginal fluid die swell functions.
13. Yong, Paul J., and Fehring, Richard J.
Calendar rules for the Marquette Model II.

1

Multi-country data on Lactational Amenorrhea Method (LAM) knowledge and practice, counseling received during routine health contacts, and challenges to implementation

Justine A. Kavle, PhD, MPH, CPH, Rebecka Lundgren, MPH, and Victoria Jennings, PhD, Institute for Reproductive Health, Georgetown University

Poor birth spacing contributes to a significant proportion of maternal, neonatal and child mortality and morbidity. Lactational Amenorrhea Method (LAM) supports optimal breastfeeding (BF) practices in the initial 6 months postpartum and contributes to healthy timing and spacing of pregnancies. Yet, providers are often poorly equipped to offer LAM. Evidence is needed on LAM messages during routine health contacts and the extent to which women are aware of and use LAM.

We examined scale-up of LAM in Mali, India and Rwanda in January-August 2009. We conducted household surveys, health facility assessments and health facility and community-based provider interviews to provide a baseline measure of LAM counseling, LAM knowledge/ attitudes/ practice, and infant feeding practices in project areas. Although most Malian and less than half of Indian women receive exclusive BF messages, few received information on LAM. Only 30% of Malian women and virtually no Indian women ever heard of

LAM. Accordingly, very few women report use of LAM in Mali and India. Early introduction of foods, late initiation of BF and low exclusive BF rates present challenges for implementing LAM in India. In Mali, breastfeeding practices were more favorable.

Emphasis on LAM in the context of child survival and maternal health messages is needed during routine health contacts. These data point to the need to promote exclusive BF and to teach amenorrheic BF women to use Natural Family Planning upon approaching 6 months post partum to maximize resources for both maternal and child health.

2

Meeting clients' needs for family planning without hormones: opportunities for introducing SDM/CycleBeads

Katherine S. Lavoie, MPH, Myriam Hernandez-Jennings, MA, Renee Marshall, MA, and Rebecka Lundgren, MPH, Institute for Reproductive Health, Georgetown University, Washington, DC

Despite their efficacy and safety, availability and use of fertility-awareness based family planning methods (FAM) are low in U.S. Title X clinics. The Standard Days Method® (SDM) is a simple yet effective FAM that can be taught in a short time. Introducing SDM into clinic programming represents a feasible way to mainstream FAM and expand client choice by providing an alternative to hormonal methods.

SDM is appropriate for women who get their periods every 26 to 32 days and is used with a color-coded visual tool called CycleBeads®. A study is being conducted to develop and test a process to introduce SDM in four clinics in California and Massachusetts. The process pioneers the World Health Organization's Strategic Approach for family planning method introduction in a U.S.-based project and calls for the integration strategy to be developed through a participatory process focusing on client needs and quality services.

This paper presents the results of the needs assessment phase that assesses the demand for SDM and identifies opportunities and obstacles for SDM introduction. Methods included community focus groups to assess potential demand for SDM; provider interviews to assess knowledge, attitudes and practices with regard to FAM and

SDM; and a site assessment to identify operational and logistical considerations to adding SDM to services.

Results suggest that SDM appeals to potential clients who desire a non-hormonal family planning method, and providers are amenable to offering it. The results from the needs assessment will be used to tailor the integration strategy to each clinic's setting.

3

First year experience with NFP instruction as a marriage requirement in the Diocese of Covington, KY

Michael D. Manhart, PhD, Couple to Couple League

Beginning in January 2009, the Diocese of Covington required a complete course of NFP instruction as part of its Catholic marriage preparation program. In the first year of this requirement, Couple to Couple League teachers instructed 262 student couples in a total of 21 class series; a five fold increase compared to the previous 3 year average. Based on published diocesan records, this represents approximately 54% of the annual weddings in the diocese. A cohort (n=219) of this student population had demographic information available for review.

Not unexpected, the vast majority of student couples were engaged (n=209, 94%) with some married (n=13, 6%). When asked reasons for attending, only 25% indicated a reason other than "required for marriage." Consistent with historical trends in the diocese, 65% of engaged couples are both Catholic. Of the engaged couples, 35% are cohabitating (based on identical address for man and woman), 54.2% are currently using hormonal birth control (HBC), 22.6% formerly used HBC (with most discontinuations within the last 12 months), and 23.6 % claimed to have never used a form of HBC. Those couples attending class solely due to the marriage requirement were significantly more likely to be current uses of HBC than those attending for reasons other than required for marriage (55% vs. 38% respectively p=0.011).

In conclusion, couples being married in Covington do not appear to differ markedly from national averages for young adults when examining HBC use and cohabitation rates although those seeking NFP instruction for reasons beyond a marriage requirement are less likely to be current users of HBC.

4

A profile of NFP students using a home study course

Michael D. Manhart PhD and Karen B. Manhart BS, Couple to Couple League

All charts from students in Couple to Couple League's Home Study course seeking assistance from a single expert reviewer (Karen B. Manhart) were collected over a 12 month period (July 2008-June 2009). In total, 98 women (mean age= 27.8 yrs) submitted 251 charts over this period; 59 were engaged, 32 married, 5 were postpartum (all married).

Forty-eight women reported taking the course as a requirement for marriage. Engaged women taking the course as a requirement (*n*=42) began charting on average 3.2 months prior to their planned wedding date (range 0-9 months) whereas engaged women taking the course voluntarily (*n*=17) began just 1.4 months (range 0-8 mos.) prior to their wedding (p<0.002). On average, women submitted 2.7 charts during the training (range 1-8); there was no difference in the number of charts per woman between those taking voluntarily versus those required to take the course. Women who continued taking Hormonal Birth Control (HBC) during the course (*n*=13) submitted significantly fewer charts (mean=1.3, range 1-3, p=0.001). Loss to follow-up (defined as < 3 charts reviewed and no response at 4 & 6 months follow-up) was comparable in those taking the course as a requirement (20/48, 42%) and those voluntarily enrolling (11/45, 24%) (p=0.08).

Overall, 58% of the charts were classified as normal by the expert reviewer; those recently discontinuing HBC (*n*=24) had a similar incidence of normal charts. The remaining charts fell into one of several classes of abnormality with no one type dominating. A weak or irregular mucus pattern was infrequent overall but significantly more common in those recently stopping HBC compared to those with no recent history of HBC (11.5% vs. 1.8% respectively, p=0.002).

5

An algorithm for identifying and treating three groups of PCOS Patients

Mary W. Martin, MD, FACOG, Billings Center For Fertility and Reproductive Medicine, Oklahoma City, OK

Polycystic ovarian syndrome (PCOS) is the most common reproductive endocrinopathy of women. Medical literature cites insulin resistance as the etiology underlying the polycystic ovary, yet admits there are patients who do not respond to insulin-reducing or sensitizing therapies.

Recent research conducted by Vigil identifies three distinct groups of PCOS patients: the insulin-resistant, the non-insulin resistant, and an intermediate group.[1] Discriminating between these three groups is clinically challenging: standard lab testing does not identify the subtle differences in insulin sensitivity or hyperprolactinemia which underlie hyperandrogenism, the unifying feature and cause of PCOS.

The purpose of this study is to clinically evaluate an algorithm to identify and treat the 3 groups of PCOS patients, utilizing the Billings Ovulation Method (BOM) chart, standard lab tests and transvaginal ultrasound. The study population is a private-practice obstetric/gynecologic/infertility patient group of 30. The desired clinical outcome is the correction of ovulation defects, as evidenced by Peak as defined by BOM, or a positive pregnancy test. Study drugs included Metformin, Decadron, or both.

Since May of 2009, more than twelve pregnancies have occurred in Decadron patients who had been previously treated unsuccessfully with Metformin. One pregnancy occurred on dual therapy group, nine patients developed ovulatory cycles, and nine patients are currently in the treatment algorithm. The algorithm represents a valid method of identifying and treating PCOS using a Natural Family Planning method.

1. Vigil P., Contreras P., Alvarado J.L., Godoy A., Salgado A.M., Cortés M.E. "Evidence of subpopulations with different levels of insulin resistance in women with polycystic ovary syndrome." *Human Reproduction*. 2007 Nov;22(11):2974-80.

6

Characteristics of the menstrual cycle after discontinuation of oral contraceptives

Claudia L. Nassaralla, PhD, MD,Medical Consultant, Marquette University, Institute for NFP; Joseph B. Stanford, MD, MSPH, University of Utah; K. Diane Daly, RN, CFCE; Saint John's Mercy Medical Center, Co-coordinator, Dept Fertility Care Service, Saint Louis, Missouri; Mary Schneider, MSN, RN, Marquette University;Karen C. Schliep, MSPH, University of Utah; and Richard J. Fehring, PhD, RN, Marquette University (presenter: Joseph Stanford, MD, MSPH)

Menstrual cycle function may continue to be altered after discontinuation of oral contraceptives (OC). Few studies have been published on the effects of recent OC use on menstrual cycle parameters.

The purpose of this retrospective matched cohort is to assess biomarkers of the menstrual cycle after discontinuation of OC. The population studied included 140 women from three clinical sites in the United States: Atlanta, Georgia; Milwaukee, Wisconsin and St Louis, Missouri.

Among a sample of women who daily recorded observations of menstrual cycle biomarkers, 70 women who had recently discontinued OC were randomly matched by age and parity with 70 women who had not used OC for at least one year. Outcomes investigated included overall cycle length, length of the luteal phase, estimated day of ovulation, duration of menstrual flow, menstrual flow score (menstrual intensity) and mucus score (mucus quality). Differences between recent OC users and controls were assessed using random effects modeling.

The results demonstrate that recent OC users had significantly lower scores for mucus quality and intensity of menstrual flow for up to 6 cycles. Additionally, OC users had longer cycle lengths for up to 6 cycles (difference=3.50 days, $p<0.05$), a later estimated day of ovulation for up to 6 cycles (3.78 days, $p<0.05$) and decreased duration of menstrual flow for up to 2 cycles (difference= -0.48 days, $p<0.05$).

The authors conlclude that menstrual cycle biomarkers are altered for at least 6 cycles after discontinuation of OC, this may help explain the temporary decrease in fecundity associated with recent OC use.

7

Natural Family Planning Archive: A valuable new resource for researchers

Christopher H. Owen, PhD, Northeastern State University

This poster describes the foundation of a promising new NFP archive which provides an important new source of information for researchers. The archive encompasses the collections of seven major American NFP scientists and organizational leaders, including the papers of Lawrence J. Kane (Human Life Foundation), Kay Ek (BOMA), Mary Shivanandan (John Paul II Institute), Konald A. Prem (University of Minnesota), Robert Kambic (USAID and WHO), Claude Lanctot (International Federation for Family Life Promotion and SERENA), Hanna Klaus (TeenSTAR), Thomasina Bjorkman (George Mason University). These seven men and women, recognized widely for their contributions to the development of NFP, have brought together their personal libraries, correspondence and research notes to build the Natural Family Planning Archive of the Canizaro Library at Ave Maria University (Florida). The archives contains key publications in NFP history including basic works by Latz, Hartman, Röetzer, and also includes complete series of important relevant journals such as *Child and Family* and the *International Review of Natural Family Planning.*

The purpose of the project is to make interested researchers aware of this resource and how they can use it. To do so, the poster will demonstrate how Lawrence J. Kane put the collection together, detail what resources it includes, show where it is located and how it may be accessed. After delving into the origins and contents of the archive, the poster will explain how the collection will help researchers both to understand the growth of NFP science and to place NFP into its proper social and historical context.

8

Identifying the peak day of fertility: peri-conceptional exposure assessment

Christina Porucznik, PhD, MSPH, Karen Schliep, MSPH, and Joseph Stanford, MD, MSPH University of Utah, Department of Family and Preventive Medicine, Salt Lake City, UT

Early intrauterine exposures may have both short- and long-term consequences on human growth and development. Monitoring should begin near the time of conception. Prospectively determining ovulation dates would allow for targeted exposure assessment during the relevant developmental windows.

The purpose of this study is to demonstrate the acceptability, accuracy and actual use of cervical secretion observation or cervical secretion observation combined with basal body temperature readings for identifying the estimated day of ovulation.

The population examined included women (n=100) between the ages of 18 and 44 who are not currently pregnant nor using hormonal contraception are being recruited using referrals from other reproductive studies, flyers, word-of-mouth and social media.

Women who consent to participate: 1) completed baseline exposure questionnaire securely online; 2) read a 3-page educational brochure; and 3) were asked to record their fertility signs and complete a 1-page exposure questionnaire for up to 6 months or pregnancy. The women were informed that they could choose to monitor cervical mucus alone or cervical mucus combined with basal body temperature.

The results demonstrate that of the 37 currently enrolled women, 97% correctly estimated day of ovulation at least once. On average, it took women 1.23 cycles (range 1-2) to correctly estimating day of ovulation. Women preferred to measure cervical secretions alone (65.4%), compared to monitoring cervical secretions along with basal body temperature.

The authors conclude that the preliminary results indicate that most women who receive little compensation can properly identify their estimated day of ovulation but require phone and/or email follow-up.

9

Trends in family planning and NFP use among U.S. Hispanic women: 1995-2002

Dana Rodriguez, MSN, PNP (PhD student) Marquette University, College of Nursing

Hispanics are the largest and the fastest growing minority population in the United States. Many Hispanics follow the Catholic faith, which only allows the use of Natural Family Planning (NFP) for avoiding pregnancy. Past studies have shown that religiosity affects sexual behaviors among the U.S. Hispanic population.

The purpose of this study was to describe the trends in family planning among U.S. Hispanic women between the age of 15-44, with particular interest in type and importance of religion and the use of NFP.

The method of the study was to review the data sets of the 2,702 Hispanic (Latina) women in the 1995 and the 1,589 Latinas in the 2002 National Survey of Family Growth. The current religious status and importance of religion were used to describe NFP use.

Results included: In 1995 only 0.1% of Hispanics were using NFP. That figure increased to 0.3% in 2002, as compared to 0.2% in all US women at both time periods. However, in both time periods, female sterilization (19-21%) followed by the pill (13.0-13.6%) were the top two family planning methods utilized. In 2002, 3.5% of Catholic Latinas ever used NFP and 3.3% who viewed religion as important but only 0.3% of Catholic Latinas and 0.5% who viewed religion as very important were currently using NFP.

It was concluded that although there is a slight increase in use of NFP among Latinas, faith and the importance of religion has little influence in family planning choice.

10

The TwoDay Method: a quick start approach

Irit Sinai, PhD, Institute for Reproductive Health, Georgetown University, Washington, DC

The TwoDay Method is a fertility awareness method of family planning based on the identification of the presence or absence of cervical secretions (of any type). An efficacy study demonstrated that the method is efficacious. Participants in the study were counseled in method use during the first week of their menstrual cycle, before the onset of secretions. However requiring women to wait until the onset of secretions before they can begin using a method presents an obstacle to access.

An Operations Research study was conducted in Peru to assess if women who are counseled in TwoDay Method use later in the cycle, can use it as successfully. Some 161 women were admitted to the study, and were followed for up to seven months of method use. Only a third were in their first week of the cycle at the time of method counseling. Participants were counseled in TwoDay method use regardless of their cycle-day, and started using the method immediately.

Results demonstrate that the time in the cycle in which users are counseled in method use does not influence correct use of the method. In addition, simulated client visits show that day of the cycle client is on does not affect the quality of counseling. We conclude that the TwoDay Method is an effective and acceptable fertility awareness-based method of family planning that can be taught to users at any time in their menstrual cycle.

11

Estimating the probability of a live birth with natural procreative technology

Joseph B. Stanford, MD, MSPH, and *Karen C. Schliep, MSPH, University of Utah, Department of Family and Preventive Medicine, Salt Lake City, UT; Tracey A. Parnell, MD, Department of Family Medicine, University of British Columbia; and Philip C. Boyle, MB, MB, Galway Clinic, Ireland*

Stanford, Parnell, and Boyle, the International Institute of Restorative Reproductive Medicine, London, United Kingdom

Infertility is a common problem, affecting approximately one in every 7 couples in their reproductive lifetime. Treatments for infertility include assisted reproductive technology, which carries potential risks for both the woman and her baby. Natural procreative technology (NPT) is an alternative approach that is less invasive and has fewer adverse perinatal outcomes.

The authors sought to devise a prediction model using logistic regression to calculate the chance of a live birth within 2 years for couples treated for infertility with NPT.

Included in the analyses were 1,072 Irish couples who had been trying for at least a year to conceive before initiating NPT treatment between 1998 and 2002.

The main outcome was live birth predictors included women's characteristics, reproductive history, and physiological parameters identified by NPT evaluation. Model selection was done manually based on iterative results and physiologic considerations. From the final model, a prediction equation was generated for the probability of a live birth.

The results include: woman's age, length of time trying to conceive, prior pregnancies and live births, prior ART attempts, the presence of an abnormality of semen analysis, decreased production of cervical mucus, suboptimal levels of estrogen and progesterone and laparascopic intervention were significant independent predictors of the probability of live birth.

The authors conclude that the prediction model is consistent with prognostic factors identified for other infertility treatments and also includes factors uniquely identified by the NPT evaluation. It requires validation studies and may prove useful for clinical counseling.

12

The fertile and infertile phases of the menstrual cycle are signaled by cervical-vaginal fluid die swell functions

Jian Wang, PhD, Graduate Student, Department of Chemical Engineering, Texas Tech University, Lubbock, TX; Stephen J. Usala, MD, PhD, Clinical Associate Professor, Department of Internal Medicine, Texas Tech University Health Sciences Center, Amarillo, TX; Faye O'Brien-Usala, DC, Clinical Coordinator, Amarillo Medical Specialists, Amarillo, TX; William C. Biggs, MD, FACE, Clinical Associate Professor, Department of Internal Medicine, Texas Tech University Health Sciences Center, Amarillo, TX; Mark W. Vaughn, PhD, Associate Professor, Department of Chemical Engineering, Texas Tech University, Lubbock, TX; and Gregory B. McKenna, PhD, Horn Professor, Department of Chemical Engineering, Texas Tech University, Lubbock, TX

Natural Family Planning is a method of fertility awareness based in part on detection of the fertile and infertile phases of the menstrual cycle through self-observation of cervical-vaginal secretions.

Cervical-vaginal fluid (CVF) contains cervical mucus, a hydrogel that undergoes cyclic changes in viscoelasticity. We constructed a die swell device to study the viscoelastic properties and establish material functions of CVF samples that women obtain by self-aspiration. Two women for a total of 8 cycles provided day-specific CVF, urine and blood samples. Day-specific CVF samples were indexed to the day of ovulation (day 0) defined as the day of the luteinizing hormone peak. These samples were analyzed by extrusion through the die swell device and measurement of the subsequent flowgrams. Die swell ratio (B) was measured as the ratio, (maximum diameter of fluid swell after extrusion)/(inner die diameter), and die swell position (DisMax) was measured as the start position of maximum swell from the die orifice. These 2 rheological material functions, B and DisMax, were found to reliably correlate with the fertile and infertile phases of the cycle. This novel die swell device and methodology enables detection of viscoelasticity and therefore the presence of cervical mucus in CVF. Furthermore, it provides rheological measurements of cervical-vaginal secretions that correlate with the fertile and infertile phases of the menstrual cycle. The die swell device and methodology may serve as an aid for Natural Family Planning. Algorithms based on B and DisMax measurements to monitor real-time fertility will be discussed.

13

Calendar rules for the Marquette Model II

Paul J. Yong, MD, PhD, University British Columbia and Richard J. Fehring, PhD, RN, Marquette University

The Marquette Model II combines the Clearblue monitor with calendar rules for NFP; however, these rules require validation.

At the Marquette Institute for Natural Family Planning, the study designed seeks to develop evidence-based calendar rules. The population examined is a retrospective sample of women using Clearblue for 3 consecutive cycles prior to the current cycle (130 women). The method employed is statistical analysis of cycle data.

Results include the following:

Rule 1: For the first 3 cycles, if the fertile window (FW) is defined as starting on *Day* 5, then 0.8% of women (1/130) had a FW that began prior to this cut-off.

Rule 2: For the current cycle, if the start of FW is defined as the earliest day of ovulation from the previous 3 cycles *minus 9 days* (with a minimum of *Day* 5), then 0.8% of women (1/130) had a FW that began prior to this cut-off.

Rule 3: For the current cycle, if the end of the FW is defined as the latest day of ovulation from the previous 3 cycles *plus 4 days,* then 0.8% of women (1/130) had a FW ending after this cut-off.

The preliminary conclusions of the findings demonstrate that conservative calendar rules are:

Rule 1: For the first 3 cycles, fertility begins on Day 5;

Rule 2: For subsequent cycles, fertility begins on the earliest day of ovulation from the previous 3 cycles minus 9 days (minimum Day 5);

Rule 3: If the monitor misses the LH surge, then the estimated day of ovulation is the latest day of ovulation from the previous 3 cycles plus 4 days.

Index

E

F

R

S

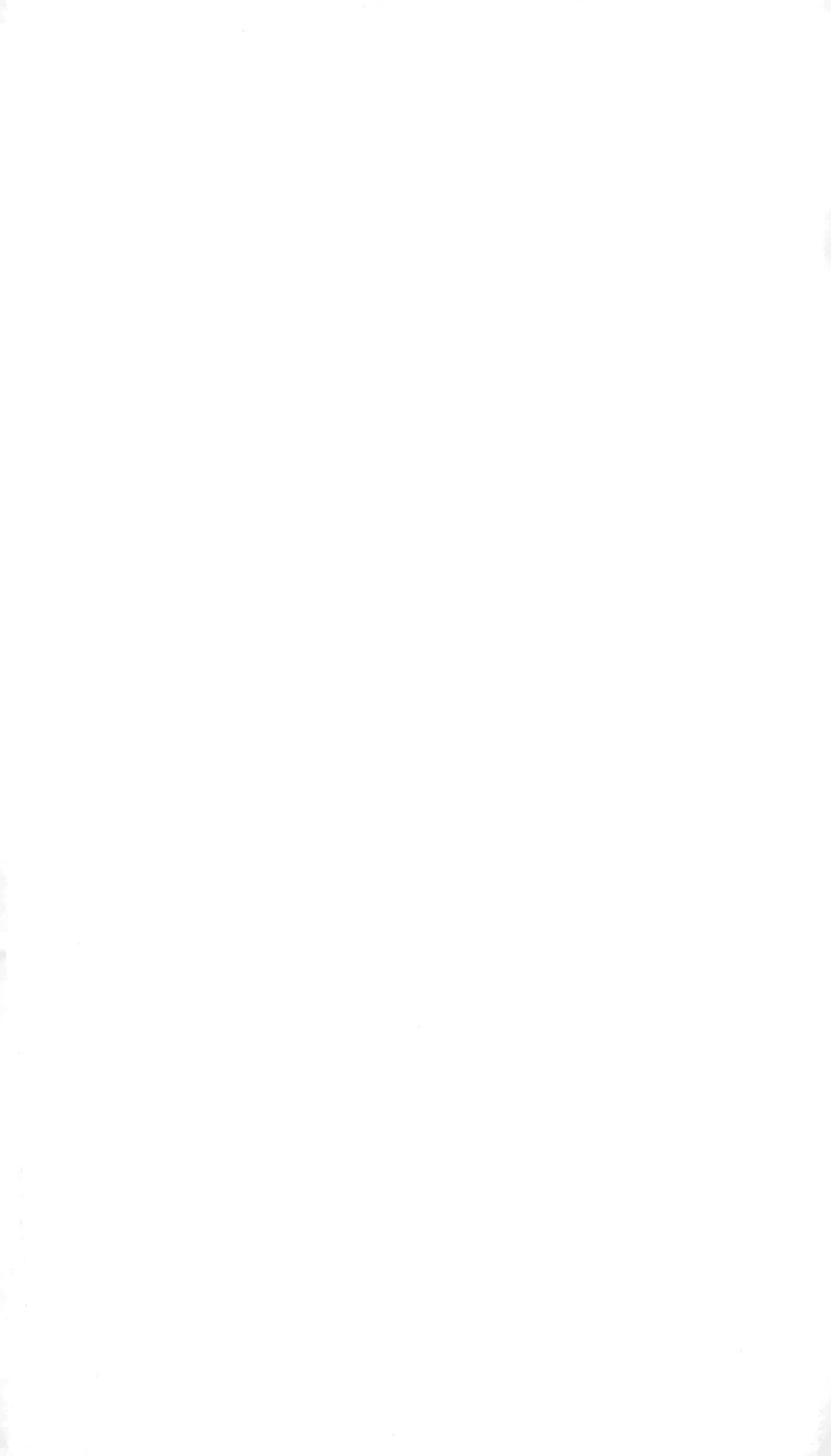